Metastasis of Breast Cancer

Metastasis of Breast Cancer

Editor: Ava Santiago

AMERICAN
MEDICAL PUBLISHERS
www.americanmedicalpublishers.com

AMERICAN
MEDICAL PUBLISHERS
www.americanmedicalpublishers.com

Cataloging-in-publication Data

Metastasis of breast cancer / edited by Ava Santiago.
p. cm.
Includes bibliographical references and index.
ISBN 979-8-88740-263-5
1. Breast--Cancer. 2. Metastasis. 3. Metastasis--Diagnosis. I. Santiago, Ava.
RC280.B8 M48 2023
616.994 49--dc23

American Medical Publishers,
41 Flatbush Avenue,
1st Floor, New York,
NY 11217, USA

ISBN 979-8-88740-263-5 (Hardback)

Contents

Preface

I am honored to present to you this unique book which encompasses the most up-to-date data in the field. I was extremely pleased to get this opportunity of editing the work of experts from across the globe. I have also written papers in this field and researched the various aspects revolving around the progress of the discipline. I have tried to unify my knowledge along with that of stalwarts from every corner of the world, to produce a text which not only benefits the readers but also facilitates the growth of the field.

Breast cancer is the cancer that develops in the tissues of the breast. The signs of breast cancer include change in the shape of breast, secretion of fluid from the nipple, scaly red patch of skin, lump in the breast, and a new inverted nipple. Metastasis is the process through which cancer cells spread. Metastatic breast cancer is the condition where cancer cells originated in the breast spread to other body parts, like brain, lungs, liver and bones. Metastatic cancer originates when cancer cells from the primary tumor break away and enter the lymphatic system or blood stream, which carry fluids across the body. The cancer cells travel from the primary tumor through these fluids, and then they settle and develop new tumors in other parts of the body. This book unravels the recent studies on the metastasis of breast cancer. It consists of contributions made by international experts. This book aims to equip students and experts with the advanced topics and upcoming concepts in this area of study.

Finally, I would like to thank all the contributing authors for their valuable time and contributions. This book would not have been possible without their efforts. I would also like to thank my friends and family for their constant support.

Editor

1

The Role of MicroRNAs in Estrogen Receptor α-Positive Human Breast Cancer

Hiroko Yamashita, Tatsuya Toyama, Nobuyasu Yoshimoto, Yumi Endo, Mai Iwasa and Yoshitaka Fujii
Oncology, Immunology and Surgery, Nagoya City University Graduate School of Medical Sciences, Japan

1. Introduction

MicroRNAs (miRNAs) are a class naturally occurring small non-coding RNAs that control gene expression by targeting mRNAs for translational repression or cleavage (Krol et al., 2010). Recent evidence has shown that miRNA mutations or mis-expression correlate with various human cancers, and that loss- or gain-of function of specific miRNAs contributes to breast epithelial cellular transformation and tumorigenesis (Esquela-Kerscher et al., 2006). miRNA expression profiling also revealed that miRNAs are differently expressed among molecular subtypes in breast cancer (Blenkiron et al., 2007; Iorio et al., 2005).

There are large-scale molecular differences between estrogen receptor (ER) α-positive and ERα-negative breast cancers (Perou et al., 2000; Sorlie et al., 2003). Endocrine therapy has become the most important treatment option for women with ERα-positive breast cancer, and approximately 70% of primary breast cancers express ERα. ERα is essential for estrogen-dependent growth, and its level of expression is a crucial determinant of response to endocrine therapy and prognosis in ERα-positive breast cancer (Dowsett et al., 2008; Harvey et al., 1999; Yamashita et al., 2006). Multiple mechanisms involved in altering ERα gene expression in breast cancer have been proposed, including ERα gene amplification (Holst et al., 2007) as well as transcriptional silencing by DNA methylation of CpG islands within the ERα promoter (Giacinti et al., 2006) and mutations within the open reading frame of ERα (Herynk et al., 2004). However, expression levels of ERα in breast cancer tissues differ widely among patients (Yamashita et al., 2011), and frequently change during disease progression and in response to systemic therapies (Yamashita et al., 2009). It was reported that the microRNA miR-206 decreases endogenous ERα mRNA and protein levels in human MCF-7 breast cancer cells via two specific target sites within the 3′-untranslated region (UTR) of the human ERα transcript (Adams et al., 2007). We found that the expression levels of miR-206 were gradually decreased as ERα protein expression increased in breast cancer tissues, suggesting that miR-206 is a key factor for the regulation of ERα expression in human breast cancer (Kondo et al., 2008). Moreover, recent studies have shown that ERα-regulating miRNAs, miR-18a, miR-18b, miR-22, miR-193b, miR-302c, and miR-221/222, as well as miR-206, directly targeted ERα in 3′UTR reporter assays, and suggested that several miRNAs regulate ERα expression.

2. Estrogen receptor (ER) α expression in human breast cancer

2.1 Expression of ERα in human breast cancer tissues

2.1.1 ERα expression in normal and malignant breast epithelial cells

ERα expression in normal and premalignant breast epithelial cells has been assessed by immunohistochemistry. It was reported that on average, normal premenopausal terminal duct lobular units contain about 30% ERα-positive cells (Allred et al., 2004). In contrast, nearly all cells express very high levels of ERα in the majority of premalignant breast lesions, including atypical ductal hyperplasia, atypical lobular hyperplasia and lobular carcinoma in situ. DCIS (Ductal carcinoma in situ) shows various levels of ERα expression ranging from high levels of lower-grade lesions to low levels of higher-grade lesions, including entirely ERα-negative. Furthermore, the wide range of ERα expression is observed in invasive ductal carcinoma. There is a substantial (~25%) subset of invasive breast cancers that does not contain any ERα-expressing cells. The majority (~75%) of invasive breast cancers, however, does contain ERα-expressing cells, but the proportion varies ranging from very low, to intermediate, to very high. We examined ERα expression in breast cancer tissues by immunohistochemistry using Allred score (Allred et al., 1998), and demonstrated that breast tumors show a wide range of ERα expression levels (Yamashita et al., 2011). Moreover, intensity of ERα expression is not equal among breast cancer cells in an individual tumor. Eastern cooperative oncology group compared the distribution of ERα protein expression by immunohistochemistry and ERα mRNA expression by quantitative reverse transcription (RT)-PCR in ECOG 2197 study (Badve et al., 2008). They reported that ERα mRNA expression in breast cancer tissues also showed continuous and the wide range.

2.1.2 Role of expression levels of ERα in human breast cancer

It is well established that expression levels of ERα govern response to endocrine therapy and prognosis in ERα-positive human breast cancer. Allred and colleagues first reported that expression levels of ERα assessed by immunohistochemistry affected prognosis (Harvey et al., 1999). ERα status using Allred score was a highly significant predictor of disease-free survival for patients who received adjuvant endocrine therapy. Recently, relationship between expression levels of ERα and prognosis was analyzed in adjuvant endocrine therapy trials for postmenopausal breast cancer, and demonstrated that disease-free survival or time to recurrence were significantly different according to expression levels of ERα (Dowsett et al., 2008; Viale et al., 2007). It was reported that the use of a cutoff of 1% staining cells for ERα indicated a better prognosis and at least some degree of endocrine responsiveness (Hammond et al., 2010). In the neoadjuvant endocrine therapy trial for postmenopausal women, correlation between expression levels of ERα assessed by Allred score and response to neoadjuvant endocrine therapy was analyzed (Ellis et al., 2001). It showed that letrozole response rates were superior to tamoxifen response rates in every ERα Allred score from 3 to 8, indicating that letrozole is more effective than tamoxifen regardless of the level of ERα expression. We also studied expression levels of ERα on pretreatment biopsies and post-treatment surgical specimens in postmenopausal patients with ERα-positive primary breast cancer who were treated with aromatase inhibitors for 6 months (Yamashita et al., 2009). We showed that ERα expression was decreased in post-treatment tumors compared to pretreatment specimens. On the other hand, we analyzed expression levels of ERα in primary breast cancer specimens from 75 metastatic breast cancer patients who received endocrine therapy on relapse, and analyzed the correlation between expression levels of ERα and response to endocrine therapy and post-relapse survival (Yamashita et al., 2006). Our results indicated that patients with higher ERα expression responded significantly to endocrine therapy, and that patients with higher ERα expression had better survival after relapse. Moreover, we recently reported that patients whose breast tumors contained high ERα expression effectively responded to aromatase inhibitors and displayed longer time to progression during first-line endocrine therapy with aromatase inhibitors and time to endocrine therapy failure (Endo et al., 2011).

2.2 Regulation of expression levels of ERα

Multiple mechanisms involved in the regulation of ERα expression in breast cancer have been identified, including mutations of ERα gene (Herynk et al., 2004) and transcriptional silencing by DNA methylation within the ERα promoter (Gaudet et al., 2009; Giacinti et al., 2006; Iwase et al., 1999). It was recently reported ERα gene amplification in breast cancer (Holst et al., 2007; Tomita et al., 2009). Holst and colleagues demonstrated that ERα gene amplification was frequent and more than 20% of breast cancers harbored genomic amplification by FISH analysis. They reported that ESR1 amplification was tightly linked to ERα protein expression, and that ESR1 amplification was also found in benign and precancerous breast diseases, such as atypical ductal hyperplasia, ductal carcinoma in situ and lobular carcinoma in situ. However, breast cancer patients show a wide range of ERα expression levels (Yamashita et al., 2011), and the levels of expression in individual patients change during disease progression and in response to systemic therapies (Yamashita et al., 2009). Therefore, other mechanisms may also regulate ERα expression in breast cancer.

2.2.1 miRNA biogenesis and function

MicroRNAs (miRNAs) comprise a large family of ~21-nucleotide-long RNAs that have emerged as key post-transcriptional regulators of gene expression (Krol et al., 2010). In mammals, miRNAs are predicted to control the activity of ~50% of all protein-coding genes. Functional studies indicate that miRNAs participate in the regulation of almost every cellular process investigated so far and that changes in their expression are associated with many human pathologies. Primary miRNA transcripts are cleaved into 70- to 80-nucleotide precursor miRNA (pre-miRNA) hairpins by RNase III Drosha in the cell nucleus and transported to the cytoplasm, where pre-miRNAs are processed by RNA Dicer into 19- to 25-nucleotide miRNA duplexes. One strand of each duplex is degraded, and the other strands become mature miRNAs, which, incorporated into the RNA-induced silencing complex, recognize sites in the 3′-UTR of the target mRNAs and cause translational repression or mRNA cleavage. miRNAs are a new player among gene regulation mechanisms, and their functions have not been fully explored but are known to include the regulation of cellular differentiation, proliferation and apoptosis. Recent evidence has shown that miRNA mutations or mis-expression are associated with various human cancers (Esquela-Kerscher et al., 2006).

2.2.2 Regulation of expression levels of ERα by miRNAs

Adams and colleagues first identified two potential miRNA miR-206 target sites within the 3'-UTR of ERα mRNA via in Silico analysis (Adams et al., 2007). The validation assay revealed that both miR-206 target sites specifically interacted with miR-206, which in turn repressed the corresponding ERα mRNA and protein expression. They also demonstrated that expression levels of endogenous miR-206 were significantly higher in ERα-negative MDA-MB-231 cells than in ERα-positive MCF-7 cells. Moreover, they showed that miR-206 repressed ERα mRNA and protein expression in MCF-7 and T47D cells. We showed that miR-206 expression assayed by quantitative RT-PCR analysis was inversely correlated with ERα but not ERβ mRNA expression in human breast cancer tissues (Kondo et al., 2008). Moreover, miR-206 expression levels were gradually decreased as ERα protein expression increased in human breast cancer. Transfection experiments revealed that introduction of miR-206 in estrogen dependent MCF-7 cells inhibited cell growth. Transfection of miR-206 into MCF-7 cells suppressed ERα expression and inhibited cell growth in a dose-dependent manner. Furthermore, introduction of miR-206 produced a dose-dependent decrease of mRNA expression of ERα-target genes, such as progesterone receptor, cyclin D1 and pS2. Adams and colleagues recently reported that miR-206 coordinately targeted mRNAs encoding the coactivator proteins SRC-1 and SRC-3, and the transcription factor GATA-3, all of which contribute to estrogenic signaling and a luminal A phenotype (Adams et al., 2009). Furthermore, they identified that miR-206 contributed to the epidermal growth factor (EGF) induced repression of ERα signaling in MCF-7 cells.

2.2.3 MiRNAs that directly target ERα in human breast cancer

Zhao and colleagues demonstrated that miR-221 and miR-222 were highly expressed in ERα-negative breast cancer cells, and that miRNA in situ hybridization analyses also showed overexpression of miR-221 and miR-222 in ERα-negative breast tumors (Zhao et al., 2008). Recently, two groups reported several miRNAs that down-regulated ERα in breast cancer cells. They identified the target sites of miRNAs, such as miR-18a and b, miR-302, miR-193b, miR-22, and miR221/222 as well as miR-206, in the ERα 3'-UTR, and showed that these miRNAs inhibited estrogen signaling by directly targeting ERα mRNA (Leivonen et al., 2009; Pandey et al., 2009) (Fig.1).

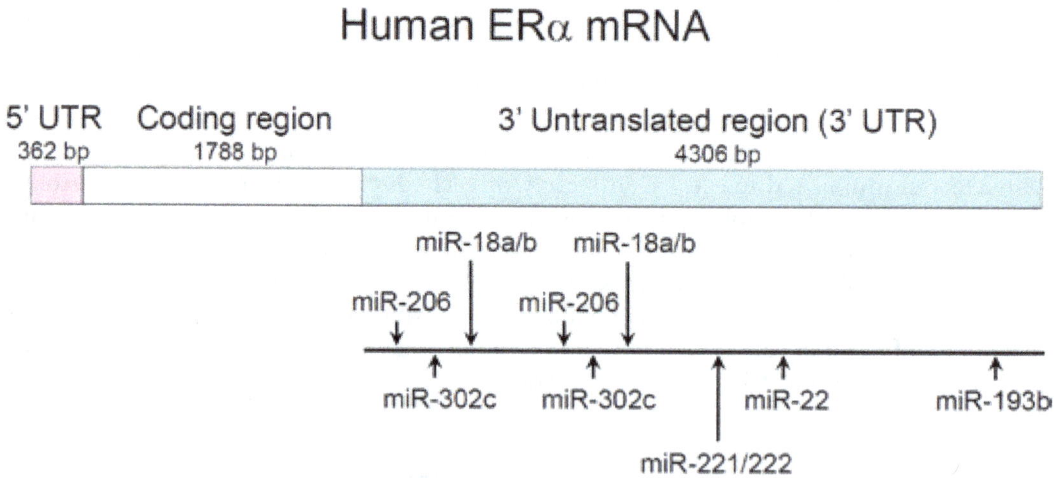

Fig. 1. Schematic representation of the human ERα mRNA and the predicted miRNA target sites.

We recently analyzed expression levels of miRNAs that directly target ERα, including miR-18a, miR-18b, miR-22, miR-193b, miR-221/222 and miR-302c in human breast cancer samples by quantitative RT-PCR analysis (Yoshimoto et al., 2011). Our results showed that miR-18a expression was much higher in ERα-negative than ERα-positive tumors, with the expression levels of miR-18a not differing in ERα-positive breast cancer as a function of ERα protein level. Surprisingly, expression levels of miR-193b and miR-221 were significantly lower in ERα-negative than ERα-positive tumors, and the levels of these miRNAs gradually increased as ERα protein expression increased. There was no statistically significant association between miR-22 and ERα expression, and miR-302c expression was minimal in human breast cancer samples. Prognostic analysis showed that low miR-18b expression was significantly associated with improved survival in HER2-negative breast cancer. Our results suggest that miRNAs that directly target ERα have distinct roles in not only regulating ERα but also regulating other target genes in human breast cancer, and that some miRNAs might be associated with characteristics of ERα-positive breast cancer.

2.3 Role of miRNAs in breast cancer

miRNAs can function as tumor suppressors and oncogenes (Esquela-Kerscher et al., 2006). The reduction or deletion of a miRNA that functions as a tumor suppressor leads to tumor formation. On the other hand, the amplification or overexpression of a miRNA that function as an oncogene results in tumor formation. Lu and colleagues first analyzed miRNA expression profiling in normal and tumor samples, and revealed global changes in miRNA expression (Lu et al., 2005). It was found that miRNA expression seems globally higher in normal tissues compared with tumors. Moreover, miRNAs are differentially expressed in various cancers. miRNA expression profiling also revealed that miRNAs are differently expressed among molecular subtypes in breast cancer (Blenkiron et al., 2007; Iorio et al., 2005). Iorio and colleagues first reported the miRNA gene expression profile in human breast cancer (Iorio et al., 2005). Compared with normal breast tissue, miRNAs are aberrantly expressed in human breast cancer. They also reported differentially expressed miRNAs associated with ERα expression, including miR-206. Blenkiron and colleagues analyzed miRNA expression in human breast cancer, and found that many miRNAs were differently expressed between breast cancer subtypes, such as luminal A, luminal B, HER2-positive, basal-like and normal-like (Blenkiron et al., 2007). They also found significant association between miRNA expression profiling and clinicopathological factors such as ERα status and tumor grade. Furthermore, recent studies have demonstrated that loss- or gain-of function of specific miRNAs contributes to breast epithelial cellular transformation and tumorigenesis. The interconnections between miRNAs and tumor suppressor genes and oncogenes in breast cancer were summarized by Zoon and colleagues (Zoon et al., 2009).

3. Conclusion

It is well recognized that individual miRNA sequences can suppress the production of hundreds of proteins (Krol et al., 2010). Reduction of protein levels in this way is often modest, however, and many such RNAs probably collectively fine-tune gene expression. Accumulating evidence supports the hypothesis that the ability of miRNAs to simultaneously regulate many target genes makes them attractive candidates for regulating normal and cancer cells. miRNAs are potential therapeutic targets for more tailored treatment strategies for breast cancer.

4. References

Adams BD, Cowee DM & White BA (2009). The role of miR-206 in the epidermal growth factor (EGF) induced repression of estrogen receptor-alpha (ERalpha) signaling and a luminal phenotype in MCF-7 breast cancer cells. *Mol Endocrinol,* Vol.23, No.8, pp. 1215-1230, ISSN 1944-9917

Adams BD, Furneaux H & White BA (2007). The micro-ribonucleic acid (miRNA) miR-206 targets the human estrogen receptor-alpha (ERalpha) and represses ERalpha messenger RNA and protein expression in breast cancer cell lines. *Mol Endocrinol,* Vol.21, No.5, pp. 1132-1147, ISSN 0888-8809

Allred DC, Brown P & Medina D (2004). The origins of estrogen receptor alpha-positive and estrogen receptor alpha-negative human breast cancer. *Breast Cancer Res,* Vol. 6, No. 6, pp. 240-245, ISSN 1465-542X

Allred DC, Harvey JM, Berardo M & Clark GM (1998). Prognostic and predictive factors in breast cancer by immunohistochemical analysis. *Mod Pathol,* Vol.11, No. 2, pp. 155-168, ISSN 0893-3952

Badve SS, Baehner FL, Gray RP, Childs BH, Maddala T, Liu ML, Rowley SC, Shak S, Perez EA, Shulman LJ, Martino S, Davidson NE, Sledge GW, Goldstein LJ & Sparano JA (2008). Estrogen- and progesterone-receptor status in ECOG 2197: comparison of immunohistochemistry by local and central laboratories and quantitative reverse transcription polymerase chain reaction by central laboratory. *J Clin Oncol,* Vol.26, No. 15, pp. 2473-2481, ISSN 1527-7755

Blenkiron C, Goldstein LD, Thorne NP, Spiteri I, Chin SF, Dunning MJ, Barbosa-Morais NL, Teschendorff AE, Green AR, Ellis IO, Tavare S, Caldas C & Miska EA (2007). MicroRNA expression profiling of human breast cancer identifies new markers of tumor subtype. *Genome Biol,* Vol.8, No. 10, pp. R214

Dowsett M, Allred C, Knox J, Quinn E, Salter J, Wale C, Cuzick J, Houghton J, Williams N, Mallon E, Bishop H, Ellis I, Larsimont D, Sasano H, Carder P, Cussac AL, Knox F, Speirs V, Forbes J & Buzdar A (2008). Relationship between quantitative estrogen and progesterone receptor expression and human epidermal growth factor receptor 2 (HER-2) status with recurrence in the Arimidex, Tamoxifen, Alone or in Combination trial. *J Clin Oncol,* Vol. 26, No. 7, pp. 1059-1065

Ellis MJ, Coop A, Singh B, Mauriac L, Llombert-Cussac A, Janicke F, Miller WR, Evans DB, Dugan M, Brady C, Quebe-Fehling E & Borgs M (2001). Letrozole is more effective neoadjuvant endocrine therapy than tamoxifen for ErbB-1- and/or ErbB-2-positive, estrogen receptor-positive primary breast cancer: evidence from a phase III randomized trial. *J Clin Oncol,* Vol. 19, No. 18, pp. 3808-3816

Endo Y, Toyama T, Takahashi S, Sugiura H, Yoshimoto N, Iwasa M, Kobayashi S, Fujii Y & Yamashita H (2011). High estrogen receptor expression and low Ki67 expression are associated with improved time to progression during first-line endocrine therapy with aromatase inhibitors in breast cancer. *Int J Clin Oncol,* ISSN 2547-7772, DOI 10.1007/s10147-011-0215-5

Esquela-Kerscher A & Slack FJ (2006). Oncomirs - microRNAs with a role in cancer. *Nat Rev Cancer,* Vol. 6, No. 4, pp. 259-269

Gaudet MM, Campan M, Figueroa JD, Yang XR, Lissowska J, Peplonska B, Brinton LA, Rimm DL, Laird PW, Garcia-Closas M & Sherman ME (2009). DNA hypermethylation of ESR1 and PGR in breast cancer: pathologic and epidemiologic associations. *Cancer Epidemiol Biomarkers Prev,* Vol. 18, No. 22, pp. 3036-3043, ISSN 1538-7755

Giacinti L, Claudio PP, Lopez M & Giordano A (2006). Epigenetic information and estrogen receptor alpha expression in breast cancer. *Oncologist,* Vol. 11, No. 1, pp. 1-8

Hammond ME, Hayes DF, Dowsett M, Allred DC, Hagerty KL, Badve S, Fitzgibbons PL, Francis G, Goldstein NS, Hayes M, Hicks DG, Lester S, Love R, Mangu PB, McShane L, Miller K, Osborne CK, Paik S, Perlmutter J, Rhodes A, Sasano H, Schwartz JN, Sweep FC, Taube S, Torlakovic EE, Valenstein P, Viale G, Visscher D, Wheeler T, Williams RB, Wittliff JL & Wolff AC (2010). American society of clinical oncology/college of american pathologists guideline recommendations for immunohistochemical testing of estrogen and progesterone receptors in breast cancer. *J Clin Oncol,* Vol. 28, No. 16, pp. 2784-2795

Harvey JM, Clark GM, Osborne CK & Allred DC (1999). Estrogen receptor status by immunohistochemistry is superior to the ligand-binding assay for predicting response to adjuvant endocrine therapy in breast cancer. *J Clin Oncol,* Vol. 17, No. 5, pp. 1474-1481, ISSN 0732-183X

Herynk MH & Fuqua SA (2004). Estrogen receptor mutations in human disease. *Endocr Rev,* Vol. 25, No. 6, pp. 869-898

Holst F, Stahl PR, Ruiz C, Hellwinkel O, Jehan Z, Wendland M, Lebeau A, Terracciano L, Al-Kuraya K, Janicke F, Sauter G & Simon R (2007). Estrogen receptor alpha (ESR1) gene amplification is frequent in breast cancer. *Nat Genet,* Vol. 39, No. 5, pp. 655-660

Iorio MV, Ferracin M, Liu CG, Veronese A, Spizzo R, Sabbioni S, Magri E, Pedriali M, Fabbri M, Campiglio M, Menard S, Palazzo JP, Rosenberg A, Musiani P, Volinia S, Nenci I, Calin GA, Querzoli P, Negrini M & Croce CM (2005). MicroRNA gene expression deregulation in human breast cancer. *Cancer Res,* Vol. 65, No. 16, pp. 7065-7070, ISSN 0008-5472

Iwase H, Omoto Y, Iwata H, Toyama T, Hara Y, Ando Y, Ito Y, Fujii Y & Kobayashi S (1999). DNA methylation analysis at distal and proximal promoter regions of the oestrogen receptor gene in breast cancers. *Br J Cancer,* Vol. 80, No. 12, pp. 1982-1986, ISSN 0007-0920

Kondo N, Toyama T, Sugiura H, Fujii Y & Yamashita H (2008). miR-206 Expression is down-regulated in estrogen receptor alpha-positive human breast cancer. *Cancer Res,* Vol. 68, No. 13, pp. 5004-5008, ISSN 1538-7445

Krol J, Loedige I & Filipowicz W (2010). The widespread regulation of microRNA biogenesis, function and decay. *Nat Rev Genet,* Vol. 11, No. 9, pp. 597-610, ISSN 1471-0064

Leivonen SK, Makela R, Ostling P, Kohonen P, Haapa-Paananen S, Kleivi K, Enerly E, Aakula A, Hellstrom K, Sahlberg N, Kristensen VN, Borresen-Dale AL, Saviranta P, Perala M & Kallioniemi O (2009). Protein lysate microarray analysis to identify microRNAs regulating estrogen receptor signaling in breast cancer cell lines. *Oncogene,* Vol. 28, No. 44, pp. 3926-3936, ISSN 1476-5594

Lu J, Getz G, Miska EA, Alvarez-Saavedra E, Lamb J, Peck D, Sweet-Cordero A, Ebert BL, Mak RH, Ferrando AA, Downing JR, Jacks T, Horvitz HR & Golub TR (2005). MicroRNA expression profiles classify human cancers. *Nature,* Vol. 435, No. 7043, pp. 834-838, ISSN 1476-4687

Pandey DP & Picard D (2009). miR-22 inhibits estrogen signaling by directly targeting the estrogen receptor alpha mRNA. *Mol Cell Biol,* Vol.29, No. 13, pp. 3783-3790, ISSN 1098-5549

Perou CM, Sorlie T, Eisen MB, van de Rijn M, Jeffrey SS, Rees CA, Pollack JR, Ross DT, Johnsen H, Akslen LA, Fluge O, Pergamenschikov A, Williams C, Zhu SX, Lonning PE, Borresen-Dale AL, Brown PO & Botstein D (2000). Molecular portraits of human breast tumours. *Nature,* Vol. 406, No. 6797, pp. 747-752

Sorlie T, Tibshirani R, Parker J, Hastie T, Marron JS, Nobel A, Deng S, Johnsen H, Pesich R, Geisler S, Demeter J, Perou CM, Lonning PE, Brown PO, Borresen-Dale AL & Botstein D (2003). Repeated observation of breast tumor subtypes in independent gene expression data sets. *Proc Natl Acad Sci U S A,* Vol. 100, No. 14, pp. 8418-8423

Tomita S, Zhang Z, Nakano M, Ibusuki M, Kawazoe T, Yamamoto Y & Iwase H (2009). Estrogen receptor alpha gene ESR1 amplification may predict endocrine therapy responsiveness in breast cancer patients. *Cancer Sci,* Vol. 100, No. 6, pp. 1012-1017, ISSN 1349-7006

Viale G, Regan MM, Maiorano E, Mastropasqua MG, Dell'Orto P, Rasmussen BB, Raffoul J, Neven P, Orosz Z, Braye S, Ohlschlegel C, Thurlimann B, Gelber RD, Castiglione-Gertsch M, Price KN, Goldhirsch A, Gusterson BA & Coates AS (2007). Prognostic and predictive value of centrally reviewed expression of estrogen and progesterone receptors in a randomized trial comparing letrozole and tamoxifen adjuvant therapy for postmenopausal early breast cancer: BIG 1-98. *J Clin Oncol,* Vol. 25, No. 25, pp. 3846-3852, ISSN 1527-7755

Yamashita H, Iwase H, Toyama T, Takahashi S, Sugiura H, Yoshimoto N, Endo Y, Fujii Y & Kobayashi S (2011). Estrogen receptor-positive breast cancer in Japanese women: trends in incidence, characteristics, and prognosis. *Ann Oncol,* Vol. 22, No. 6, pp. 1318-1325, ISSN 1569-8041

Yamashita H, Takahashi S, Ito Y, Yamashita T, Ando Y, Toyama T, Sugiura H, Yoshimoto N, Kobayashi S, Fujii Y & Iwase H (2009). Predictors of response to exemestane as primary endocrine therapy in estrogen receptor-positive breast cancer. *Cancer Sci,* Vol. 100, No. 11, pp. 2028-2033, ISSN 1349-7006

Yamashita H, Ando Y, Nishio M, Zhang Z, Hamaguchi M, Mita K, Kobayashi S, Fujii Y & Iwase H (2006). Immunohistochemical evaluation of hormone receptor status for predicting response to endocrine therapy in metastatic breast cancer. *Breast Cancer,* Vol. 13, No. 1, pp. 74-83, ISSN 1340-6868

Yoshimoto N, Toyama T, Takahashi S, Sugiura H, Endo Y, Iwasa M, Fujii Y & Yamashita H (2011). Distinct expressions of microRNAs that directly target estrogen receptor α in human breast cancer. *Breast Cancer Res Treat,* online, DOI 10.1007/s10549-011-1672-2

Zhao JJ, Lin J, Yang H, Kong W, He L, Ma X, Coppola D & Cheng JQ (2008). MicroRNA-221/222 negatively regulates estrogen receptor alpha and is associated with tamoxifen resistance in breast cancer. *J Biol Chem,* Vol. 283, No. 45, pp. 31079-31086, ISSN 0021-9258

Zoon CK, Starker EQ, Wilson AM, Emmert-Buck MR, Libutti SK & Tangrea MA (2009). Current molecular diagnostics of breast cancer and the potential incorporation of microRNA. *Expert Rev Mol Diagn,* Vol. 9, No. 5, pp. 455-467, ISSN 1744-8352

2

EGF Regulation of HRPAP20: A Role for Calmodulin and Protein Kinase C in Breast Cancer Cells

Manasi N. Shukla, Donna J. Buckley and Arthur R. Buckley
Division of Pharmaceutical Sciences, James L. Winkle College of Pharmacy, University of Cincinnati, Cincinnati, OH, United States of America

1. Introduction

The breast cancer cell genome is remarkably unstable, most likely due to early dysfunction of DNA replication, repair or recombination (Roskelley and Bissel, 2002). Accumulation of genetic alterations in the cells and/or stroma lead to development of a genetically diverse cell population characterized by uncontrolled cell proliferation (Witz, 2002; Gupta et al., 2006). Therefore, identification of genes that may be responsible for pre-disposition or facilitate progression of the disease may contribute to improvement of currently available therapeutic approaches in treatment of breast cancer.

We previously reported the identification, cloning and functional characterization of HRPAP20, which encodes for protein designated Hormone Regulated Proliferation-Associated Protein 20 (accession number: NM_ 014165; Karp et al., 2004). Our observations indicated that HRPAP20 is a regulator of proliferation, survival, and invasion in hormone-responsive breast cancer cells. Moreover, highly invasive, hormone unresponsive breast cell lines, such as MDA-MB-231 and tumor specimens of invasive breast adenocarcinomas from patients exhibited constitutively elevated levels of HRPAP20 (Karp et al., 2007). Results from an independent study conducted by another group suggested that HRPAP20 is a promising marker of tamoxifen resistance in women with ER alpha-positive breast tumors (Tozlu-Kara et al., 2007). Together, these observations suggested that elevated HRPAP20 may facilitate breast cancer progression toward a more malignant phenotype.

Other studies from our group suggested that an interaction between HRPAP20 and calmodulin (CaM) may contribute to HRPAP20-mediated biological effects in tumor cells. Furthermore, a basic amino acid residue (K73) within the putative CaM-binding domain of HRPAP20 appeared to be important for CaM-binding to the protein. CaM has been shown to influence cell cycle control and proliferation in human breast cancer cells by activating CaM-kinase II (CaMK II) and MAPK-mediated signaling pathways (Cheung , 1980; Wang et al., 1983; Rodriguez-Mora et al., 2005). The recent identification of the ErbB2/HER2/Neu, ER-α, and androgen receptor (AR) as CaM-binding proteins, has opened new areas of investigation in the regulation of signaling by CaM, particularly in hormone-responsive cancer (Cifuentes et al., 2004; Li et al., 2006; Maximciuc et al., 2006).

Overexpression or constitutive activation of the epidermal growth factor receptor (EGFR) is frequently associated with the development and progression of a number of human cancers, including breast cancer (Garcia et al., 2006). HER-2, a member of this receptor tyrosine kinase family is overexpressed in 20% -30% of aggressive breast cancers, making it an appealing target for prognosis and therapy of the disease (Meric-Bernstam et al., 2006). These and other observations have shed light on the fact that the complex role of EGF signaling in development and progression of breast cancer is incompletely understood, and suggests that gaps exist in our knowledge of its signaling mechanisms. Therefore, experiments were conducted to evaluate a potential role of HRPAP20 in EGF-mediated signaling in hormone-dependent breast cancer cells.

Protein kinase C (PKC) is a signaling intermediate that has been linked to EGF stimulation in cancer cells. The PKC family of at least 12 serine/threonine protein kinase isoforms, has been extensively studied in the regulation of intracellular signaling in response to stimuli such as growth factors and hormones (Dekker et al., 1994; Nishizuka et al., 1995; Newton 1995, and 1997; Mellor et al., 1998). The classical and novel isoforms of PKC are targets for phorbol ester compounds, such as TPA, which are a widely studied tumor promoters that mimic the actions of diacylglycerol on PKC activation (Barry et al., 2001). Altered expression and activity of several PKC isoenzymes has been observed in numerous cancers including those affecting the lung, colon, and breast (Gordge et al., 1996; McCracken et al., 2003; Gokmen-Polar et al., 2001). It has been reported that PKC-α, -δ and -ε activate several substrates that promote breast tumor cell migration and invasion (Pan et al., 2005; Tan et al., 2006; Ways et al., 1995). Therefore, it appears that PKC isoforms have distinct roles, which relate to their unique localization and/or access to substrates upon activation (Nakagawa et al., 2005). Here we show results from experiments conducted to evaluate whether HRPAP20 is a substrate for PKC. We also demonstrate whether specific PKC isoforms activated by EGF stimulation are possibly involved in HRPAP20 phosphorylation and invasion. The observations presented in this chapter support the hypothesis that HRPAP20 is an important regulator of tumor cell signaling, which may direct malignant progression in breast cancer.

2. Experimental procedures

2.1 Cell culture and treatments

The human mammary adenocarcinoma cell line MCF-7 was maintained in DMEM supplemented with 10% FBS and penicillin/streptomycin. MCF-7 cells were serum starved for 24 hrs in DMEM supplemented with 1% ITS+ (BD Biosciences, Bedford, MA) or 0.1% BSA. Quiescent MCF-7 cells were treated with EGF (100 ng/ml) or TPA (20 nM). Treatment of MCF-7 cells with Gö6976 (1μM) or Rottlerin (10μM) was carried out 60 min prior to stimulation with EGF (100 ng/ml for 30 min). All cells were harvested by washing with ice-cold PBS and centrifugation.

2.2 HRPAP20 plasmid construction and site-directed mutagenesis

The full length HRPAP20 cDNA was ligated into the mammalian expression vector pcDNA3.1 using the restriction sites Hind III (5′ end) and Eco-RI (3′ end). The construct was sequenced and used for transfection of MCF-7 cells. For bacterial expression of recombinant HRPAP20-GST fusion protein, the restriction sites Bam-H1 and Eco-RI were engineered on the 5′ and 3′ terminals of the protein frame of HRPAP20 respectively. This oligonucleotide was generated by PCR and ligated into the bacterial expression vector PGEX-4T1 (Amersham Biosciences, Piscataway, NJ). The vectors pcDNA 3.1 and PGEX-4T1 encoding

HRPAP20 were used as templates for site-directed mutagenesis. Alanine substitutions were performed using the Quick-Change point-mutation kit (Stratagene, La Jolla, CA.). The following primers were synthesized to generate the variant HRPAP20 oligonucleotides. K73A: 5′-GAGATGTATATGTCAATTCCGCAGATCCGGTGCCTTCCT-3′. R66A: 5′-ACAAGCTGTTGTCCTTACTAGCAGATGTATATGTCAATTCC-3′. Reverse primers were synthesized complementary to the forward primers. The HRPAP20 sequence harboring both K73A and R66A site-mutations was generated by using HRPAP20/K73A as a template using primers encoding for the R66A mutation. A PCR reaction using cycling conditions recommended by the manufacturer was performed. Digestion of the parental plasmid template was accomplished using Dpn I. The site mutants were transformed into E-coli, and colonies selected on ampicillin-containing soft agar. The individual colonies were grown and the plasmid constructs isolated using Qiagen plasmid Mini-prep kit protocol. All constructs were sequenced at the University of Cincinnati DNA core facility to confirm the amino acid substitutions. The appropriate plasmids were then used for stable transfection of cells, or for bacterial expression of variant HRPAP20-GST fusion proteins.

2.3 Recombinant HRPAP20-GST protein expression and purification

Recombinant HRPAP20-GST fusion protein was produced by transformation of the Escherichia coli strain BL21-Star/p-RARE with the plasmid vector PGEX-4T1 encoding for wild-type or variant HRPAP20. The construct was sequenced at the University of Cincinnati's DNA Core Facility prior to transformation. Bacteria transformed with the empty vector alone were used to express recombinant GST alone, which was used as an assay control. The transformants were grown in complete LB broth, and IPTG (5mM) was used to induce protein expression at 27°C. Following 4 hrs of induction, the cells were lyzed by freeze-thawing (3X) and sonication (60V, 5 cycles). Sonicates were centrifuged and GST or HRPAP20-GST fusion proteins in the supernatants were purified using glutathione-agarose (Amersham). Bound GST or HRPAP20-GST protein was eluted by reduced glutathione (20mM) and quantitated using Bradford reagent (Biorad, Hercules, CA). The purity and molecular weights of the proteins were confirmed by SDS-PAGE followed by Coomassie blue staining.

2.4 CaM-Sepharose binding analysis

The assay was performed as described previously (Boehning et. al, 2004; Karp et al., 2007). Briefly, 20 µl of CaM-Sepharose-4B beads (1.3 mg/ml, Amersham) were equilibriated with Buffer A. The equilibriated beads were then blocked for 1 h at room temperature with 1% BSA, followed by washing 1X with 500 µl of buffer A. Binding of HRPAP20-GST to CaM was evaluated by incubating 5 µg of HRPAP20-GST (wild-type or variant) or GST-only with CaM-Sepharose for 1 h at 4°C in buffer A ± $CaCl_2$ (5 mM). Bound protein was eluted using SDS sample buffer, followed by SDS-PAGE analysis. Immunoblotting with α-GST or α-HRPAP20 was used to identify HRPAP20 binding to CaM.

2.5 *In vitro* PKC kinase assay employing HRPAP20 as a substrate

The assay was performed as described in (Li and McNulty et al., 2005). Briefly, 5 µg of the fusion protein HRPAP20-GST or GST in 100 µl of PKC buffer containing 20 mM HEPES (pH: 7.4), 1.67 mM $CaCl_2$,10 mM $MgCl_2$, 1 mM DTT, 1mM ATP and 10 µCi of [γ-^{32}P] ATP was used for the kinase reaction. Myristoylated peptide PKC inhibitor (Promega, Madison, WI) was used at a concentration of 100 mM. The kinase reaction was initiated by adding 1 µl of PKC (Promega), followed by incubation at 30 °C for 30 min. A duplicate set of the above reactions with the substitution of [γ-^{32}P] ATP with non-radioactive ATP was performed in parallel for immunoblotting analysis. The reactions were stopped by placing on ice. The fusion proteins were isolated using glutathione agarose, followed by washing, elution and SDS-PAGE. The resolved proteins were transfered to PVDF membranes and subjected to autoradiography, or immunoblotting with α-GST. The immunoblotted membranes were subsequently stripped and reprobed with α-HRPAP20.

2.6 Immune-complex kinase assay

Cells were harvested and lyzed using phosphorylation lysis buffer containing 50 mM HEPES (pH: 7.5), 150 mM NaCl, 200 µM sodium orthovanadate, 10 mM sodium pyrophosphate, 100 mM sodium fluoride, 1 mM EDTA, 1.5 mM $MgCl_2$, 10% glycerol, 1% Triton X-100, and protease inhibitors (Rahman et al., 2001). Lysates were immunoprecipitated using α-PKC-A3 (Santa Cruz Biotechnology, Santa Cruz, CA) and protein-G agarose. Immune-complexes were washed with kinase wash buffer: Tris HCl (50 mM , pH 7.4), NaF (10 mM), sodium orthovanadate (1 mM), EDTA (0.5 mM), EGTA (0.5 mM), magnesium chloride (2 mM), leupeptin (10 µg/ml), PMSF (1mM) as previously described (Arya et al., 2004). 5 µg of recombinant HRPAP20-GST or GST protein, in a kinase reaction buffer containing 20 mM Tris-HCl (pH: 7.4), 10 mM $MgCl_2$ and 1 mM DTT was incubated with ATP (1 µM), γ-^{32}P-ATP (10 µCi) for 30 min at 30°C. The reactions were terminated by placing on ice, followed by SDS-PAGE and autoradiography as described in previous section.

2.7 Cell transfection

MCF-7 cells were transfected with wild-type HRPAP20, R66A, K73A+R66A, or empty vector (pcDNA 3.1) alone, according to manufacturer's protocol using Lipofectamine® (Invitrogen, Carlsbad, CA). Following transfection, all cells were subjected to G418 selection (250 µg/ml) to generate stably transfected cell lines. Cells were transiently transfected with wild-type and dominant-negative PKC-δ constructs or empty vector pcDNA3.1, and used in experiments 72 hrs after transfection (previously described in Kruger et al., 2003).

2.8 Co-immunoprecipitation/immunoblotting (co-IP/IB)

Following treatments, cells were harvested using ice-cold PBS and centrifugation; then lysed in a buffer containing 10 mM Tris (pH 7.4), 0.15 M NaCl, 5 mM EDTA and 1% Triton X-100. The lysates were pre-cleared with normal rabbit serum and protein G (Upstate, Lake Placid, NY), then immunoprecipitated using α-HRPAP20 antiserum (Karp et. al, 2004) and protein G. The immunoprecipitates, together with lysates, were resolved using 12% SDS-PAGE gels, then immunoblotted with α-CaM (Upstate, Charlottesville, VA.). The membranes were subsequently stripped using a buffer containing 62.5 mM Tris (pH 6.8) and 2% SDS, then reprobed with α-HRPAP20.

2.9 Cell invasion analysis

The invasive capacity of the breast tumor cell lines was measured utilizing an in vitro transwell assay (Repesh et al., 1989, Karp et al., 2007). Briefly, 2.5 x 10^5 cells, in DMEM containing 0.1% BSA, were added to the upper well of transwell chambers (Corning Inc.,

Corning, NY) containing an 8 μm porous membrane, previously coated with type I collagen, fibronectin, and Matrigel ® (Becton Dickinson Biosciences, San Diego, CA). Lower chambers contained DMEM containing 0.1% BSA and 10% FBS as a chemoattractant. Following 24 hrs, invading cells were fixed with 4% paraformaldehyde, stained with crystal violet, and counted microscopically (20X magnification) in five random fields/membrane.

3. Results

3.1 EGF regulates the interaction between HRPAP20 and CaM in MCF-7 cells

We previously showed that HRPAP20 interacts with Ca^{2+}/CaM in purified preparations and in MCF-7 cells (Karp et al., 2007). To determine whether this interaction was influenced by mitogenic stimulation such by EGF, co-immunoprecipitation/ immunoblotting (co-IP/IB) experiments were conducted using MCF-7 cells. As shown in Fig. 1, CaM co-immunoprecipitated with HRPAP20 in lysates from control cell suggesting that the two proteins existed as a complex in unstimulated cells (time 0) consistent with our previous observations. Stimulation with EGF (100 ng/ml) rapidly disrupted the HRPAP20:CaM ($p<0.05$). Thus, mitogenic stimulation appeared to cause dissociation of the protein complex that was observed in unstimulated cells. These observations suggest that HRPAP20 may function as a signaling intermediate coupled to activation of the EGFreceptor.

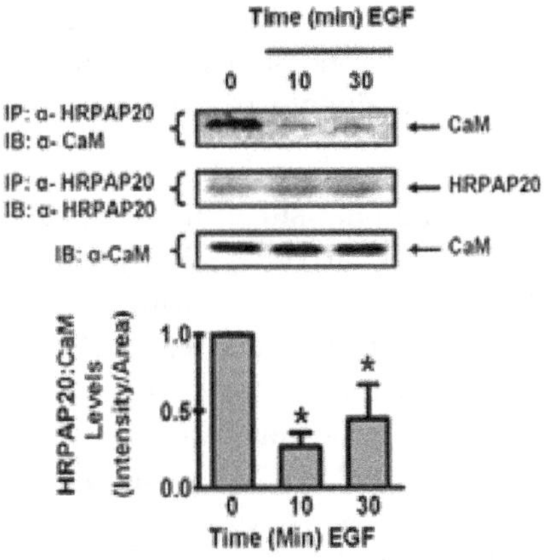

Fig. 1. EGF stimulation disrupts HRPAP20:CaM in MCF-7 cells. MCF-7 cells, previously cultured for 24 hr in serum-free medium, were treated with h-EGF (100 ng/ml). The cells were harvested at the indicated times following EGF stimulation. Cell lysates were immuno precipitated with α-CaM (upper panel). Membranes were stripped and reprobed with α-HRPAP20 (middle panel). 10% of total protein used for immunoprecipitation was resolved in parallel as an input control and Immunoblotted with α-CaM (lower panel). Densitometric analysis of three separate experiments is presented. *$p<0.05$ vs CTL.

HRPAP20:CaM interaction requires basic residues K73 and R66 in MCF-7 cells. Experiements were conducted to determine which amino acid residues within HRPAP20 were required for its interaction with CaM. Studies by others (Bagchi et al., 1992) showed that certain basic residues within the CaM-binding domains of several interacting proteins were required for their interaction. K73, R66, and V70 (hydrophobic) were identified as potential critical residues within HRPAP20 for its interaction with CaM based upon comparison with other binding proteins (Fig. 2).

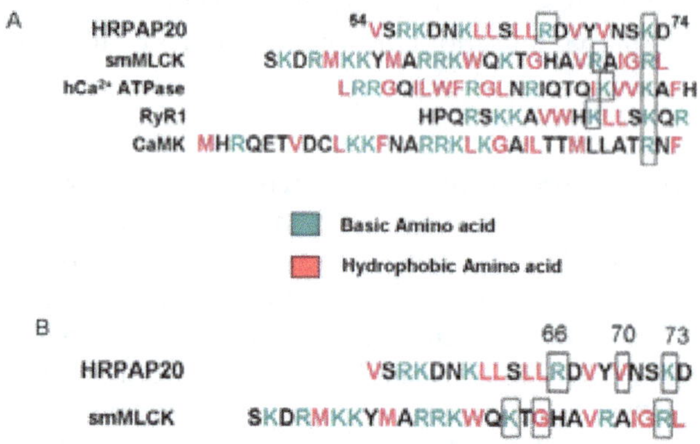

Fig. 2. Sequence of the HRPAP20 CaM-binding domain. (A) The amino acid sequence of HRPAP20 (residues 54-74) consisting of the predicted CaM-binding motif, was aligned with those of other well-characterized CaM-binding proteins. While there is no sequence conservation observed in most of the CaM-binding domain, they are characterized by a typical positioning of a C-terminal basic residue, preceded by 2-3 hydrophobic residues. (B) Sequence alignment of the CaM-binding motif of HRPAP20 with that present in smMLCK indicating positions of basic and hydrophobic residues on smMLCK that are critical for CaM-binding (Bagchi et al., 1992). Analogous residues within HRPAP20 are boxed and the positions numbered.

Previously, we showed that alanine (ala) substitution of K73 resulted in diminished CaM-binding of HRPAP20 in MCF-7 cells (Karp et al., 2007). Using site-directed mutagenesis, we generated a series of HRPAP20 variants harboring ala substitutions at these residues (HRPAP20-K73A, HRPAP20/R66A or HRPAP20/K73A+R66A, and HRPAP20/V70A). The proteins were expressed as GST-fusion proteins, then the purified recombinant proteins were evaluated by CaM-Sepharose pull-down analysis to assess their capacity to bind to CaM. The results indicated that HRPAP20-K73A exhibited ~50% reduction in CaM-binding compared to the wild-type protein (Fig. 3). Moreover, ala substitutions at K73 and R66 in combination inhibited the HRPAP20:CaM interaction to the same extent as R66A, indicating that each of these residues may contribute to CaM-binding (Fig. 3). Alanine substitution of the hydrophobic residue V70 did not significantly affect CaM-binding of HRPAP20, suggesting that this residue may not be required for in HRPAP20:CaM complex formation (results not shown).

To determine whether the HRPAP20/R66A or HRPAP20/K73A+R66A exhibited a diminished interaction with CaM in MCF-7 cells, we conducted co-IP/IB experiments using cells stably transfected with HRPAP20, R66A, K73A+R66A, or the empty vector as a control. The results demonstrated that CaM co-immunoprecipitated using α-HRPAP20, in MCF-7/HRPAP20 cells, consistent with our previous observations. In contrast, significantly reduced CaM binding was observed in cells transfected with HRPAP20/R66A or HRPAP20/K73A+R66A compared to the level observed in wildtype HRPAP20 (Fig. 4A and D). The membranes from Fig. 4A were subsequently stripped and reprobed with

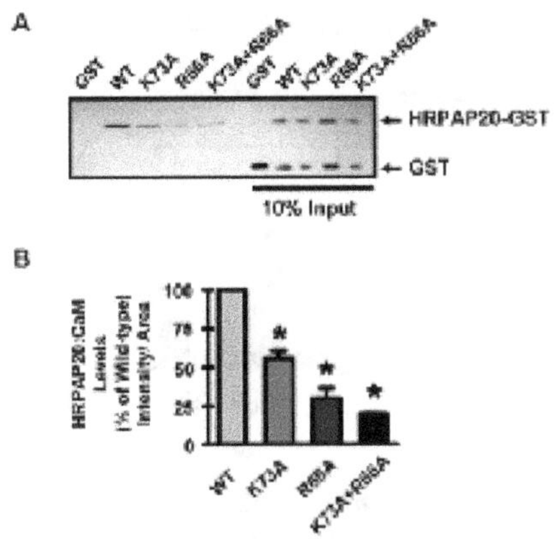

Fig. 3. K73 and R66 regulate HRPAP20:CaM interact1on in vitro. (A) 5 µg of recombinant HRPAP20-GST [wildtype-WT, or HRPAP20 harboring the substitutions K73A, R66A, or K73A+R66A] or GST alone were incubated with CaM-Sepharose in the presence of Ca^{2+} (5 mM). Eluted proteins were resolved bySDS-PAGE, then immunoblotted with α-GST. 10% of each protein used in pull-down assays was evaluated in parallel as an input control. (B) Cumulative results of densitometric analysis of three separate experiments is presented. *$p<0.05$ vs. WT.

α-HRPAP20 to confirm HRPAP20 immunoprecipitation in each of the samples (Fig. 4B). Equal concentrations of lysate protein from each of the transfectants were immunoblotted using α-CaM as an additional control (Fig. 4C). Together, these results suggested that the basic residues K73 and R66 in the CaM-binding motif of HRPAP20 may regulate its interaction with CaM in MCF-7 breast cancer cells.

Shown in Fig. 4E are results from in vitro invasion analysis of cells transfected with HRPAP20 and and its variants. Here wildtype HRPAP20 significantly ($p<0.\ 01$) increased invasion through Matrigel® coated filters in transwell chambers. In contrast, invasion observed by the cells expressing the HRPAP20 variants R66A or K73A+R66A did not differ from empty vector-transfected controls. These observations indicated that even a partial disruption of the HRPAP20:CaM interaction by mutation of the basic residues K73 and R66 blocked HRPAP20-mediated increase in invasion. Therefore, it is suggested that K73 and R66 are likely required to maintain integrity of the HRPAP20:CaM complex, which appears to be a requisite for MCF-7 invasion.

3.2 HRPAP20 is a substrate for PKC

We previously showed that HRPAP20 is a phosphoprotein and that pharmacological inhibition of PKC reduced its phosphorylation in Nb2-11 cells (Karp et al., 2004). Experiments to evaluate whether HRPAP20 is phosphorylated by PKC were conducted utilizing recombinant HRPAP20-GST fusion protein and catalytically active rat brain PKC, in the presence of cofactors and ^{32}P-ATP. As shown in Fig. 5A, HRPAP20 was phosphorylated in the presence of PKC (lane 1), but not in its absence (lane 2). Addition of a myristoylated peptide substrate, serving as a competitive inhibitor of PKC, inhibited PKC-mediated phosphorylation of HRPAP20 (lane 3). An equal amount of recombinant GST

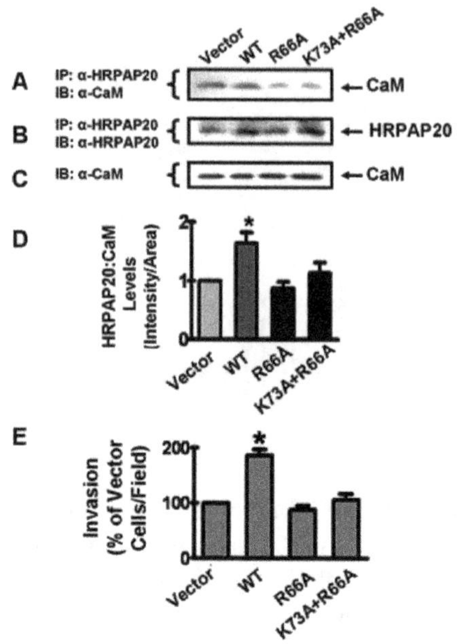

Fig. 4. Effect of HRPAP20 amino acid substitution (R66A, K73A+R66A) on HRPAP20:CaM association and invasion in MCF-7 cells. (A) MCF-7 cells, transfected with empty vector (Vector), wildtype HRPAP20 (WT), HRPAP20/R66A (R66A) or HRPAP20/K73A+R66A (K73A + R66A) were immunoprecipitated with α-HRPAP20 and immunoblotted with α-CaM. (B) Membranes were stripped and reprobed with α-HRPAP20. (C) 10% of total protein used for immunoprecipitation was resolved in parallel as an input control and immunoblotted with α-CaM. (D) Densitometric analysis of three separate experiments is presented. *$p<0.01$ WT vs Vector; $p<0.05$ WT vs K73A. (E) Cumulative results obtained from three separate in vitro invasion experiments. *$p<0.01$ WT vs Vector.

incubated with PKC represents a control reaction demonstrating the inability of PKC to phosphorylate GST (lane 4). To ensure equal loading of samples, duplicates of the above reactions with the substitution of ^{32}P-ATP with non radioactive ATP were resolved in parallel and subjected to immunoblotting with α-HRPAP20 (Fig. 5B) or α-GST (Fig. 5C). Together, these results suggest that HRPAP20 is a substrate for PKC in vitro.

3.3 HRPAP20 is phosphorylated by EGF-activated PKC

There is abundant evidence indicating an important role for EGFR and its ligands in the development and progression of human neoplasia (Johnston et al., 2006; Ji et al., 2006; Speake et al., 2005; D'Alessio et al., 2010). To evaluate whether PKC-mediated HRPAP20 phosphorylation is an event that occurrs downstream of EGF stimulation, immune-complex kinase assays were performed utilizing PKC immunoprecipitated from lysates of EGF-treated MCF-7 cells and HRPAP20-GSTas a substrate. The reactions were performed in the presence of ^{32}P-ATP, but in the absence of cofactors. As illustrated in Fig. 6A and B, HRPAP20 phosphorylation was significantly elevated upon its incubation with PKC immunoprecipitated from EGF-treated cells, compared to the level observed in control samples from untreated cells. These results suggest that PKC, activated by EGF stimulation catalyzed HRPAP20 phosphorylation.

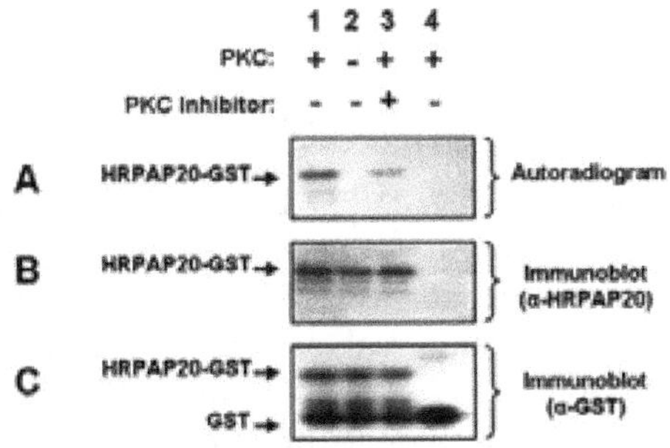

Fig. 5. Phosphorylation of HRPAP20 by PKC. (A) Recombinant HRPAP20-GST (lanes 1-3) or GST alone (lane 4) were incubated at 30°C in the presence (+) or absence (-) of purified rat brain PKC or a PKC inhibitor (myristoylated PKC peptide inhibitor, 100 μM) in the presence of [γ-^{32}P] ATP. Samples were resolved by SDS-Page followed by autoradiography. (B) Duplicates of reactions in (A), but without [γ-^{32}P] ATP, were immunoblotted with α-HRPAP20. (C) Membranes from (B) were stripped, then reprobed with α-GST.

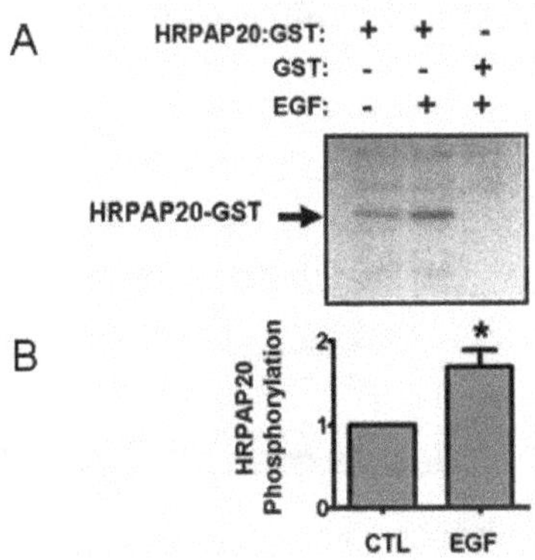

Fig. 6. HRPAP20 is phosphorylated by PKC activated subsequent to EGF stimulation in MCF-7 cells. (A) PKC from quiescent or EGF-treated MCF-7 cells was immunoprecipitated, then incubated with recombinant HRPAP20-GST or GST in the presence of γ-^{32}P-ATP, followed by SDS-PAGE and autoradiography. A representative autoradiograph indicating the level of HRPAP20 phosphorylation is shown. (B) Cumulative results from three independent experiments analyzed by densitometry are presented. *$p<0.01$ vs CTL.

3.4 PKC-δ phosphorylates HRPAP20 subsequent to EGF stimulation and is required for invasion in MCF-7 cells

The role of various PKC isoforms in the process of tumor progression in the mammary epithelium is only partially understood. However, several studies support a role for PKC-δ in breast tumor progression (McCracken et al., 2003; Nabha et al., 2005). Moreover, PKC-δ has been shown to regulate the activation of MMP-9 in breast tumor cells; an effect also observed in MCF-7 cells stably expressing elevated levels of HRPAP20 (Karp et al., 2007). Therefore, experiments were conducted to determine whether PKC-δ phosphorylated of HRPAP20 following EGF stimulation in this cell line. Quiescent MCF-7 cells were subjected to treatment with Gö6976, a pharmacological inhibitor of classic PKC isozymes, or Rottlerin, with specificity directed toward the PKC-δ isoform. The results from immunecomplex kinase analysis indicated that while Gö6976 did not affect EGF-stimulated HRPAP20 phosphorylation, Rottlerin nearly completely blocked this effect (Fig. 7A). These results suggested that PKC-δ, activated by EGF stimulation, may be responsible for the downstream phosphorylation of HRPAP20.

To further investigate whether PKC-δ catalyzed HRPAP20 phosphorylation, MCF-7 cells were transiently transfected with constructs encoding a constitutively active wild-type (WT) PKC-δ, a kinase inactive/dominant negative PKC-δ (DN), or with the empty vector. Transfectants were treated with EGF and evaluated using immune-complex kinase analysis. The results indicated that EGF stimulated substantial HRPAP20 phosphorylation in cells expressing WT-PKC-δ (Fig. 7B). However, expression of DN- PKC-δ almost completely abolished this effect. Together, these results support the hypothesis that PKC-δ mediates phosphorylation of HRPAP20 and that this effect may underlie EGF stimulated actions.

To determine whether HRPAP20 phosphorylation affected cell invasion in vitro, invasion analysis was conducted using MCF-7 cells co-transfected with HRPAP20 and dominant negative PKC-δ. As shownin Fig. 7C, co-expression of dominant negative PKC-δ with HRPAP20, caused a significant reduction of MCF-7 cell invasion, compared to the level observed in cells transfected with HRPAP20 alone. These results suggested that activated PKC-δ is required to regulate HRPAP20, ultimately resulting in stimulating increased invasiveness in breast cancer cells.

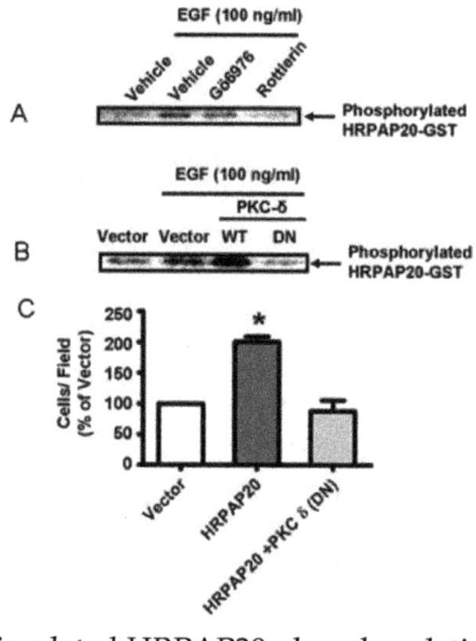

Fig. 7. PKC-δ catalyzes EGF-stimulated HRPAP20 phosphorylation and contributes to invasion. (A) Quiescent MCF-7 cells were pre-treated with PKC inhibitors Gö6976 (1 μM) or Rottlerin (10 μM), followed by the addition of EGF (100 ng/ml). PKC was immunoprecipitated and incubated with recombinant HRPAP20-GST in the presence of γ-^{32}P-ATP. A representative autoradiograph showing HRPAP20 phosphorylation is presented. (B) MCF-7 cells were transiently transfected with empty vector (Vector), wild-type (WT) or dominant negative PKC-δ (DN). Cells were then treated with EGF, followed by immunecomplex kinase analysis. (C) MCF-7 cells were transfected with empty vector (Vector), HRPAP20, or HRPAP20 and PKC-δ (DN), then evaluated by in vitro invasion assay. Cumulative results from three independently performed experiments are presented. *$p<0.01$ (HRPAP20 vs. Vector or HRPAP20 + DN-PKC-δ).

3.5 Effect of phosphorylation on HRPAP20: CaM interaction

Numerous previous studies have reported that post-translational modification may alter protein-protein interactions. Therefore, whether HRPAP20 phosphorylation affected its interaction with CaM was investigated. Experiments were conducted using MCF-7 cells treated with the phorbol ester, TPA, an activator of PKC. The HRPAP20:CaM interaction in these cells was evaluated by co-IP analysis. As demonstrated in Fig. 8A, TPA rapidly stimulated a significant ($p<0.01$) reduction in HRPAP20:CaM complex suggesting that PKC-catalyzed phosphorylation of HRPAP20 may reduce its binding capacity to CaM. Moreover, this observation correlated with the pattern of HRPAP20:CaM disruption observed upon EGF stimulation in these cells.

Furthermore, CaM Sepharose pull-down experiments were conducted to determine whether PKC-mediated phosphorylation of HRPAP20 affected its CaM-binding in vitro. The results obtained indicated that HRPAP20, phosphorylated by PKC prior to incubation with CaM, exhibited markedly reduced HRPAP20:CaM complex formation, in contrast to that observed with the native protein (Fig. 8B). This observation is consistent with our previous results suggesting that PKC likely regulates HRPAP20:CaM association. Taken together, the results suggest that HRPAP20 may modulate signaling involved in growth factor/hormone-responsive cancers by associating with PKC and CaM.

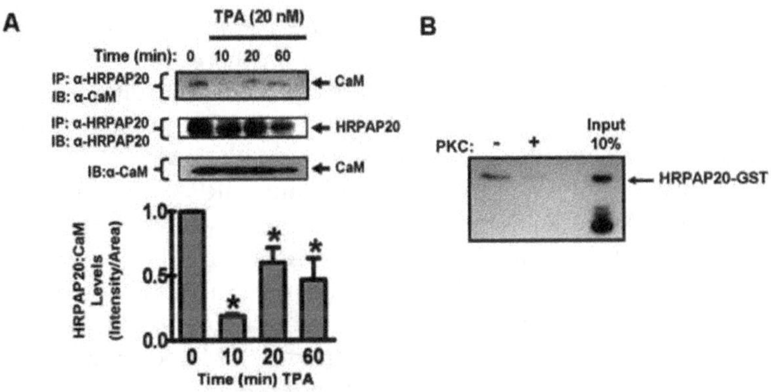

Fig. 8. HRPAP20:CaM is likely regulated by PKC-catalyzed phosphorylation. (A) Serum starved MCF-7 cells were treated with TPA (20 nM). Cells were harvested at the indicated time points, followed by immunoprecipitation of lysates using α-HRPAP20, then immunoblotted with α-CaM (upper panel). Membranes were stripped and reprobed with α-HRPAP20 (middle panel). 10% of total protein used for immunoprecipitation was resolved in parallel as an input control and immunoblotted with α-CaM (lower panel). Densitometric analysis of three separate experiments is presented. *$p<0.05$ vs. 0 min. (B) 5 μg of recombinant HRPAP20-GST was phosphorylated in vitro using rat brain PKC, then subjected to CaM- pulldown assay. A representative immunoblot using α- is shown.

4. Discussion

Tumor cell responses to extracellular stimuli includes activation of kinase pathways and alteration of protein-protein interactions, ultimately resulting in modulation of biological responses leading to progression of the disease. Since previous observations implicated a role for HRPAP20 in breast tumor proliferation and invasion, it was important to investigate the mechanisms by which this protein participated in tumor cell signaling.

Previously we showed that HRPAP20 and CaM interacted in vitro and in MCF-7 cells (Karp et al., 2007). We therefore sought to investigate whether this interaction contributed to tumor signaling and whether it was subject to regulation by growth factor stimulation.

Recent studies have broadened the view of signal transduction to encompass a complex networks, which allow interaction between discrete signaling pathways with EGFR as a key unit for integration of multiple stimuli (Prenzel et al., 2000). CaM has been shown to bind to the EGFR, as well as modulate EGF-stimulated signaling leading to tumor progression. It was therefore important to investigate whether HRPAP20 was subject to regulation downstream of EGFR activation in tumor cells. Using co-IP/IB, we showed that HRPAP20 resides within a complex with CaM in quiescent MCF-7 cells. Stimulation with EGF caused a significant reduction in HRPAP20:CaM association. These results suggest that the HRPAP20:CaM complex is likely regulated by EGF, and may serve as a potentially important step in growth factor-stimulated cell signaling.

To investigate which specific amino acid residues within HRPAP20 participate in its interaction with CaM, we compared the sequence of the CaM-binding domain of HRPAP20 to binding domains present in other CaM interacting proteins. This assessment revealed that several basic and hydrophobic amino acids were interspersed within the HRPAP20 CaM-binding motif at positions analogous to those found to be important for other CaM-binding proteins (Bagchi et al., 1992; Fitzsimons et al., 1992). Following generation of HRPAP20 variants harboring ala substitutions at suspected key locations, experiments were conducted to evaluate HRPAP20:CaM binding of the altered proteins. Results from these suggested that the basic residues, K73 and R66, located near the C-terminus of the CaM-binding domain of HRPAP20, may be critical for its interaction with CaM.

Bioinformatic analysis of the wildtype and variant HRPAP20 amino acid sequences indicated that both K73A and R66A substitutions most likely altered the length and stability of α-helices within the protein. Notably, K73 was predicted to be responsible for a bend in the strand following the α-helix that constituted the CaM-binding motif of HRPAP20 (www.igb.uci.edu/tools/scratch.html; http://npsa-pbil.ibcp.fr/cgi-bin/secpred_hnn.pl; NNPredict Query server; and http://distill.ucd.ie/porter/). Moreover, alanine substitution of R66 reduced the number of its residue contacts, hence potentially destabilizing the helix and potentially affecting its ability to bind CaM.

To investigate whether abrogation of HRPAP20:CaM interaction by R66A or K73A+R66A substitutions affected tumor cell invasion, we compared the invasive capacity of MCF-7 cells transfected with either wildtype HRPAP20 or its variants. In contrast to the wildtype protein, HRPAP20/R66A or HRPAP20/K73A+R66A failed to increase invasion. Therefore, consistent with our previous observations, the results suggest reports an upstream requirement for CaM-binding of HRPAP20 that is coupled to tumor invasiveness.

Protein phosphorylation has been known to play a significant role in the regulation of numerous aspects of cellular function such as growth, metabolism, motility, survival, and apoptosis. Moreover, numerous protein-protein interactions have been shown to be regulated by phosphorylation (Cho et al., 2004). Since HRPAP20 appears to complex with CaM and contains three consensus motifs for PKC catalyzed phosphorylation, it was hypothesized that HRPAP20 function may be regulated by CaM-binding and phosphorylation. EGF has been reported to activate PKC in MCF-7 cells (Mueller et al., 1997). Increased levels of PKC expression and activation have been associated with malignant transformation in a number of cell lines including breast, lung and gastric carcinomas (O'Brian et al., 1989; Takenaga et al., 1986; Schwartz et al., 1993). These observations suggest that PKC contributes to tumor progression and may serve as a therapeutic target for treatment of breast cancer.

We proposed that EGF stimulation in MCF-7 cells may subsequently induce HRPAP20 phosphorylation, following activation of PKC. To test this hypothesis, we conducted immune-complex kinase assays utilizing recombinant HRPAP20 and PKC immunoprecipitated from MCF-7 cells treated with/without EGF. Indeed, the results generated suggest that PKC immunoprecipitated from EGF-treated MCF-7 cells catalyzed HRPAP20 phosphorylation. Therefore, it appeared likely that EGF stimulation, which subsequently activates PKC, may lead to downstream phosphorylation of HRPAP20.

Results provided by others have suggested that the PKC-δ isoform is a positive regulator of metastatic progression and a survival factor in breast cancer (McCracken et al., 2003). Several reports now suggest that PKC-δ plays an important role in EGFR-mediated breast tumor progression as an important contributor to the later stages of cell migration (Kruger et al., 2003). Results presented here from immune-complex kinase assays suggested that while PKC-δ inhibition by rottlerin abrogated EGF-stimulated HRPAP20 phosphorylation, inhibition of conventional PKC isoforms with Gö6976 had no effect. This suggests that PKC-δ but not -α, -β, or -γ may mediate EGF-induced HRPAP20 phosphorylation. To further investigate HRPAP20 phosphorylation, immune-complex kinase assays were conducted using PKC immunoprecipitated from MCF-7 cells transiently transfected with wildtype or dominant negative PKC-δ. The results indicated that while expression of wildtype PKC-δ enhanced EGF-mediated HRPAP20 phosphorylation, the dominant negative PKC-δ variant failed to produce this effect. Together, the results strongly indicate that PKC-δ, activated upon EGF stimulation, may be responsible for HRPAP20 phosphorylation.

In breast cancer cell lines and fibroblasts, EGF stimulation has been shown to induce chemotactic migration with significant involvement of PKC α, ζ, δ and ε (Rabinovitz et al., 1999; Joberty et al., 2000; Iwabu et al., 2004). To determine whether PKC-δ is required for the observed HRPAP20-mediated increase in MCF-7 cell invasion, in vitro invasion experiments were conducted using cells co-expressing HRPAP20 and the dominant negative PKC-δ construct. It was observed that cells co-expressing DN PKC-δ with HRPAP20, failed to increase invasion above levels found in empty vector transfectants. These observations suggest that HRPAP20 phosphorylation by PKC-δ may be required for breast tumor cell invasion. Together, the results suggest that HRPAP20 may participate in EGF-stimulated signaling pathways in tumor cells, and that the effects of HRPAP20 may be regulated at least in part by CaM and PKC-catalyzed phosphorylation.

Phosphorylation has been shown to affect the CaM-binding affinity of several proteins. The myristoylated alanine rich C kinase substrate (MARCKS) protein and its homologue, MARCKS related protein (MRP), have been shown to bind CaM in a Ca^{2+}-dependent manner. Importantly, their interaction with CaM was diminished upon phosphorylation by PKC (Porumb et. al, 1997; Mc Ilroy et al., 1991). Several hormones produce an increase in intracellular Ca^{2+}, which facilitates CaM-binding to its target proteins and the consequent activation of PKC. These and the previous observations implicate that activation of PKC by various external stimuli may result in release of its substrates from CaM-bound pools by virtue of their phosphorylation. On the other hand, this may, in effect, result in the increase in intracellular levels of freely accessible CaM, leading to amplification of CaM-dependent processes.

Based on these observations and results indicating that HRPAP20 was a substrate for PKC downstream of EGF stimulation, we investigated whether phosphorylation affected CaM-binding of HRPAP20. Our results indicated that TPA caused a disruption of the HRPAP20:CaM complex in MCF-7 cells, in a manner similar to that observed upon EGF stimulation. In addition results from CaM-Sepharose pull-down assays illustrated that the phosphorylated form of HRPAP20 exhibited diminished CaM-binding in vitro, compared to the unphosphorylated protein.

We suggest that EGF stimulation, which activates PKC, may subsequently result in HRPAP20 phosphorylation. Furthermore, our observations clearly indicate that PKC-catalyzed phosphorylation of HRPAP20 regulates HRPAP20:CaM complex formation, and may potentially serve as an activation intermediate that leads to tumor invasion. Finally, our results suggest that a requirement of PKC-δ together with elevated HRPAP20 as factors that enhance breast cancer cell invasion. These observations provide additional clues with regard to the mechanism of regulation of HRPAP20 function and invasion in breast cancer. Thus, further studies on the role of HRPAP20 in tumor progression may reveal a hitherto unsuspected target for therapy of breast cancer.

5. Acknowledgements

We thank Dr. Jae-Won Soh at the Biomedical Research Center for Signal Transduction Networks, Inha University, Incheon, Korea, for generously providing constructs encoding wildtype and dominant negative PKC-δ.

6. References

Bagchi, I. C., Q. H. Huang, et al. (1992). "Identification of amino acids essential for calmodulin binding and activation of smooth muscle myosin light chain kinase." J Biol Chem 267(5): 3024-9.

Barry, O. P. and M. G. Kazanietz (2001). "Protein kinase C isozymes, novel phorbol ester receptors and cancer chemotherapy." Curr Pharm Des 7(17): 1725-44.

Cheung, W. Y. (1980). "Calmodulin plays a pivotal role in cellular regulation." Science 207(4426): 19-27.

Cho, S., S. G. Park, et al. (2004). "Protein-protein interaction networks: from interactions to networks." J Biochem Mol Biol 37(1): 45-52.

Cifuentes, E., J. M. Mataraza, et al. (2004). "Physical and functional interaction of androgen receptor with calmodulin in prostate cancer cells." Proc Natl Acad Sci U S A 101(2): 464-9.

D'Alessio, A., A. De Luca, et al. (2010). "Effects of the combined blockade of EGFR and ErbB-2 on signal transduction and regulation of cell cycle regulatory proteins in breast cancer cells." Breast Cancer Res Treat 123(2): 387-96.

Dekker, L. V. and P. J. Parker (1994). "Protein kinase C--a question of specificity." Trends Biochem Sci 19(2): 73-7.

Fitzsimons, D. P., B. P. Herring, et al. (1992). "Identification of basic residues involved in activation and calmodulin binding of rabbit smooth muscle myosin light chain kinase." J Biol Chem 267(33): 23903-9.

Garcia, R., R. A. Franklin, et al. (2006). "EGF induces cell motility and multi-drug resistance gene expression in breast cancer cells." Cell Cycle 5(23): 2820-6.

Gokmen-Polar, Y., N. R. Murray, et al. (2001). "Elevated protein kinase C betaII is an early promotive event in colon carcinogenesis." Cancer Res 61(4): 1375-81.

Gordge, P. C., M. J. Hulme, et al. (1996). "Elevation of protein kinase A and protein kinase C activities in malignant as compared with normal human breast tissue." Eur J Cancer 32A(12): 2120-6.

Gupta, G. P. and J. Massague (2006). "Cancer metastasis: building a framework." Cell 127(4): 679-95.

Iwabu, A., K. Smith, et al. (2004). "Epidermal growth factor induces fibroblast contractility and motility via a protein kinase C delta-dependent pathway." J Biol Chem 279(15): 14551-60.

Ji, H., D. Li, et al. (2006). "The impact of human EGFR kinase domain mutations on lung tumorigenesis and in vivo sensitivity to EGFR-targeted therapies." Cancer Cell 9(6): 485-95.

Joberty, G., C. Petersen, et al. (2000). "The cell-polarity protein Par6 links Par3 and atypical protein kinase C to Cdc42." Nat Cell Biol 2(8): 531-9.

Johnston, J. B., S. Navaratnam, et al. (2006). "Targeting the EGFR pathway for cancer therapy." Curr Med Chem 13(29): 3483-92.

Karp, C. M., H. Pan, et al. (2004). "Identification of HRPAP20: a novel phosphoprotein that enhances growth and survival in hormone-responsive tumor cells." Cancer Res 64(3): 1016-25.

Karp, C. M., M. N. Shukla, et al. (2007). "HRPAP20: a novel calmodulin-binding protein that increases breast cancer cell invasion." Oncogene 26(12): 1780-8.

Kruger, J. S. and K. B. Reddy (2003). "Distinct mechanisms mediate the initial and sustained phases of cell migration in epidermal growth factor receptor-overexpressing cells." Mol Cancer Res 1(11): 801-9.

Li, L. and D. B. Sacks (2007). "Functional interactions between calmodulin and estrogen receptor-alpha." Cell Signal 19(3): 439-43.

Maximciuc, A. A., J. A. Putkey, et al. (2006). "Complex of calmodulin with a ryanodine receptor target reveals a novel, flexible binding mode." Structure 14(10): 1547-56.

McCracken, M. A., L. J. Miraglia, et al. (2003). "Protein kinase C delta is a prosurvival factor in human breast tumor cell lines." Mol Cancer Ther 2(3): 273-81.

McIlroy, B. K., J. D. Walters, et al. (1991). "Phosphorylation-dependent binding of a synthetic MARCKS peptide to calmodulin." J Biol Chem 266(8): 4959-64.

Mellor, H. and P. J. Parker (1998). "The extended protein kinase C superfamily." Biochem J 332 (Pt 2): 281-92.

Meric-Bernstam, F. and M. C. Hung (2006). "Advances in targeting human epidermal growth factor receptor-2 signaling for cancer therapy." Clin Cancer Res 12(21): 6326-30.

Mueller, H., R. Liu, et al. (1997). "Selective modulation of protein kinase A and protein kinase C activities in epidermal growth factor (EGF)-stimulated MCF-7 breast cancer cells." Biol Chem 378(9): 1023-9.

Nabha, S. M., S. Glaros, et al. (2005). "Upregulation of PKC-delta contributes to antiestrogen resistance in mammary tumor cells." Oncogene 24(19): 3166-76.

Nakagawa, M., J. L. Oliva, et al. (2005). "Phorbol ester-induced G1 phase arrest selectively mediated by protein kinase Cdelta-dependent induction of p21." J Biol Chem 280(40): 33926-34.

Newton, A. C. (1995). "Protein kinase C: structure, function, and regulation." J Biol Chem 270(48): 28495-8.

Newton, A. C. (1997). "Regulation of protein kinase C." Curr Opin Cell Biol 9(2): 161-7.

Nishizuka, Y. (1995). "Protein kinase C and lipid signaling for sustained cellular responses." FASEB J 9(7): 484-96.

O'Brian C. (1989). "Elevated protein kinase C expression in human breast tumor biopsies relative to normal breast tissue." Cancer Res. 49(12):3215-7

Pan, Q., L. W. Bao, et al. (2005). "Protein kinase C epsilon is a predictive biomarker of aggressive breast cancer and a validated target for RNA interference anticancer therapy." Cancer Res 65(18): 8366-71.

Porumb, T., A. Crivici, et al. (1997). "Calcium binding and conformational properties of calmodulin complexed with peptides derived from myristoylated alanine-rich C kinase substrate (MARCKS) and MARCKS-related protein (MRP)." Eur Biophys J 25(4): 239-47.

Prenzel, N., E. Zwick, et al. (2000). "Tyrosine kinase signalling in breast cancer. Epidermal growth factor receptor: convergence point for signal integration and diversification." Breast Cancer Res 2(3): 184-90.

Rabinovitz, I., A. Toker, et al. (1999). "Protein kinase C-dependent mobilization of the alpha6beta4 integrin from hemidesmosomes and its association with actin-rich cell protrusions drive the chemotactic migration of carcinoma cells." J Cell Biol 146(5): 1147-60.

Rodriguez-Mora, O. G., M. M. LaHair, et al. (2005). "Calcium/calmodulin-dependent kinase I and calcium/calmodulin-dependent kinase kinase participate in the control of cell cycle progression in MCF-7 human breast cancer cells." Cancer Res 65(12): 5408-16.

Roskelley, C. D. and M. J. Bissell (2002). "The dominance of the microenvironment in breast and ovarian cancer." Semin Cancer Biol 12(2): 97-104.

Schwartz, G. K., J. Jiang, et al. (1993). "Protein kinase C: a novel target for inhibiting gastric cancer cell invasion." J Natl Cancer Inst 85(5): 402-7.

Speake, G., B. Holloway, et al. (2005). "Recent developments related to the EGFR as a target for cancer chemotherapy." Curr Opin Pharmacol 5(4): 343-9.

Takenaga, K. and K. Takahashi (1986). "Effects of 12-O-tetradecanoylphorbol-13-acetate on adhesiveness and lung-colonizing ability of Lewis lung carcinoma cells." Cancer Res 46(1): 375-80.

Tan, M., P. Li, et al. (2006). "Upregulation and activation of PKC alpha by ErbB2 through Src promotes breast cancer cell invasion that can be blocked by combined treatment with PKC alpha and Src inhibitors." Oncogene 25(23): 3286-95.

Tozlu-Kara S. et al. (2007). "Oligonucleotide microarray analysis of estrogen receptor alpha-positive postmenopausal breast carcinomas: identification of HRPAP20 and TIMELESS as outstanding candidate markers to predict the response to tamoxifen". J Mol Endocrinol. 2007 Oct;39(4):305-18.

Wang, K. C., B. Mutus, et al. (1983). "On the mechanism of interaction between calmodulin and calmodulin-dependent proteins." Can J Biochem Cell Biol 61(8): 911-20.

Ways, D. K., C. A. Kukoly, et al. (1995). "MCF-7 breast cancer cells transfected with protein kinase C-alpha exhibit altered expression of other protein kinase C isoforms and display a more aggressive neoplastic phenotype." J Clin Invest 95(4): 1906-15

Witz, I. P. (2002). "The tumour microenvironment--introduction." Semin Cancer Biol 12(2): 87-8.

3

ER-Alpha36 Mediates Non-Genomic Estrogen and Anti-Estrogen Signaling in Breast Cancer Cells

ZhaoYi Wang, XianTian Zhang and LianGuo Kang
Department of Medical Microbiology & Immunology,
Creighton University Medical School, Omaha, NE,
USA

1. Introduction

Estrogen signaling is essential in the initiation and development of neoplasia in mammary gland. In the past several decades, extensive efforts have been dedicated to understand the underlying mechanisms of this important signaling pathway in mammary carcinogenesis, which have facilitated the development of anti-estrogen therapy, the first targeted therapy for human cancer.

It has been well documented that the diverse activities of estrogens and anti-estrogens are mediated by specific receptors designated as estrogen receptors (ERs). Currently, there are two identified ERs, ER-α and ER-β, both of which are ligand-activated transcription factors that stimulate target gene transcription. Compelling evidence indicates that estrogens, especially 17β-estradiol (E2β), up-regulate the expression and function of c-Myc and cyclin D1, activate cyclin E-Cdk2 complexes and promotes cell cycle progression from G1 to S phase in mammary epithelial cells. Thus, stimulation of target gene expression by ERs in response to estrogens is prevailingly thought to be responsible for estrogen-stimulated mammary carcinoma initiation and progression.

Despite the clarity with which ERs have been shown to act as ligand-dependent transcription factors, it became apparent now that not all of the activities mediated by ERs are accomplished through a direct effect on gene transcription. Another signaling pathway (also known as a non-classic, non-genomic, extra-nuclear or membrane-initiated signaling pathway) exists that involves cytoplasmic signaling proteins, growth factor receptors and other membrane-initiated signaling pathways. Several intracellular signaling pathways have been shown cross-talking with the membrane-initiated estrogen signaling: the adenylate cyclase pathway, the phospholipase C pathway, the G-protein-coupled receptor-activated pathways, the PI3K/AKT and the MAPK pathways.

Currently, the identity of the membrane-based estrogen receptor that mediates non-genomic estrogen effects has not been fully established. ER-β, two forms of ER-α, full-length (66-kDa) and short form (46-kDa) have been found on or near the plasma membrane and mediates membrane-initiated estrogen signaling. In addition, there is also evidence indicating that GPR30, an orphan G-protein-coupled-receptor, mediates the rapid, non-genomic responses to estrogens. In 2005, our laboratory identified and cloned a novel variant of ER-α, which has a molecular weight of 36-kDa and thus we have termed it ER-α36. This ER-α variant differs from the original 66 kDa ER-α (ER-α66) by lacking both transcriptional activation domains (AF-1 and AF-2) but retaining the DNA-binding domain and partial dimerization and ligand-binding domains. ER-α36 is predominantly expressed on the plasma membrane of both ER-positive and -negative breast cancer cells, mediates membrane-initiated estrogen and anti-estrogen signaling such as activation of the MAPK/ERK and PI3K/AKT signaling pathways and stimulation of cell proliferation. Thus, ER-α36 is a novel membrane-associated estrogen receptor that mediates membrane-initiated estrogen and anti-estrogen signaling in both ER-positive and -negative breast cancer cells.

In this chapter, we highlight the historical understanding of non-genomic estrogen signaling and its role in cell survival and proliferation, and specifically illustrate the biological function and the possible underlying mechanisms of ER-α36 in non-genomic estrogen and anti-estrogen signaling in both ER-positive and –negative breast cancer cells. We also discuss the integral roles of EGFR, Src and STAT5 in the non-genomic estrogen signaling mediated by ER-α36 and the complex regulatory network among ER-α66, 46 and 36. In addition, the novel biology of non-genomic estrogen signaling mediated by ER-α36 also has significance for understanding the physiology of bone remodeling. Thus, ER-α36-mediated signaling has a broad appeal in physiology of non-classical estrogen targeting tissues and general cancer research.

2. Estrogen receptors and genomic estrogen signaling

Estrogen signaling is pivotal in the establishment and maintenance of reproductive function in men and women. It is also involved in normal development and physiology of bone, liver, cardiovascular and neuronal systems. Inappropriate estrogen signaling is involved in osteoporosis, atherosclerosis and Alzheimer's disease and is essential in the initiation and development of neoplasia in breast and endometrial cancers (Nilsson et al., 2001). Hence, it is important to understand the molecular mechanisms by which this important signaling pathway functions, so its participation in a wide variety of different biological processes can be clarified, including how its dysregulation contributes to different diseases and even neoplastic transformation.

The diverse physiological and pathological functions of estrogens are mediated by specific receptors designated as estrogen receptors (ERs). In 1986, the cloning of the estrogen receptor (ER) was first reported (Green et al., 1986; Greene et al., 1986). Until 1996, it was assumed that there was only one ER responsible for all of the physiological and pharmacological effects of natural and synthetic estrogens and anti-estrogens. However, in 1996, a second ER was cloned (Kuiper et al., 1996). Currently, the first ER discovered is referred to as ER-α, while the second is called ER-β.

ER-α and ER-β share a common structural architecture (Reviewed by Kong et al., 2003; Zheng et al., 2003). Both are composed of three independent but interacting functional domains: the N-terminal A/B domain, the C or DNA-binding domain, and the D/E/F or ligand-binding domain. The N-terminal domain of ERs encodes a ligand-independent activation function (AF-1), a region involved in interaction with co-activators, and transcriptional activation of target genes. The DNA-binding domain or C domain contains a two zinc-finger structure, which is involved in receptor dimerization and binding to specific DNA sequences. The C-terminal E/F domain is a ligand-binding domain that mediates ligand binding, receptor dimerization, nuclear translocation, and a ligand-dependent transactivation function (AF-2). The relative contributions that both AF-1 and AF-2 exert on transcriptional control vary in a cell-specific and DNA promoter-specific manner (Berry et al., 1990; Tzukerman et al., 1994).

It is well established that estrogen receptors are members of the nuclear receptor superfamily of ligand-activated transcription factors that control various physiological processes. It is prevailingly thought that this control often occurs through the regulation of gene transcription (Reviewed by Katzenellenbogen & Katzenellenbogen, 2000; McDonnell & Norris, 2002). The estrogen receptor utilizes multiple mechanisms to either activate or repress transcription of its target genes. These mechanisms include: (a) direct interaction of the ligand-occupied receptor with DNA at a consensus estrogen response elements (ERE, GGTCAnnnTGACC) followed by recruitment of transcriptional coregulator or mediator complexes (Reviewed by Klinge, 2001), (b) interaction of the ligand-occupied ER with other transcription factors such as AP-1 (Kushner at al., 2000), Sp1 (Safe, 2001) or NF-κB (McKay & Cidlowski, 1999), or (c) indirect modulation of gene transcription via sequestration of general/common transcriptional components (Harnish et al., 2000; Speir et al., 2000). In addition, the ability of an estrogen receptor to regulate transcription through these mechanisms appears to be cell-type specific, perhaps due to differences in the complement of transcriptional co-regulatory factors available in each cell type (Cerillo et al., 1998; Evans et al., 2001; Maret et al., 1999). Also, transcriptional regulation is dependent upon the nature of the ligand, with various natural and synthetic selective estrogen receptor modulators (SERM) acting as either estrogen receptor agonists or antagonists through these various mechanisms (Shang & Brown, 2002; Katzenellenbogen & Katzenellenbogen, 2002; Margeat et al., 2003).

3. Estrogen signaling and breast cancer

Experimental and clinical evidence for the role of endogenous estrogens in normal development of mammary glands and breast cancer etiology has been well documented (Reviewed by Feigelson & Henderson, 1996). Estrogen signaling is involved in mammary epithelial cell proliferation and differentiation. Dysregulated estrogen signaling increases the rate of cell proliferation and thus the risk for development of breast cancer.

ER-α is expressed in approximately 15-30% of luminal epithelial cells and not at all in any other cell types in the normal human breast (Clarke *et. al.,* 1997). However, dual label immunofluorescent technique revealed that ER-α expressing cells are separate from those labeled with proliferation markers such as Ki67 and cyclin A in both normal human and rodent mammary glands (Clarke et al., 1997; Zeps et al., 1999). This is in direct contrast to estrogen action in breast cancer cells, where estrogens, especially 17β-estradiol (E2β), functions as potent mitogens through promoting cell cycle progression from G1 to S phase (Prall et al., 1998; Altucci et al., 1996 & 1997). Thus, it is thought that estrogens directly interact with ERs in ER-positive human breast cancer cells, where they induce transcriptional activation of "immediate early" and cyclin genes, and promote cell cycle progression. Consistent with its role in mammary carcinogenesis, ER-α expression is increased at the earliest stages of ductal hyperplasia and increases even more with increasing atypia, such that most cells in atypical ductal hyperplasias and in ductal cancer in situ of low and intermediate grade contain ER-α (Khan et. al., 1994). As ER-α expression increases during breast cancer development, the inverse relationship between ER-α expression and cell proliferation become dysregulated (Shoker *et. al.,* 1999 a and b).

Approximately 70% of invasive breast carcinomas express the ER-α and most of these tumors contain ER-α positive proliferating cells (Clarke *et. al.,* 1997).

Currently, ER-α is the most widely used marker in diagnosis of human breast cancer. Breast cancers are diagnosed either as ER-positive or -negative depending on the existence or absence of ER-α. At the onset, 46%-77% of breast cancers are ER-positive (Robertson *et. al.,* 1996). The ER-positive tumors are histologically well differentiated and diploid, and patients with ER-positive tumors generally have a better prognosis since they respond well to anti-estrogen treatment (Clark *et. al.,* 1984; Osborne *et. al.,* 1980). ER-negative breast cancers that account for about one third of breast cancers diagnosed, however, are more malignant and aggressive through a still unknown mechanism (Sheikh *et. al.,* 1994), and they generally respond poorly to anti-estrogen treatment.

ER-negative breast cancers are often considered to be the result of tumor progression from ER-positive premalignant lesions or ER-positive breast cancers by epigenetic alterations such as promoter methylation (Ferguson et. al., 1995) or ER-α protein degradation by the proteasome system after hypoxia in non-vascularized tumors (Stoner et. al., 2002). However, immunohistochemical studies in human breast cancers showed that some proliferative ductal lesions and many high-grade ductal carcinomas in situ (DCIS) are ER-α-negative (Roger et. al., 2000), suggesting some ER-negative breast cancers may be progressed directly from ER-negative premalignant lesions.

4. Non-genomic estrogen signaling

It become clear now that estrogens elicit two signaling pathways; the first requires hours to days to result in transcriptional changes of target genes and is known as genomic, classic or nuclear signaling pathway while the second occurs in seconds to minutes after estrogen treatment and usually initiates at the plasma membrane. Thus, the second signaling pathway is also known as a non-classic, non-genomic, extra-nuclear or membrane-initiated signaling pathway which is mediated by estrogen binding proteins associated with the plasma membrane and employs various cytoplasmic signaling proteins, growth factor receptors and G-protein-coupled-receptor signaling pathways (Segars & Driggers, 2002; Driggers & Segars, 2002; Kelly & Levin, 2001; Levin, 2002; Hammes & Levin, 2007).

Pietras and Szego first described the rapid estrogen signaling more than 30 years ago (Pietras & Szego, 1975 &1977), noting immediate calcium fluxes in endometrial cells induced by estrogen and specific binding sites at the outer surfaces of isolated endometrial cells. Quick estrogen responses were also recorded in neuroendocrine tissue such as a rapid rise of intracellular calcium in pituitary cells, which leads to cell depolarization within 1 min (Dufy et al., 1979). Rapid estrogen signaling also induces prolactin secretion from pituitary tumor cells (Watson et al., 1999). Such signaling of estrogens has also been described in uterine (Aronica et al., 1994) and ovarian cells (Morley et al., 1992; Tesarik & Mendoza, 1997) as well as bone (Endoh et al., 1997; Longo et al., 2004; Sylvia et al., 2001), vascular endothelial (Russell et al., 2000; Lu et al., 2004) and neuronal cells (Kelly et al., 1977; Mermelstein et al., 1996), indicating that the rapid, non-genomic estrogen signaling is involved in various physiological and pathological estrogen activities.

Non-genomic estrogen signaling has been also documented in breast cancer cells for cell proliferation and survival (Song et al., 2002; Migliaccio et al., 1996; Ahmad et al., 1999; Lobenhofer et al., 2000; Castoria et al., 1999 & 2001). These findings strongly suggest that the rapid, non-genomic estrogen signaling is involved in estrogen-induced proliferation in breast cancer cells.

5. Nature of membrane-based estrogen receptor

While it is clear that membrane-initiated estrogen signaling exists, the identity of the membrane-based estrogen receptor that mediates these rapid estrogen effects, especially the effects in mammary epithelial cell proliferation and survival, has not been fully established. Laboratory evidence indicated that both ER-α and ER-β are involved in the rapid, non-genomic estrogen signaling (Razandi et al., 1999). However, evidence also suggests that more than one membrane-initiated signaling pathway is associated with estrogen action. Data from several laboratories using the membrane-impermeable compound 17β-estradiol-bovine serum albumin (E2β-BSA) indicates the existence of two functionally distinct membrane-associated pathways: one sensitive to anti-estrogens and one resistant (Chen et al., 1999; Russell et al., 2000; Watters et al., 1997). For example, ER-α/knockout mice retained rapid estrogen-stimulated membrane effects in neurons, which were not blocked by anti-estrogen ICI-182, 780 (Gu, et. al., 1999). These findings suggest that another membrane-based ER may exist since all known ERs are sensitive to anti-estrogen inhibition. As a consequence, an orphan G-protein coupled receptor, GPCR30, and some other unknown proteins have been reported to mediate this anti-estrogen resistant non-genomic estrogen signaling.

6. ER-α

A large body of experimental evidence indicated that ER-α is involved in both genomic and non-genomic estrogen signaling. Immunofluorescent staining of non-permeabilized pituitary tumor cells with anti-ER-α antibodies revealed a punctuated staining pattern on cell surface although most ER-α were localized in cell nuclei (Watson et al., 1999). ER-α associated with the plasma membrane is also detected by a panel of antibodies targeting different domains of ER-α in intact breast cancer cells and in breast cancer specimens (Pietras et al., 2005; Kim et al., 2006). The findings that transfection of the nuclear ER-α cDNA into ER-"null" Chinese hamster ovary (CHO) cells leads to expression of both membrane and nuclear ER-α further support the notion that membrane-associated ER-α is derived from the same transcript as nuclear ER-α (Razandi et al., 1999). However, recent evidence indicates that the CHO-K1, Rat2-fibroblasts and COS7 cells previously considered as ER "null' cells and extensively used to transfect ER cDNAs in order to demonstrate rapid estrogen signaling actually exhibit strong non-genomic estrogen signaling such as activation of the MAPK/ERK before transfection (Nethrapalli et al., 2005), suggesting these cells already posses some unknown proteins other than classical ERs that mediate the rapid estrogen signaling.

It is widely accepted that estrogen signaling promotes cell proliferation in target cells. However, the explanation of this effect of estrogen signaling simply by the function of ER-α is confounding. When ER-α was expressed in ER-"null" CHO cells (Kushner *et. al.*, 1990), and human cervical cancer HeLa cells (Touitou *et. al.*, 1990), E2β failed to stimulate cell growth. On the contrary, E2β inhibited cell proliferation and even induced cell apoptosis. Likewise, the ER-negative immortal MCF10A breast epithelial cells (Pilat *et. al.*, 1996), and MDA-MB-231 breast cancer cells (Jiang & Jordan, 1992) were both growth inhibited by estrogen when stably transfected with ER-α cDNA. These experimental results argue against a positive function of the well-known ER-α alone in mitogenic estrogen signaling.

7. ER-β

ER-β acts as a classical ligand-induced transcription factor. Like ER-α, ligand-bound ER-β functions by regulating downstream target genes. ER-β also heterodimerizes with ER-α and modulates ER-α function (Reviewed by Harris, 2007; Deroo & Buensuceso, 2010). ER-β has been shown to be S-palmitoylated, which facilitates the localization of ER-β at the plasma membrane to mediate the rapid, non-genomic estrogen effects (Marino & Ascenzi, 2008). Indeed, the involvement of ER-β in rapid, non-genomic estrogen signaling has been documented when ER-β cDNA was introduced into CHO cells (Razandi et al., 1999). In colon cancer, pro-apoptotic activities of ER-β have been reported to be mediated by membrane-initiated signaling; induction of ER-β via the MAPK/p38 signaling pathway, which in turn leads to downstream apoptotic events (Caiazza et al., 2007), indicating a potential role of ER-β as a tumor suppressor. In addition, inhibition of ER-β palmitoylation in colon cancer cells abrogated the pro-apoptotic activity of ER-β (Galluzzo et al., 2007), suggesting that non-genomic effects mediated by membrane–associated ER-β is important for its pro-apoptotic function.

The biological significance of ER-β in breast cancer has not been well established. Approximately 70% of breast tumor express ER-β and most tumor co-express both ER-α and -β (Dotzlaw et al., 1997; Fuqua et al., 1999 & 2003). Studies indicated that ER-β expression in human breast cancer is associated with a poorer prognosis, compared with tumors that only express ER-α (Speirs et al., 1999). ER-β expression is associated with elevated levels of proliferation markers, Ki67 and cyclin A, in human breast cancer (Jensen et al., 2001) These studies suggested that ER-β may promote cell proliferation and breast cancer progression.

In contrast, accumulating evidence indicated that ER-β acts as a tumor suppressor in breast cancer. ER-β is expressed in both normal and malignant mammary glands (Warner et al., 2000; Speirs et al., 2002). In the rodent mammary gland, ER-β expressing cells can proliferate but the majority cells that express proliferation markers do not express either ER (Saji et al., 2001). The levels of ER-β expression are highest in normal mammary gland and are decreased as tumors progress from pre-invasive to invasive (Leygue et al., 1998; Iwao et al., 2000; Roger et al., 2001). The presence of ER-β in breast cancer confers a more favorable prognosis and is associated with node-negative, low-grade tumors (Jarvinen et al., 2000) as well as a greater disease-free survival rate (Omoto et al., 2001). Several laboratory studies demonstrated that ER-β inhibited angiogenesis and malignant growth of T47D breast tumor xenograft and malignant growth of MCF7 breast cancer cells *in vitro* and in nude mice (Hartman et al., 2006; Paruthiyil et al., 2004). Intriguingly, ER-β also inhibited proliferation of ER-negative breast cancer MDA-MB-231 cells in a ligand-independent manner whereas ER-α inhibition of MDA-MB-231 cell proliferation is estrogen-dependent (Lazennec et al., 2001). These results indicate that ER-β negatively regulates mitogenic estrogen signaling.

8. ER-α46

Previously, it was reported that a 46-kDa antigen is tightly associated with ER-α in human breast cancer samples (Diaz-Chico *et. al.*, 1988). This 46-kDa antigen is enriched in the cell cytosol and could be recognized by an isolated monoclonal antibody, E476, raised against the human ER-α (Diaz-Chico *et. al.*, 1988). Similarly, Jozan (1991) later reported that there are two species of ER with different molecular weight (65 and 47 kDa), and three species of tumors (36% containing the highest form of ER alone, 49% bearing the two forms in variable amounts, and 15% bearing only the minor form). These results strongly suggest that two different forms of ER-α exist at different ratios in human breast cancer.

In 2000, Flouriot *et. al.* cloned a 46-kDa isoform of ER-α and demonstrated that the 46-kDa isoform lacks the first 173 amino acids (A/B or AF-1 domain) and is derived from alternative splicing of the ER-α gene by skipping exon 1. This alternative splicing event generates an mRNA that has an AUG in a favorable Kozak sequence for translation initiation in frame with the remainder of the open reading frame of ER-α (Flouriot et. al., 2000). This new isoform of ER-α is named as ER-α46 and the original one as ER-α66. ER-α46 forms homo-dimers and binds to an ERE, and it can also form heterodimers with ER-α66 (Flouriot et. al., 2000). Furthermore, the ER-α46/66 heterodimers form preferentially over the ER-α66 homodimers and ER-α46 acts competitively to inhibit transactivation mediated by AF-1 domain of ER-α66 but without effect on AF-2-dependent transactivation (Floutiot et. al., 2000). Therefore, ER-α46 is a naturally occurring isoform of ER-α that regulates genomic estrogen signaling mediated by the AF-1 domain of ER-α66.

Previously, two forms of ER-α, full-length (66-kDa) and short form (46-kDa) were co-purified with 5′ nucleotidase, a plasma membrane-marker enzyme (Marquez & Pietras, 2001), suggesting a possible role of ER-α46 in the rapid, non-genomic estrogen signaling. Recently, ER-α46 was localized on the plasma membrane, in the cytosol, and nucleus of endothelial cells and mediated rapid estrogen signaling such as activation of the Src/PI3K/AKT signaling and stimulation of NO synthesis (Kim & Bender, 2005; Li *et. al.*, 2003; Reviewed by Moriarty et al., 2006), further confirming that the ER-α46 isoform functions as a membrane-associated estrogen receptor.

Although it is clear now that ER-α46 is involved in both genomic and non-genomic estrogen signaling, its function in breast cancer has been less investigated. Forced expression of ER-α46 inhibited proliferation of MCF-7 breast cancer cells and cyclin D1 promoter activity (Penot et al., 2005). Overexpression of both ER-α46 and ER-α66 in ER-negative MDA-MB-231 cells revealed that ER-α46 inhibited basal transcription of the estrogen responsive gene pS2 while estrogen treatment released this inhibition (Metivier et al., 2004). Recently, expression levels of ER-α46 was found to be down-regulated in tamoxifen-resistant breast cancer cells and re-introduction of ER-α46 into these cells inhibited cell proliferation and ER-α66-regulated gene transcription (Klinge et al., 2010). Thus, these results suggest that ER-α46 may function as a negative-regulator of mitogenic estrogen signaling in ER-positive breast cancer cells.

9. ER-α36

In 2005, our laboratory identified a 5.4 kb cDNA clone from a normal human edometrium cDNA library (RZPD clone number: DKFZp686N23123) and later cloned this cDNA from a human placenta cDNA library (Wang et al., 2005). This cDNA clone harbors a 310 amino acid open-reading frame that can produce a protein with a predicted molecular weight of 35.7 kDa. To differentiate it from ER-α66 and 46, and apply consistent nomenclature, this novel isoform of ER-α was named as ER-α36.

The cDNA sequence of the open-reading frame matches 100% to the DNA sequence of the exons 2 to 6 of the ER-α66 gene. The 5′untraslated region (5′UTR) of the cDNA showed 100% homology to the DNA sequence of the first intron of the ER-α66 gene. Thus, the transcript of this ER-α isoform is initiated from a previously unidentified promoter in the first intron of the ER-α66 gene (Figure 1, Zou et al., 2009). A small, non-coding novel exon in the first intron of the ER-α66 gene was designated as exon 1′. The exon 1′ is then spliced directly into the exon 2 of the ER-α66 gene and continues from exon 2 to exon 6 of the ER-α66 gene. Exon 6 is then spliced to an exon located 64,141 bp downstream of the ER-α66 gene (Figure 1). The cDNA sequence encoding the last 27 amino acids and the 4,293 bp 3′untranslated region (3′UTR) was matched 100% to a continuous sequence from the genomic sequence of clone RP1-1304 on chromosome 6q24.2-25.3 (GeneBank accession number AL78582), indicating the remaining cDNA sequence of this novel ER-α isoform is transcribed from one big exon of 4,374 bp located downstream of the ER-α66 gene. This exon is thus designated as exon 9 to reflect the extra exon beyond the previous reported eight exons for ER-α66 gene (Figure 1). All of these splicing events are supported by the identification of perfect splice donors and acceptors at the splice juncture. The protein ER-α36 can be produced from a perfect Kozak sequence located in the second exon, the same initiation codon used to produce ER-α46 (Flouriot *et. al.,* 2000). ER-α36 differs from the ER-α66 by lacking both transcriptional activation domains (AF-1 and AF-2) but retaining the DNA-binding and dimerization domains, and partial ligand-binding domains. It also possesses an extra, unique 27 amino acid domain to replace the last 138 amino acids encoded by exon 7 and 8 of the ER-α66 (Figure 2). Thus, ER-α36 is another naturally occurring novel isoform of ER-α that may play an important role in both genomic and non-genomic estrogen signaling. Currently, there are three major ER-α isoforms observed in ER-positive breast cancer MCF7 cells that correspond to three mRNA variants generated from different promoter usage and alternative splicing (Figure 2).

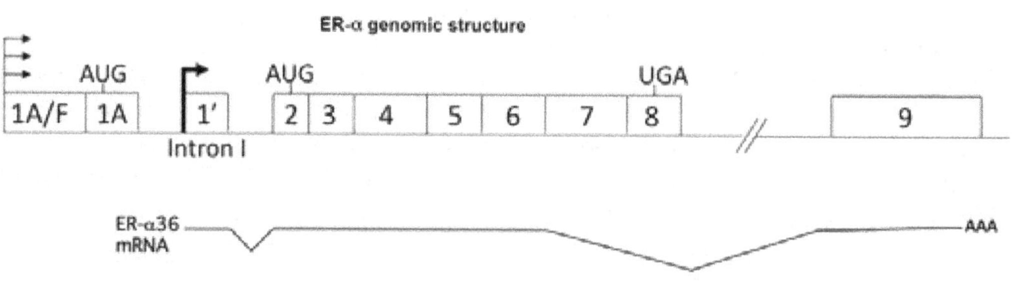

Fig. 1. Genomic organization of the human ER-α36 gene. The locations of multiple promoters of human ER-α66 gene are shown as arrows. The translation start and stop codons are indicated as AUG and UGA. The common exons are shown as numbered open boxes. The extra exon that is beyond the 8 exons of the human ER-α66 gene is numbered as 9 in the open box. The intron 1 is also shown with the exon 1′ in the open box. The lower panel shows mRNA structure of human ER-α36 isoform.

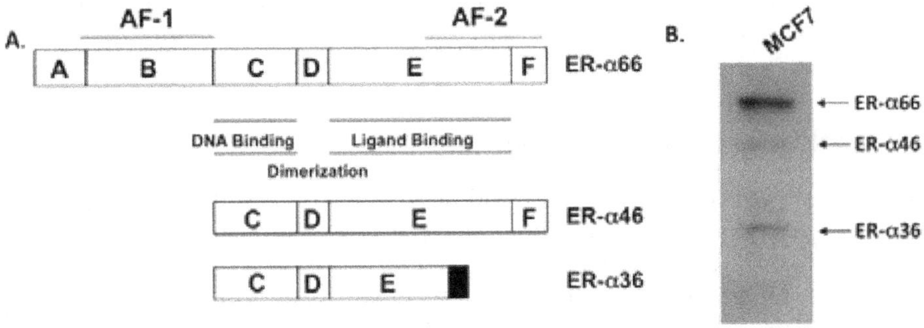

Fig. 2. Domain structure and expression of human estrogen receptor-α variants in ER-positive breast cancer MCF7 cells. (A). Domain structure representation of human ER-α isoforms. Domains (labeled A–F), and activation function domains (AF-1 and -2) are shown. The function of each domain is indicated. The last 27 amino acids of human ER-α36 are indicated as a filled box. (B). Western blot analysis of three human ER-α isoforms in MCF7 cells with an anti-ER-α66 antibody (H222).

10. GPR30

Previously, different laboratories demonstrated the existence of two distinct membrane-associated pathways: one sensitive to anti-estrogens and one resistant (Chen et al., 1999; Russell et al., 2000; Watters et al., 1997). These results suggest that another membrane-associated estrogen receptor may exist since both ER-α and -β are sensitive to anti-estrogen inhibition.

An orphan G protein-coupled receptor, GPR30 was reported to mediate the rapid, non-genomic estrogen signaling that was insensitive to ICI 182,780; estrogen stimulates changes of Ca^{2+} currents and cAMP signaling in cells expressing GPR30 (Revankar et al., 2005) and activates the MAPK/ERK phosphorylation and the PI3K/Akt signalling pathways via transactivation of the EGFR pathway in ER-negative but GPR30-positive breast cancer cells (Filardo et al., 2000 & 2007). Thus, GPR30 was considered as a novel type of membrane-associated estrogen receptor that mediates the rapid, non-genomic estrogen signaling.

There are also reports that challenge the role of GPR30 as a novel estrogen receptor. A study showed that introduction of GPR30 anti-sense oligonucleotides failed to block the MAPK/ERK activation and cell growth induced by estrogen in ER-positive breast cancer cells (Ahola et al., 2002). Pedram *et al.* (2006) failed to observe the cAMP or ERK activation in GPR30-positive, ER-negative breast cancer cells. Another study demonstrated that the GPR30 selective agonist G1 failed to exert estrogenic effect in two classical estrogen target organs, the uterus and the mammary gland (Otto et al., 2008). Recently, Otto *et al.* generated GPR30-deficient mice and demonstrated that the development of reproductive organs was unimpaired in these mice and the estrogenic responses in the uterus and the mammary gland were completely maintained in GPR30-deficient animals (Otto et al., 2009).

Recently, our group reported that knockdown of GPR30 expression in ER-negative breast cancer SK-BR-3 cells down-regulated the expression levels of ER-α36 (Kang et al., 2010b). Introduction of a GPR30 expression vector into GPR30 non-expressing cells induced endogenous ER-α36 expression and GPR30 activated the promoter activity of ER-α36 via an AP-1 binding site located in the 5′-flanking region of ER-α36 (Kang et al., 2010b). Thus, ERα36 is a downstream target gene of GPR30-mediated signaling and the previously reported activities of GPR30 as a membrane-based estrogen receptor are through its ability to induce ER-α36 expression.

11. Other putative estrogen receptors

Other unknown proteins that may be involved in the rapid, non-genomic estrogen signaling have been also reported. For an example, a report that E2β activated the MAPK/ERK signaling in un-trasnfected CHO-K1, COS7 and Rat2-fibroblasts (Nethrapalli et al., 2005) suggested the existence of an unidentified membrane-associated mER. Recently, we reported that un-transfected COS7 cells express high levels of endogenous ER-α36 (Kang et al., 2010b) and found that CHO-K1 cells also express ER-α36 (Kang et al., unpublished observations), suggesting that ER-α36 may mediates the rapid, non-genomic estrogen signaling observed in these cells.

Another unique membrane-associated ER with an estimated molecular weight of 63-65 kDa, referred to as ER-X, is developmentally regulated differently from both ER-α and -β. Its pharmacological profile was also different from ER-α and -β, even with some features opposite to those shown for these two receptors (Toran-Allerand et al., 2002). For examples, ER-X mediated rapid estrogen signaling was not sensitive to anti-estrogen, and the association of Hsp90 is required for the inactive state of ER-α while ER-X requires to be associated with hsp90 for its activity (Toran-Allerand et al., 2002). Whereas ER-X shares limited similarities with ER-α36, such as reaction with antibodies to the ligand-binding domain of ER-α66 and responding equally to 17α- and β-estradiol, the molecular similarity of these two receptors awaits for the cloning and sequencing of ER-X.

Additionally, a heterodimeric estrogen-binding protein, referred to as the putative ER (pER), was reported to bind to E2β at a sub-nanomolar affinity but was unable to bind other estrogens or anti-estrogens. Depending on cell types, pER is expressed on the plasma and/or nuclear membranes or in the cytoplasm and nucleus (Rao et al., 1998). Since the polyclonal anti-pER antibody failed to react with estrogen receptors and was unable to detect pER expression in reproductive organs (Rao et al., 1998), the role of this putative estrogen receptor in non-genomic estrogen signaling of breast cancer cells remains elusive.

12. Negative regulation of genomic estrogen signaling by ER-α36

Comparison of protein structures of ER-α66 and ER-α36 indicated that ER-α36 lacks both AF-1 and -2 transcription activation domains but retains the DNA-binding domain and dimerization domain. Transient co-transfection assays using a luciferase-expressing reporter construct that contains two Estrogen Response Element (ERE) placed upstream of the thymidine kinase promoter (2 X ERE-tk-Luc) revealed that ER-α36 has no intrinsic transcriptional activity in the presence and absence of E2β (Wang et al., 2006). However, ER-α36 strongly inhibited the transactivation activities mediated by the AF-1 and -2 domains of both ER-α66 and ER-β (Wang et al., 2006). These data indicate that ER-α36 itself is unable to mediate genomic estrogen signaling by regulate target gene expression. However, ER-α36 acts as a naturally occurring dominant-negative regulator of the genomic estrogen signaling mediated by the AF1 and AF2 domains of ER-α66 and ER-β.

13. Membrane-association and mitogenic signaling of ER-α36

The fact that ER-α36 posses no intrinsic transcription regulatory activity suggests that ER-α36 may be a membrane-associated estrogen receptor. The sub-cellular fractionation assay in ER-α36 transfected HEK293 cells revealed that a high percentage of ER-α36 (~50%) is localized on or near the plasma membrane and a low percentage of it in cytosol (~40%) and nucleus (~10%) (Wang *et al.*, 2006). Immuno-fluorescence staining of intact breast cancer MCF7 cells and endometrial cancer Hec1A cells using the ER-α36 specific antibody recognizing the last 20 amino acids that are unique to ER-α36 exhibits a membrane expression pattern that is co-localized with caviolin-1, a typical cell-surface protein (Lin et al., 2010). Immunohistochemistry analysis of specimens from breast cancer patients also demonstrated an expression pattern of ER-α36 predominantly on the breast cancer cell surface (Lee et al., 2008; Vranic et al., 2011). This anti-ER-α36 specific antibody also blocked ER-α36-mediated non-genomic estrogen signaling such as activation of the MAPK/ERK signaling in breast cancer cells presumably through steric hindrance of estrogen accesses to its binding pocket (Kang *et. al.*, 2010b), indicating that the antibody is accessible to the C-terminal region of the plasma membrane-associated ER-α36 in intact cells. These results thus demonstrated that ER-α36 is expressed on or near the plasma membrane and suggested that ER-α36 may be also shuttled to the cell cytoplasm and nucleus depending on cell context and extracellular signals.

Both 17β-estradiol (E2β) and BSA-conjugated E2β elicit the rapid, membrane-initiated estrogen signaling such as activation of the MAPK/ERK signaling pathway and stimulation of cell proliferation in ER-α36 transfected HEK293 cells, which is not blocked by anti-estrogens such as tamoxifen, 4-hydroxy-tamoxifen and ICI 182, 780 (Wang et al., 2006). In addition, other estrogens including estrone (E1), 17α-estradiol (E2α), estriol (E3) and estetrol (E4) all activate the ERK1/2 phosphorylation at a very similar level (Wang et al., 2006). Recently, it was reported that ER-α36 even mediated testosterone-stimulated activation of the MAPK/ERK and PI3K/Akt signaling pathways in endometrial cancer Hec1A cells (Lin et al., 2009). ER-α36 also mediates estrogen activation of the PKCδ/ERK signaling pathway (Tong et al., 2010). The finding that the non-genomic estrogen signaling mediated by ER-α36 was insensitive to anti-estrogens suggests that ER-α36 may be a receptor involved in the anti-estrogen-insensitive estrogen signaling described in different systems before. Taken together, ER-α36 is a membrane-associated estrogen receptor that mediates rapid and mitogenic estrogen signaling.

14. ER-α36 in anti-estrogen signaling and anti-estrogen resistance

Since mitogenic estrogen signaling plays a pivotal role in development and maintenance of ER-positive breast cancer, treatment with anti-estrogens such as tamoxifen (TAM) has become a first-line therapy for advanced ER-positive breast cancer. However, laboratory and clinical evidence indicated that TAM and its metabolites such as 4-hydroxytamoxifen (4-OHT) have mixed agonist/antagonist or estrogenic/anti-estrogenic actions depending on cell and tissue context, and the agonist activity of tamoxifen may contribute to tamoxifen resistance observed in almost all patients treated with tamoxifen. As a consequence, a more potent and "pure" anti-estrogen, ICI 182, 780 (Fulvestrant, Faslodex) has been developed (Reviewed by Howell et al., 2000).

TAM and 4-OHT are thought to function as antagonists by competing with E2β and other estrogens for binding to ERs. Further structural studies revealed that TAM induces an ER-α conformation that does not recruit coactivators to trans-activate target genes but recruits co-repressors (Shang *et. al.*, 2000), suggesting that TAM- and 4-OHT-bounded ER-α66 is unable to effectively activate genes involved in cell growth and breast cancer development. On the other hand, ICI 182, 780, a 'pure' antiestrogen without estrogenic activity, works in a different mechanism. ICI 182, 780 binds to ERs, impairs receptor dimerization and inhibits nuclear localization of receptor (Fawell, *et. al.*, 1990; Dauvois *et. al.*, 1992). Furthermore, ICI 182, 780 also accelerates degradation of the ER-α66 protein without a reduction of ER-α66 mRNA (Nicholson *et. al.*, 1995). Thus, ICI 182, 780 binds ER-α66 and accelerates degradation of ER-α66 protein, resulting in a complete inhibition of estrogen signaling mediated by ER-α66.

Although ICI 182, 780 has been depicted as a non-agonist or 'full' or 'pure' anti-estrogen, different laboratories documented estrogenic agonist activities of ICI 182, 780 in different systems. Estrogenic agonist activity of ICI 182, 780 has been found in hippocampal neurons and in bone cells where ICI 182, 780 promoted bone growth (Zhao et al., 2006; Sibonga et al., 1998). Agonist-like activities of ICI 182, 780 have also been reported in tamoxifen-resistant KPL-1 breast cancer cells (Kurebayashi et al., 1998) and Yeast (Dudley et al., 2000). Both tamoxifen and ICI 182, 780 were also reported to induce phosphorylation of the adhesion molecules p130Cas/BCR1, FAK and Src in ER-positive breast cancer MCF7 cells (Cowell et al., 2006). The molecular mechanisms by which ICI 182, 780 acts as an estrogenic agonist have never been elucidated. Studies from a number of laboratories suggested that a membrane associated estrogen-binding receptor mediates the agonist actions of ICI 182, 780 in neurons (Reviewed by Brinton 2001; Zhao et al., 2005; McEwen, 2002).

As described above, ER-α36 mediated non-genomic estrogen signaling is insensitive to anti-estrogens such as TAM and ICI 182, 780 (Wang et al., 2006). ER-α36 also mediates agonist activities of tamoxifen and ICI 182, 780 such as activation of the MAPK/ERK and the PI3K/AKT signaling pathways in breast and endometrial cancer cells (Wang *et. al.*, 2006; Lin *et. al.*, 2010). ICI 182, 780 failed to induce degradation of ER-α36 (Kang et al., 2010a) presumably because ER-α36 has a truncated ligand-binding domain that lacks the last 4 helixes (helix 9–12) of ER-α66 (Wang et al., 2005). The helix-12 domain is critical in protein degradation induced by ICI 182, 780 and different positioning of the helix 12 and the F domain of ER-α66 regulates functional differences between agonists and antagonists (Mahfoudi et al., 1995; Pearce et al., 2003). Thus, it is possible that ER-α36 is a receptor that mediates agonist activities of TAM and ICI 182, 780 recorded in different systems.

Despite the significant anti-neoplastic activities of anti-estrogens, most breast tumors are eventually resistant to anti-estrogen therapy. Essentially, two forms of anti-estrogen resistance occur: *de novo* and acquired resistance (Reviewed by Clarke *et. al.*, 2001 & 2003; Ring & Dowestt, 2004). Although absence of ER-α66 expression is the most common *de novo* resistance mechanism, about 40-50% ER-positive tumors are already resistant to anti-estrogens by the time of diagnosis; this *de novo* resistance mechanism in these ER-positive tumors is largely unknown (Reviewed by Clarke *et. al.*, 2001 & 2003; Ring & Dowestt, 2004). Furthermore, most initially responsive breast tumors gradually acquire anti-estrogen resistance by loss of anti-estrogen responsiveness. The underlying mechanism of breast tumors loss their anti-estrogen responsiveness remains unknown. Breast tumors with acquired TAM resistance frequently but not always retain levels of ER-α66 expression that would still define them as ER-positive tumors (Reviewed by Clarke *et. al.,* 2001 & 2003). Therefore, a loss of ER-α66 expression is not the major mechanism driving acquired anti-estrogen resistance. Up-regulation of Erb-B2 (Her2/Neu) and activation of the MAPK signaling pathways are usually associated with development of anti-estrogen resistance (Reviewed by Clarke *et. al.,* 2001 & 2003; Ring & Dowsett, 2004).

A recent retrospective study of 896 cases of breast cancer patients revealed that about 40% cases of human breast cancer patients were positive for ER-α36; about 40% cases ER-positive breast cancer co-expressed ER-α66 and ER-α36 and about 40% cases of ER-negative breast cancer that lacked ER-α66 expression were positive for ER-α36 (Shi et al., 2009). The breast cancer patients with tumors expressing high levels of ER-α36 were less benefited from tamoxifen therapy than those with low levels of ER-α36 expression did, and ER-α36 expression is significantly associated with Her2/Neu expression (Shi *et. al.,* 2009). These data suggest that high levels of ER-α36 expression in breast cancer cells is one of the underlying mechanisms of *de novo* tamoxifen resistance found in ER-positive breast cancer patients.

The aromatase inhibitors (AIs), on the other hand, inhibit the action of the enzyme aromatase, which converts testosterone to E2 (estradiol) and androstenedione to E1 (estrone). The third generation AIs exemplified by anastrazole and letrozole, provides a second line therapeutic strategy in advanced ER-positive patients (Reviewed by Santen, 2003). However, breast cancer cells that express high levels of ER-α36 are super sensitive to estrogen; activation of the MAPK/ERK in response to an extreme low concentration of estrogen, 1×10^{-16} M/L (Zhang et al., 2011). The anastrozole usually suppresses a plasma level of E2β to a mean of 2.6 pmol/L and letrozole to a mean of 2.1 pmol/L (Geisler et al., 2002). These data suggest that breast cancer patients with tumors expressing high levels of ER-α36 may also be refractory to the third generation of AIs.

15. ER-α36 in ER-negative breast cancer

Because of the lack of ER-α66 expression, it is prevailingly thought that estrogen signaling is not involved in development and progression of ER-negative breast cancer. However, early study showed that ovariectomy prevents formation of both ER-positive and -negative breast cancers (Nissen-Meyer, 1964). In addition, BRCA1 mutation related tumors, the vast majority of which are ER-negative, are also effectively prevented by prophylactic ovariectomy (Rebbeck et al., 1999). The increased risk developing breast cancer following pregnancy is assumed due to the ability of pregnancy-associated hormones such as estrogen to stimulate mammary epithelial cell proliferation. Surprisingly, however, the majority of breast cancers that develop following pregnancy are negative for either estrogen and progesterone receptors. To explain this contradictory findings, Gupta et al., (2007) proposed that estrogen may promote the growth of ER-negative breast cancer via a systemic increase in host angiogenesis.

Rapid activation of the PI3K/Akt pathway in ER-negative breast cancer MDA-MB-231 cells that could not be blocked by estrogen antagonists was reported (Tsai *et. al.,* 2001), which was explained as estrogen signaling through an ER-independent pathway. Taken together, these data suggest that subsets of ER-negative breast cancer cells may retain non-genomic estrogen signaling, which may contribute to development and progression of ER-negative breast cancers. Several studies demonstrated that ER-α36 variant is expressed in established

ER-negative breast cancer cell lines such as MDA-MB-231 and MDA-MB-436 and about 40% specimens from ER-negative breast cancer patients (Wang et al., 2006; Lee et al., 2008; Shi et al., 2009). Our group recently reported that E2β treatment activated the MAPK/ERK signaling pathway, induced expression of growth-promoting genes, c-Myc and cyclin D1, stimulated cell proliferation and accelerated tumor growth *in vivo* in ER-negative breast cancer MDA-MB-231 and MDA-MB-436 cells, all of which could be abrogated by knock-down of ER-α36 expression using ER-α36 specific shRNA (Zhang et al., 2011). Thus, ER-α36-mediated mitogenic estrogen signaling contributes malignant growth of ER-negative breast cancer cells.

16. Underlying mechanism of mitogenic estrogen signaling mediated by ER-α36

Compelling evidence demonstrated that estrogens up-regulate the expression and function of c-Myc and cyclin D1, and activate cyclin E-Cdk2 complexes, all of which are rate limiting factors for cell cycle progression from G1 to S phase (Prall *et. al.*, 1998; Altucci *et. al.*, 1996 & 1997). Based on these findings, it is believed that estrogens directly interact with ERs in ER-positive human breast cancer cells, where they induce transcriptional activation of "immediate early" and cyclin genes and promote cell cycle progression. However, membrane-initiated estrogen signaling, including rapid changes of the signal transduction cascades, has been proposed to be also essential for the mitogenic action of estrogen signaling. Castoria *et. al.*, (1999) reported that NIH3T3 fibroblasts are made equally E2β-responsive in terms of DNA synthesis by transient transfection with either the wild-type or the transcriptionally inactive ER-α66 mutant. Castoria *et. al.*, (2001) later demonstrated that the PI3K/Akt signaling pathway and Src together mediates activation of cyclin D1 promoter activity and promotion of the S-phase entry in estrogen–stimulated ER-positive breast cancer MCF7 cells. These findings together with other reports (Song et al., 2002; Migliaccio et al., 1996; Ahmad et al., 1999; Lobenhofer et al., 2000) highlight the importance of the non-genomic action of estrogen signaling in estrogen-stimulated cell proliferation and mammary tumorigenesis.

The epidermal growth factor receptor (EGFR) is essential for ductal morphogenesis during normal mammary gland development and its overexpression either at the gene or protein levels is well documented in human breast cancer (Reviewed by Troyer & Lee, 2001). Overexpression of EGFR alone usually does not constitute efficient transformation and tumorigenesis in breast cancer models. However, co-expression with the non-receptor kinase c-Src dramatically increases tumorigenesis (Maa et al., 1995; Tice et al., 1999; Biscardi et al., 1998). Co-expression of EGFR and c-Src in breast cancer cell lines results in their association and c-Src-mediated phosphorylation of the EGFR at tyrosine 845 (Tyr845) within its catalytic domain, which contributes to enhanced proliferation *in vitro* and tumor formation *in vivo* (Biscardi et al., 1998; Maa et al., 1995; Tice et al., 1999; Biscardi et al., 2000). Accumulating evidence indicated that c-Src is involved in non-genomic estrogen signaling by interacting with ER-α66 in ER-positive breast cancer cells (Shupnik, 2004). In ER-negative breast cancer cells, E2β induced the MAPK/ERK activation through a mechanism that involves the interaction between ER-α36 and the EGFR/Src/Shc complex (Zhang et al, 2011). Intriguingly, ER-α36 interacts strongly with EGFR in the absence of estrogen and is progressively dissociated from EGFR after estrogen treatment (Zhang et al., 2011), which is in contradictory to the finding that estrogen stimulates recruitment of ER-α66 to the EGFR complex (Reviewed by Levin, 2003). Like ER-α66 (Song et al., 2002), interaction between ER-α36 and the Src/Shc was estrogen-dependent (Zhang et al., 2011), which results in Src-Tyr-416 phosphorylation and phosphorylation of the EGFR-Tyr-845 but not the major auto-phosphorylation sites of EGFR such as Tyr-992, -1068 and -1073. Tyr-845 in the EGFR is not an auto-phosphorylation site and is not required for EGFR kinase activity but is phosphorylated by Src (Biscardi et al., 1998).

Signal transducer and activator of transcription 5b (STAT5b), c-Src and EGFR play important roles in estrogen-stimulated proliferation of ER-positive breast cancer cells (Fox et al., 2008). Estrogen-induced Src activation and Src-dependent phosphorylation of EGFR-Tyr-845 recruit STAT5b as a downstream effector of phosphorylated EGFR-Tyr-845 to induce c-Myc and cyclin D1 expression (Fox et al., 2008). Introduction of a dominant-negative STAT5a into ER-positive T47D breast cancer cells inhibits E2β-stimulated cell proliferation and induces apoptosis (Yamashita et al., 2003). The involvement of STAT5 in ER-α36-mediated estrogen activation of the cyclin D1 promoter activity has been established (Zhang et al., unpublished data). Thus, it is possible that ER-α36 mediates mitogenic estrogen signaling through the EGFR/Src/STAT5 pathway in breast cancer cells.

17. Transcriptional regulation of ER-α36

Transcription of ER-α36 is initiated from a previously unidentified promoter in the first intron of the ER-α66 gene (Figure 1). The putative 5′-flanking region of the ER-α36 has been cloned and sequenced (Zou et al., 2009). Computer analysis revealed a TATA binding protein (TBP) recognition sequence upstream of the cDNA start site and several Sp1, NF-κB and Ap1 binding sites in the 5′-flanking region of ER-α36. A perfect half ERE site was identified at the promoter region of ER-α36 that is involved in suppression of ER-α36 promoter activity by ER-α66, indicating that ER-α36 expression is subjected to negative regulation of ER-α66 (Zou et al., 2009). This is consistent with the finding that ER-positive breast cancer cells tend to express lower levels of ER-α36 compared to ER-negative breast cancer cells (Wang et al., 2006; Zou et al., 2009). ER-α46 that lacks the AF-1 domain, however, had no effect on ER-α36 promoter activity while ER-α46 released the suppression activity of ER-α66 when co-expressed with ER-α66 (Zou et al., 2009). Thus ER-α66 suppresses the promoter activity of ER-α36 presumably through ligand-independent activity mediated by its AF1 domain, which can be blocked by ER-α46. In addition, co-expression of ER-α36 also released the suppression activity mediated by ER-α66 (Zou et al., 2009), suggesting that ER-α36 may be regulated by a positive-feedback mechanism.

BRCA1 mutations and downregulation are found in familial and sporadic breast cancers and BRCA1-related tumors are more likely to be ER-negative than are non-BRCA1 related breast cancers. It is still unknown why dysfunctional BRCA1 only predispose to cancers of estrogen responsive tissues and why these BRCA1-related breast tumors are often ER-negative. BRCA1 mediates the ligand-independent transcriptional repression activity of the ER-α66 through its AF-1 domain (Zheng *et. al.*, 2003). Since ER-α66 represses the promoter activity of ER-α36 through its AF-1 domain, it is reasonable to postulate that loss of BRCA1 function either by mutations or downregulation may activate ER-α36 expression, which then activates ER-α36-mediated mitogenic estrogen signaling that eventually leads to development of breast cancers characterized as ER-negative since they lack ER-α66 expression.

The analysis of ER-α36 promoter revealed several important features of transcriptional regulation of this potentially important player in estrogen signaling. The finding of several NF-κB binding sites indicates that ER-α36 is subject to regulation by the NF-κB signaling pathway and by different cytokines that activate the NF-κB signaling pathway. The existence of Ap-1 binding sites in the ER-α36 promoter region raised the possibility that growth factor signaling may regulate ER-α36 expression, which was confirmed by our recent report that EGFR-mediated signaling induces ER-α36 expression via one of the Ap-1 binding sites (Zhang et al., 2011). Thus, further study of the transcription regulation of ER-α36 will provide more information about the mechanisms underlying regulation of ER-α36 mediated non-genomic estrogen signaling in cells and tissues other than mammary gland.

18. Cross-regulation of ER-α36 and members of the EGFR family

In ER-positive breast cancer cells, it has been well documented that the cross-communication between EGFR and ER-α66 leads to serine phosphorylation of ER-α66 and ligand-independent activation of the ER-α66-mediated transcription (Kato et al., 1995; Bunone et al., 1996). Conversely, EGF signaling is strongly enhanced by the ER-α66 in ER-positive MCF7 cells and anti-estrogen ICI 182, 780 was able to block the EGF signaling (Migliaccio et al., 2006). In addition, our group has reported another level of cross-talk mechanism by which EGFR and ER-α36 positively regulate each other's expression in triple-negative breast cancer cells (Zhang et al., 2011); EGFR signaling activates the promoter activity of ER-α36 and ER-α36 stabilizes the steady state levels of EGFR protein. This positive feedback loop provides a molecular explanation to the aggressiveness of triple-negative breast cancer. A similar cross-regulation between Her2/Neu and ER-α36 was also found (Kang et al., unpublished observations). However, unlike EGFR, ER-α36-mediated estrogen signaling up-regulates the promoter activity of Her2/Neu gene, suggesting that ER-α36 positively regulates Her2/Neu expression. This data is consistent with the finding that ER-α36 expression is significantly correlated with Her-2/Neu expression in specimens from breast cancer patients (Shi et al., 2009). Thus, the interplay between growth factor receptors and ER-α36 may play an important role in development and progression of subsets of breast cancer that highly express ER-α36.

19. ER-α36 in osteoporosis

Non-genomic estrogen signaling plays an important role in bone protection; estrogen is able to protect the adult skeleton against bone loss by maintaining a focal balance between bone formation and resorption, which mainly results from the opposite effects of osteoblasts (OBs) and osteoclasts (OCs). Estrogen has anti-apoptotic effects on OBs and pro-apoptotic effects on OCs through an extra-nuclear signaling that leads to activation of the MAPK/ERK signaling pathway and kinase-dependent changes in transcription activities (Reviewed by Manolagas, 2000; Manolagas et al., 2004). However, the underlying mechanisms of this opposite effects of estrogen signaling have not been established. Xie et al., (2011) recently reported that the postmenopausal level of E2β induces mitogenic, anti-apoptotic and anti-osteogenic effects in postmenopausal OBs and pro-apoptotic effects in postmenopausal OCs, respectively. ER-α36 mediates the effects of post-menopausal-level E2β on proliferation, apoptosis, and differentiation of OBs through transient activation of the MAPK/ERK pathway, whereas ER-α36 mediates post-menopausal-level E2β induced apoptosis of OCs through prolonged or sustained activation of the MAPK/ERK pathway. The levels of ER-α36 expression in bone are positively associated with bone mineral density in post-menopausal women. Thus, the high levels of ER-α36 expression are required for preserving bone mass in post-menopausal and menopausal women.

20. Conclusions

Most previous studies of estrogen signaling in human breast cancer were focused on the ER-α66, the only known estrogen receptor for many years. The discovery of ER-α36 in our laboratory, combined with the previous reports of membrane-based ER-α46, raised the intriguing possibility that ER-α36 and ER-α46 are also involved in estrogen signaling. Net estrogen response in a specific target cell thus depends on absolute and relative levels of the regulated expression of full-length and alternatively processed estrogen receptor-α isoforms.

It is well established that estrogen stimulates mammary epithelial cell proliferation. However, the function of ER-α66, ER-β and ER-α46 in mitogenic estrogen signaling is confounding. A plethora of experimental evidence indicates that ER-α66, ER-α46, and ER-β negatively regulate mitogenic estrogen signaling in transfected cells, which argue against the positive role of these receptors in estrogen-stimulated cell proliferation. Thus far, ER-α36 is the only reported estrogen receptor that mediates mitogenic estrogen signaling and stimulates cell proliferation in transfected cells and in ER-negative breast cancer cells that lack expression of ER-α66, ER-α46 and ER-β but express high level of endogenous ER-α36. In addition, the finding that ER-α36 functions as a potent dominant-negative regulator of the genomic estrogen signaling mediated by ER-α66 and ER-β implicates that when ER-α36 mediates mitogenic estrogen signalling, it may require the silence of genomic estrogen signaling. This again challenges the well-known role of genomic estrogen signaling in estrogen-stimulated cell proliferation.

Accumulating evidence highlights the importance of ER-α36-mediated non-genomic estrogen signaling in malignant growth of breast cancer and endometrial cancer cells. The expression of ER-α36 has also been detected in other types of human cancer such as human colon cancer and liver cancer (Jiang et al., 2008; Miceli et al., 2011), suggesting that ER-α36 may also involved in initiation and development of human malignancy in non-classical estrogen targeting organs. Elucidating the functions of ER-α36-mediated non-genomic estrogen signaling in different types of human malignancy could provide more informed approaches to better understand the underlying mechanisms of mitogenic estrogen signaling in mammary carcinogenesis. We hope that further investigation of the function and underlying mechanisms of this ER variant in different subtypes of human breast cancer and even in the putative breast cancer stem/progenitor cells will lead to development of high efficacy, less toxic therapeutic agents for patients affected with mammary malignancies.

21. Acknowledgments

We regret the inability to cite many fine papers that contribute to this field due to space limitations. This work was supported by grants from the National Institute of Health, Susan G. Komen for the Cure and the Nebraska Tobacco Settlement Biomedical Research Program.

22. References

Ahmad, S., Singh, N. & Glazer, RI. (1999). Role of AKT1 in 17beta-estradiol- and insulin-like growth factor I (IGF-I)-dependent proliferation and prevention of apoptosis in MCF-7 breast carcinoma cells. *Biochem Pharmacol* 58:425-430.

Ahola, TM., Alkio, N., Manninen, T. & Ylikomi, T. (2002). Progestin and G protein-coupled receptor 30 inhibit mitogen-activated protein kinase activity in MCF-7 breast cancer cells. *Endocrinology.* 143:4620-4626.

Altucci, L., Addeo, R., Cicatiello, L., Dauvois, S., Parker, MG., Truss, M., Beato, M., Sica, V., Bresciani, F. & Weisz, A. (1996). 17beta-Estradiol induces cyclin D1 gene transcription, p36D1-p34cdk4 complex activation and p105Rb phosphorylation during mitogenic stimulation of G1-arrested human breast cancer cells. *Oncogene.* 12:2315-2324.

Altucci, L., Addeo, R., Cicatiello, L., Germano, D., Pacilio, C., Battista, T., Cancemi, M., Petrizzi, VB., Bresciani, F. & Weisz, A. (1997). Estrogen induces early and timed activation of cyclin-dependent kinases 4, 5, and 6 and increases cyclin messenger ribonucleic acid expression in rat uterus. *Endocrinology.* 138:978-984.

Aronica, SM., Kraus, WL. & Katzenellenbogen, BS. (1994). Estrogen action via the cAMP signaling pathway: stimulation of adenylate cyclase and cAMP-regulated gene transcription. *Proc Natl Acad Sci U S A.* 91:8517-8521.

Berry, M., Metzger, D. & Chambon, P. (1990). Role of the two activating domains of the oestrogen receptor in the cell-type and promoter-context dependent agonistic activity of the anti-oestrogen 4-hydroxytamoxifen. *EMBO J.* 9:2811-2818.

Biscardi, JS., Belsches, AP. & Parsons, SJ. (1998). Characterization of human epidermal growth factor receptor and c-Src interactions in human breast tumor cells. *Mol. Carcinog.* 21:261-272.

Biscardi, JS., Ishizawar, RC., Silva, CM. & Parsons, SJ. (2000). Tyrosine kinase signalling in breast cancer: epidermal growth factor receptor and c-Src interactions in breast cancer. *Breast Cancer. Res.* 2:203-210.

Brinton, RD. (2001). Cellular and molecular mechanisms of estrogen regulation of memory function and neuroprotection against Alzheimer's disease: recent insights and remaining challenges. *Learn Mem.* 8:121-133.

Bunone, G., Briand, PA., Miksicek, RJ. & Picard, D. (1996). Activation of the unliganded estrogen receptor by EGF involves the MAP kinase pathway and direct phosphorylation. *EMBO J.* 15:2174-2183.

Caiazza F, Galluzzo P, Lorenzetti S, Marino M (2007) 17Beta-estradiol induces ERbeta up-regulation via p38/MAPK activation in colon cancer cells. *Biochem Biophys Res Commun* 359:102-107.

Castoria, G., Barone, M.V, Di Domenico, M., Bilancio, A., Ametrano, D., Migliaccio, A. & Auricchio, F. (1999). Non-transcriptional action of oestradiol and progestin triggers DNA synthesis. *EMBO J.* 18:2500-2510.

Castoria, G., Migliaccio, A., Bilancio, A., Di Domenico, M., de Falco, A., Lombardi, M., Fiorentino, R., Varricchio, L., Barone, MV. & Auricchio, F. (2001). PI3-kinase in concert with Src promotes the S-phase entry of oestradiol-stimulated MCF-7 cells. *EMBO J.* 20:6050-6059.

Cerillo, G., Rees, A., Manchanda, N., Reilly, C., Brogan, I., White, A. & Needham, M. (1998). The oestrogen receptor regulates NFkappaB and AP-1 activity in a cell-specific manner. *J Steroid Biochem. Mol. Biol.* 67:79-88.

Chen, Z., Yuhanna, IS., Galcheva-Gargova, Z., Karas, RH., Mendelsohn, ME. & Shaul, PW. (1999.) Estrogen receptor alpha mediates the nongenomic activation of endothelial nitric oxide synthase by estrogen. *J Clin. Invest.* 103:401-406.

Clark, GM., Osborne, CK. & McGuire, WL. (1984). Correlations between estrogen receptor, progesterone receptor, and patient characteristics in human breast cancer. *J Clin Oncol.* 2:1102-1109.

Clark, GM. (2000). Prognostic and predictive factors. *Diseases of the breast,* Lippincott Williams & Wilkins, Vol. 2:489-514.

Clarke, R., Leonessa, F., Welch, JN. & Skaar, TC. (2001). Cellular and molecular pharmacology of antiestrogen action and resistance. *Pharmacol. Rev.* 53:25-71.

Clarke, R., Liu, MC., Bouker, KB., Gu, Z., Lee, RY., Zhu, Y., Skaar, TC., Gomez, B., O'Brien, K., Wang, Y. & Hilakivi-Clarke, LA. (2003). Antiestrogen resistance in breast cancer and the role of estrogen receptor signaling. *Oncogene.* 22:7316-7339.

Clarke, R., Howell, A., Potten, CS. & Anderson, E. (1997). Dissociation between steroid receptor expression and cell proliferation in the human breast. *Cancer Res.* 57:4987-4991.

Cowell, LN., Graham, JD., Bouton, AH., Clarke, CL. & O'Neill, GM. (2006). Tamoxifen treatment promotes phosphorylation of the adhesion molecules, p130Cas/BCAR1, FAK and Src, via an adhesion-dependent pathway. *Oncogene.* 25:7597-7607.

Dauvois, S., Danielian, PS., White, R. & Parker, MG. (1992.) Antiestrogen ICI 164,384 reduces cellular estrogen receptor content by increasing its turnover. *Proc Natl Acad Sci U S A.* 89:4037-4041.

Deroo, BJ. & Buensuceso, AV. (2010.) Minireview: Estrogen receptor-beta: mechanistic insights from recent studies. *Mol. Endocrinol.* 24:1703-1714.

Diaz-Chico, BN., Ogasawara, Y., Chamness, GC., Salman, M. & McGuire, WL. (1988). A 46-kDa antigen associated with estrogen receptor in human breast cancer. *J Steroid Biochem.* 30:315-320.

Dotzlaw, H., Leygue, E., Watson, PH. & Murphy, LC. (1997). Expression of estrogen receptor-beta in human breast tumors. *J Clin. Endocrino.l Metab.* 82:2371-2374.

Driggers, PH. & Segars, JH. (2002). Estrogen action and cytoplasmic signaling pathways. Part II: the role of growth factors and phosphorylation in estrogen signaling. *Trends Endocrinol. Metab.* 13:422-427.

Dudley, MW., Sheeler, CQ., Wang, H. & Khan, S. (2000). Activation of the human estrogen receptor by the antiestrogens ICI 182,780 and tamoxifen in yeast genetic systems: implications for their mechanism of action. *Proc Natl Acad Sci U S A.* 97:3696-3701.

Dufy, B., Vincent, JD., Fleury, H., Du Pasquier, P., Gourdji, D & Tixier-Vidal, A. (1979). Membrane effects of thyrotropin-releasing hormone and estrogen shown by intracellular recording from pituitary cells. *Science.* 204:509-511.

Endoh, H., Sasaki, H., Maruyama, K., Takeyama, K., Waga, I., Shimizu, T., Kato, S. & Kawashima, H. (1997). Rapid activation of MAP kinase by estrogen in the bone cell line. *Biochem. Biophys. Res. Commun.* 235:99-102.

Evans, MJ., Eckert, A., Lai, K., Adelman, SJ. & Harnish, DC. (2001). Reciprocal antagonism between estrogen receptor and NF-kappaB activity in vivo. *Circ. Res.* 89:823-830.

Fawell, SE., White, R., Hoare, S., Sydenham, M., Page, M. & Parker, MG. (1990). Inhibition of estrogen receptor-DNA binding by the "pure" antiestrogen ICI 164,384 appears to be mediated by impaired receptor dimerization. *Proc Natl Acad Sci U S A.* 87:6883-6887.

Feigelson, HS. & Henderson, BE. (1996). Estrogens and breast cancer. *Carcinogenesis.* 17:2279-2284.

Ferguson, AT., Lapidus, RG., Baylin, SB. & Davidson, NE. (1995). Demethylation of the estrogen receptor gene in estrogen receptor-negative breast cancer cells can reactivate estrogen receptor gene expression. *Cancer Res.* 55:2279-2283.

Filardo, EJ., Quinn, JA., Bland, KI. & Frackelton, AR. Jr. (2000). Estrogen-induced activation of Erk-1 and Erk-2 requires the G protein-coupled receptor homolog, GPR30, and occurs via trans-activation of the epidermal growth factor receptor through release of HB-EGF. *Mol. Endocrinol.* 14:1649-1660.

Filardo, E., Quinn, J., Pang, Y., Graeber, C., Shaw, S., Dong, J. & Thomas, P. (2007). Activation of the novel estrogen receptor G protein-coupled receptor 30 (GPR30) at the plasma membrane. *Endocrinology* 148:3236-3245.

Flouriot, G, Brand, H., Denger, S., Metivier, R., Kos, M., Reid, G., Sonntag-Buck, V. & Gannon, F. (2000). Identification of a new isoform of the human estrogen receptor-alpha (hER-alpha) that is encoded by distinct transcripts and that is able to repress hER-alpha activation function 1. *EMBO J.* 19:4688-4700.

Fox, EM., Bernaciak, TM., Wen, J., Weaver, AM., Shupnik, MA. & Silva, CM. (2008). Signal transducer and activator of transcription 5b, c-Src, and epidermal growth factor receptor signaling play integral roles in estrogen-stimulated proliferation of estrogen receptor-positive breast cancer cells. *Mol. Endocrinol.* 22:1781-1796.

Fuqua, SA., Schiff, R., Parra, I., Friedrichs, WE., Su, JL., McKee, DD., Slentz-Kesler, K., Moore, LB., Willson, TM. & Moore, JT. (1999). Expression of wild-type estrogen receptor beta and variant isoforms in human breast cancer. *Cancer Res.* 59:5425-5428.

Fuqua, SA., Schiff, R., Parra, I., Moore, JT., Mohsin, SK., Osborne, CK., Clark, GM & Allred, DC. (2003). Estrogen receptor beta protein in human breast cancer: correlation with clinical tumor parameters. *Cancer Res.* 63:2434-2439.

Galluzzo, P., Caiazza, F., Moreno, S. & Marino, M. (2007). Role of ER-beta palmitoylation in the inhibition of human colon cancer cell proliferation. *Endocr. Relat. Cancer.* 14:153-167.

Geisler, J., Haynes, B., Anker, G., Dowsett, M. & Lonning, PE. (2002). Influence of letrozole and anastrozole on total body aromatization and plasma estrogen levels in postmenopausal breast cancer patients evaluated in a randomized, cross-over study. *J Clin. Oncol.* 20:751-757.

Green, S., Walter, P., Kumar, V., Krust, A., Bornert, JM., Argos, P. & Chambon, P. (1986). Human oestrogen receptor cDNA: sequence, expression and homology to v-erb-A. *Nature.* 320:134-139.

Greene, GL., Gilna, P., Waterfield, M., Baker, A, Hort, Y. & Shine, J. (1986). Sequence and expression of human estrogen receptor complementary DNA. *Science.* 231:1150-1154.

Gu, Q., Korach, KS. & Moss, RL. (1999). Rapid action of 17beta-estradiol on kainate-induced currents in hippocampal neurons lacking intracellular estrogen receptors. *Endocrinology.* 140:660-666.

Gupta, PB., Proia, D., Cingoz, O., Weremowicz, J., Naber, SP., Weinberg, RA. & Kuperwasser, C. (2007). Systemic stromal effects of estrogen promote the growth of estrogen receptor-negative cancers. *Cancer Res.* 67:2062-2071.

Hammes, SR. & Levin, ER. (2007). Extranuclear steroid receptors: nature and actions. *Endocr. Rev.* 28:726-741.

Harnish, DC., Scicchitano, MS., Adelman, SJ., Lyttle, CR. & Karathanasis, SK. (2000). The role of CBP in estrogen receptor cross-talk with nuclear factor-kappaB in HepG2 cells. *Endocrinology.* 141:3403-3411.

Harris, HA. (2007). Estrogen receptor-beta: recent lessons from in vivo studies. *Mol. Endocrinol* .21:1-13.

Hartman, J., Lindberg, K., Morani, A., Inzunza, J., Strom, A & Gustafsson, JA. (2006). Estrogen receptor beta inhibits angiogenesis and growth of T47D breast cancer xenografts. *Cancer Res.* 66:11207-11213.

Howell, A., Osborne, CK., Morris, C. & Wakeling, AE. (2000). ICI 182,780 (Faslodex): development of a novel, "pure" antiestrogen. *Cancer.* 89:817-825.

Iwao, K., Miyoshi, Y., Egawa, C., Ikeda, N. & Noguchi, S. (2000). Quantitative analysis of estrogen receptor-beta mRNA and its variants in human breast cancers. *Int. J Cancer.* 88:733-736.

Jarvinen, TA., Pelto-Huikko, M., Holli, K. & Isola, J. (2000). Estrogen receptor beta is coexpressed with ER-alpha and PR and associated with nodal status, grade, and proliferation rate in breast cancer. *Am. J Pathol.* 156:29-35.

Jensen, EV., Cheng, G., Palmieri, C., Saji, S., Makela, S., Van Noorden, S., Wahlstrom, T., Warner, M., Coombes, RC & Gustafsson, JA. (2001). Estrogen receptors and proliferation markers in primary and recurrent breast cancer. *Proc Natl Acad Sci U S A.* 98:15197-15202.

Jiang, H., Teng, R., Wang, Q., Zhang, XT., Wang, H., Wang, ZY., Cao, J. & Teng, L. (2008). Transcriptional analysis of estrogen receptor alpha variant mRNAs in colorectal cancers and their matched normal colorectal tissues. *J Steroid Biochem. Mol. Biol.* 112:20-24.

Jiang, SY. & Jordan, VC. (1992). Growth regulation of estrogen receptor-negative breast cancer cells transfected with complementary DNAs for estrogen receptor. *J Natl. Cancer Inst.* 84:580-591.

Jozan, S., Julia, AM., Carretie, A., Eche, N., Maisongrosse, V., Fouet, B., Marques, B. & David, JF. (1991). 65 and 47 kDa forms of estrogen receptor in human breast cancer: relation with estrogen responsiveness. *Breast Cancer Res. Treat.* 19:103-109.

Kang, LG. & Wang, ZY. (2010a). Breast cancer cell growth inhibition by phenethyl isothiocyanate is associated with down-regulation of oestrogen receptor-alpha36. *J Cell Mol. Med.* 14:1485-1493.

Kang, LG., Zhang, XT., Xie, Y., Tu, YP., Wang, D., Liu, ZM. & Wang, ZY. (2010b). Involvement of estrogen receptor variant ER-alpha36, not GPR30, in nongenomic estrogen signaling. *Mol. Endocrinol.* 24:709-721.

Kato, S., Endoh, H., Masuhiro, Y., Kitamoto, T., Uchiyama, S., Sasaki, H., Masushige, S., Gotoh, Y., Nishida, E., Kawashima, H., Metzger, D. & Chambon, P. (1995). Activation of the estrogen receptor through phosphorylation by mitogen-activated protein kinase. *Science.* 270:1491-1494.

Katzenellenbogen, BS. & Katzenellenbogen, JA. (2000). Estrogen receptor transcription and transactivation: Estrogen receptor alpha and estrogen receptor beta: regulation by selective estrogen receptor modulators and importance in breast cancer. *Breast Cancer Res.* 2:335-344.

Katzenellenbogen, BS. & Katzenellenbogen, JA. (2002). Biomedicine. Defining the "S" in SERMs. *Science.* 295:2380-2381.

Kelly, MJ. & Levin, ER. (2001). Rapid actions of plasma membrane estrogen receptors. *Trends Endocrinol. Metab.* 12:152-156.

Kelly, MJ., Moss, RL., & Dudley, CA. (1976) Differential sensitivity of preoptic-septal neurons to microelectrophoresed estrogen during the estrous cycle. *Brain Res* 114:152-157.

Kelly, MJ., Moss, RL., Dudley, CA. & Fawcett, CP. (1977). The specificity of the response of preoptic-septal area neurons to estrogen: 17alpha-estradiol versus 17beta-estradiol and the response of extrahypothalamic neurons. *Exp. Brain Res.* 30:43-52.

Khan, SA., Rogers, MA., Obando, JA. & Tamsen, A. (1994). Estrogen receptor expression of benign breast epithelium and its association with breast cancer. *Cancer Res.* 54:993-997.

Kim, KH. & Bender, JR. (2005). Rapid, estrogen receptor-mediated signaling: why is the endothelium so special? *Sci. STKE.* 2005:pe28.

Kim, R., Kaneko, M., Arihiro, K., Emi, M., Tanabe, K., Murakami, S., Osaki, A. & Inai, K. (2006). Extranuclear expression of hormone receptors in primary breast cancer. *Ann Oncol* 17:1213-1220.

Klinge, CM. (2001). Estrogen receptor interaction with estrogen response elements. *Nucleic Acids Res.* 29:2905-2919.

Klinge, CM., Riggs, KA., Wickramasinghe, NS., Emberts, CG., McConda, DB., Barry, PN. &, Magnusen, JE. (2010). Estrogen receptor alpha 46 is reduced in tamoxifen resistant breast cancer cells and re-expression inhibits cell proliferation and estrogen receptor alpha 66-regulated target gene transcription. *Mol. Cell Endocrinol.* 323:268-276.

Kong, EH., Pike, AC. & Hubbard, RE. (2003). Structure and mechanism of the oestrogen receptor. *Biochem. Soc. Trans.* 31:56-59.

Kuiper, GG., Enmark, E., Pelto-Huikko, M., Nilsson, S. & Gustafsson, J.A. (1996). Cloning of a novelreceptor expressed in rat prostate and ovary. *Proc. Natl. Acad. Sci. USA.* 93: 5925-5930.

Kurebayashi J, Otsuki T, Yamamoto S, Kurosumi M, Nakata T, Akinaga S, Sonoo H (1998) A pure antiestrogen, ICI 182,780, stimulates the growth of tamoxifen-resistant KPL-1 human breast cancer cells in vivo but not in vitro. *Oncology* 55 Suppl 1:23-34.

Kushner, PJ., Agard, DA., Greene, GL., Scanlan, TS., Shiau, AK., Uht, RM. & Webb, P. (2000). Estrogen receptor pathways to AP-1. *J Steroid Biochem. Mol. Biol.* 74:311-317.

Kushner, PJ., Hort, E., Shine, J., Baxter, JD. & Greene, GL. (1990). Construction of cell lines that express high levels of the human estrogen receptor and are killed by estrogens. *Mol. Endocrinol.* 4:1465-1473.

Lazennec, G., Bresson, D., Lucas, A., Chauveau, C. & Vignon, F. (2001). ER beta inhibits proliferation and invasion of breast cancer cells. *Endocrinology.* 142:4120-4130.

Lee, LM., Cao, J., Deng, H., Chen, P., Gatalica, Z. & Wang, ZY. (2008). ER-alpha36, a novel variant of ER-alpha, is expressed in ER-positive and -negative human breast carcinomas. *Anticancer Res.* 28:479-483.

Levin, ER. (2002). Cellular functions of plasma membrane estrogen receptors. *Steroids.* 67:471-475.

Levin, ER. (2003). Bidirectional signaling between the estrogen receptor and the epidermal growth factor receptor. *Mol. Endocrinol.* 17:309-317.

Leygue, E., Dotzlaw, H., Watson, PH. & Murphy, LC. (1998). Altered estrogen receptor alpha and beta messenger RNA expression during human breast tumorigenesis. *Cancer Res.* 58:3197-3201.

Li, L., Haynes, MP. & Bender, JR. (2003.) Plasma membrane localization and function of the estrogen receptor alpha variant (ER46) in human endothelial cells. *Proc Natl Acad Sci U S A.* 100:4807-4812.

Lin, SL., Yan, LY., Liang, XW., Wang, ZB., Wang, ZY., Qiao, J., Schatten, H. & Sun, QY. (2009). A novel variant of ER-alpha, ER-alpha36 mediates testosterone-stimulated ERK and Akt activation in endometrial cancer Hec1A cells. *Reprod. Biol. Endocrinol.* 7:102.

Lin, SL., Yan, LY., Zhang, XT., Yuan, J., Li, M., Qiao, J., Wang, ZY. & Sun, QY. (2010). ER-alpha36, a variant of ER-alpha, promotes tamoxifen agonist action in endometrial cancer cells via the MAPK/ERK and PI3K/Akt pathways. *PLoS One.* 5:e9013.

Lobenhofer, EK., Huper, G., Iglehart, JD. & Marks, JR. (2000). Inhibition of mitogen-activated protein kinase and phosphatidylinositol 3-kinase activity in MCF-7 cells prevents estrogen-induced mitogenesis. *Cell Growth Differ.* 11:99-110.

Longo, M., Brama, M., Marino, M., Bernardini, S., Korach, KS., Wetsel, WC., Scandurra, R., Faraggiana, T., Spera, G., Baron, R., Teti, A. & Migliaccio, S. (2004). Interaction of estrogen receptor alpha with protein kinase C alpha and c-Src in osteoblasts during differentiation. *Bone.* 34:100-111.

Lu Q, Pallas DC, Surks HK, Baur WE, Mendelsohn ME, Karas RH (2004) Striatin assembles a membrane signaling complex necessary for rapid, nongenomic activation of endothelial NO synthase by estrogen receptor alpha. *Proc Natl Acad Sci U S A* 101:17126-17131.

Maa, MC., Leu, TH., McCarley, DJ., Schatzman, RC. & Parsons, SJ. (1995). Potentiation of epidermal growth factor receptor-mediated oncogenesis by c-Src: implications for the etiology of multiple human cancers. *Proc Natl Acad Sci U S A.* 92:6981-6985.

Mahfoudi, A., Roulet, E., Dauvois, S., Parker, MG. & Wahli, W. (1995). Specific mutations in the estrogen receptor change the properties of antiestrogens to full agonists. *Proc Natl Acad Sci U S A.* 92:4206-4210.

Manolagas, SC. (2000). Birth and death of bone cells: basic regulatory mechanisms and implications for the pathogenesis and treatment of osteoporosis. *Endocr. Rev.* 21:115-137.

Manolagas, SC., Kousteni, S., Chen, JR., Schuller, M., Plotkin, L. & Bellido, T. (2004). Kinase-mediated transcription, activators of nongenotropic estrogen-like signaling (ANGELS), and osteoporosis: a different perspective on the HRT dilemma. *Kidney Int. Suppl*: S41-49.

Maret, A., Clamens, S., Delrieu, I., Elhage, R., Arnal, JF. & Bayard, F. (1999). Expression of the interleukin-6 gene is constitutive and not regulated by estrogen in rat vascular smooth muscle cells in culture. *Endocrinology.* 140:2876-2882.

Margeat, E., Bourdoncle, A., Margueron, R., Poujol, N., Cavailles, V. & Royer, C. (2003). Ligands differentially modulate the protein interactions of the human estrogen receptors alpha and beta. *J Mol. Biol.* 326:77-92.

Marino, M. & Ascenzi, P. (2008). Membrane association of estrogen receptor alpha and beta influences 17beta-estradiol-mediated cancer cell proliferation. *Steroids.* 73:853-858.

Marquez, DC. & Pietras, RJ. (2001). Membrane-associated binding sites for estrogen contribute to growth regulation of human breast cancer cells. *Oncogene.* 20:5420-5430.

McDonnell, DP. & Norris, JD. (2002). Connections and regulation of the human estrogen receptor. *Science.* 296:1642-1644.

McEwen, B. (2002). Estrogen actions throughout the brain. *Recent Prog. Horm. Res.* 57:357-384.

McKay LI, Cidlowski JA (1999) Molecular control of immune/inflammatory responses: interactions between nuclear factor-kappa B and steroid receptor-signaling pathways. *Endocr Rev* 20:435-459.

Mermelstein, PG., Becker, JB. & Surmeier, DJ. (1996). Estradiol reduces calcium currents in rat neostriatal neurons via a membrane receptor. *J Neurosci.* 16:595-604.

Metivier, R., Penot, G., Carmouche, RP., Hubner, MR., Reid, G., Denger, S., Manu, D., Brand, H., Kos, M., Benes, V. & Gannon, F. (2004). Transcriptional complexes engaged by apo-estrogen receptor-alpha isoforms have divergent outcomes. *EMBO J.* 23:3653-3666.

Miceli, V., Cocciadiferro, L., Fregapane, M., Zarcone, M., Montalto, G., Polito, LM., Agostara, B., Granata, OM. & Carruba, G. (2011). Expression of Wild-Type and Variant Estrogen Receptor Alpha in Liver Carcinogenesis and Tumor Progression. *OMICS.* [Epub ahead of print].

Migliaccio, A., Castoria, G., Di Domenico, M., Ciociola, A., Lombardi, M., De Falco, A., Nanayakkara, M., Bottero, D., De Stasio, R., Varricchio, L. & Auricchio, F (2006). Crosstalk between EGFR and extranuclear steroid receptors. *Ann N Y Acad Sci* 1089:194-200.

Migliaccio, A., Di Domenico, M., Castoria, G., de Falco, A., Bontempo, P., Nola, E. & Auricchio, F. (1996). Tyrosine kinase/p21ras/MAP-kinase pathway activation by estradiol-receptor complex in MCF-7 cells. *EMBO J* 15:1292-1300.

Moriarty, K., Kim, KH. & Bender, JR (2006). Minireview: estrogen receptor-mediated rapid signaling. *Endocrinology.* 147:5557-5563.

Morley, P., Whitfield, JF., Vanderhyden, BC., Tsang, BK. & Schwartz, JL. (1992). A new, nongenomic estrogen action: the rapid release of intracellular calcium. *Endocrinology.* 131:1305-1312.

Nethrapalli, IS., Tinnikov, AA., Krishnan, V., Lei, CD. & Toran-Allerand, CD. (2005). Estrogen activates mitogen-activated protein kinase in native, nontransfected CHO-K1, COS-7, and RAT2 fibroblast cell lines. *Endocrinology.* 146:56-63.

Nicholson, RI., Gee, JM., Manning, DL., Wakeling, AE., Montano, MM. & Katzenellenbogen, BS. (1995). Responses to pure antiestrogens (ICI 164384, ICI 182780) in estrogen-sensitive and -resistant experimental and clinical breast cancer. *Ann. N Y Acad. Sci.* 761:148-163.

Nilsson, S., Makela, S., Treuter, E., Tujague, M., Thomsen, J., Andersson, G., Enmark, E., Pettersson, K., Warner, M. & Gustafsson, JA. (2001). Mechanisms of estrogen action. *Physiol. Rev.* 81:1535-1565.

Nissen-Meyer, R. (1964). "Prophylactic" ovariectomy and ovarian irradiation in breast cancer. *Acta. Unio. Int. Contra. Cancrum.* 20:527-530.

Omoto, Y., Inoue, S., Ogawa, S., Toyama, T., Yamashita, H., Muramatsu, M., Kobayashi, S. & Iwase, H. (2001). Clinical value of the wild-type estrogen receptor beta expression in breast cancer. *Cancer Lett.* 163:207-212.

Osborne, CK., Yochmowitz, MG., Knight, WA., 3rd. & McGuire, WL. (1980). The value of estrogen and progesterone receptors in the treatment of breast cancer. *Cancer.* 46:2884-2888.

Otto, C, Fuchs, I., Kauselmann, G., Kern, H., Zevnik, B., Andreasen, P., Schwarz, G., Altmann, H., Klewer, M.,, Schoor M., Vonk, R. & Fritzemeier, KH. (2009). GPR30 does not mediate estrogenic responses in reproductive organs in mice. *Biol. Reprod.* 80:34-41.

Otto, C., Rohde-Schulz, B, Schwarz, G., Fuchs, I., Klewer, M., Brittain, D., Langer, G., Bader, B., Prelle, K., Nubbemeyer, R. & Fritzemeier, KH. (2008). G protein-coupled receptor 30 localizes to the endoplasmic reticulum and is not activated by estradiol. *Endocrinology.* 149:4846-4856.

Paruthiyil, S., Parmar, H., Kerekatte, V., Cunha, GR., Firestone, GL. & Leitman, DC. (2004). Estrogen receptor beta inhibits human breast cancer cell proliferation and tumor formation by causing a G2 cell cycle arrest. *Cancer Res.* 64:423-428.

Pearce, ST., Liu, H. & Jordan, VC. (2003). Modulation of estrogen receptor alpha function and stability by tamoxifen and a critical amino acid (Asp-538) in helix 12. *J Biol. Chem.* 278:7630-7638.

Pedram, A., Razandi, M. & Levin, ER. (2006). Nature of functional estrogen receptors at the plasma membrane. *Mol. Endocrinol.* 20:1996-2009.

Penot, G., Le Peron, C., Merot, Y., Grimaud-Fanouillere, E., Ferriere, F., Boujrad, N., Kah, O., Saligaut, C., Ducouret, B., Metivier, R. & Flouriot, G. (2005). The human estrogen receptor-alpha isoform hERalpha46 antagonizes the proliferative influence of hERalpha66 in MCF7 breast cancer cells. *Endocrinology.* 146:5474-5484.

Pietras, RJ., Marquez, DC., Chen, HW., Tsai, E., Weinberg, O. & Fishbein, M. (2005). Estrogen and growth factor receptor interactions in human breast and non-small cell lung cancer cells. *Steroids.* 70:372-381.

Pietras, RJ. & Szego, CM. (1975). Endometrial cell calcium and oestrogen action. *Nature.* 253:357-359.

Pietras, RJ. & Szego, CM. (1977). Specific binding sites for oestrogen at the outer surfaces of isolated endometrial cells. *Nature.* 265:69-72.

Pilat, MJ., Christman, JK. & Brooks, SC. (1996). Characterization of the estrogen receptor transfected MCF10A breast cell line 139B6. *Breast Cancer Res. Treat.* 37:253-266.

Prall, OW., Rogan, EM. & Sutherland, RL. (1998). Estrogen regulation of cell cycle progression in breast cancer cells. *J Steroid Biochem. Mol. Biol.* 65:169-174.

Rao, BR. (1998). Isolation and characterization of an estrogen binding protein which may integrate the plethora of estrogenic actions in non-reproductive organs. *J Steroid Biochem, Mol Biol.* 65:3-41.

Razandi, M., Pedram, A., Greene GL & Levin, ER. (1999). Cell membrane and nuclear estrogen receptors (ERs) originate from a single transcript: studies of ER-alpha and ER-beta expressed in Chinese hamster ovary cells. *Mol Endocrinol.* 13:307-319.

Rebbeck, TR., Levin, AM., Eisen, A., Snyder, C., Watson, P., Cannon-Albright, L., Isaacs, C., Olopade, O., Garber, JE., Godwin, AK., Daly, MB., Narod, SA., Neuhausen, SL., Lynch, HT & Weber, BL. (1999). Breast cancer risk after bilateral prophylactic oophorectomy in BRCA1 mutation carriers. *J Natl. Cancer Inst.* 91:1475-1479.

Revankar, CM., Cimino, DF., Sklar, LA., Arterburn, JB. & Prossnitz, ER. (2005). A transmembrane intracellular estrogen receptor mediates rapid cell signaling. *Science.* 307:1625-1630.

Ring, A. & Dowsett, M. (2004.) Mechanisms of tamoxifen resistance. *Endocr. Relat. Cancer.* 11:643-658.

Robertson, JF. (1996). Oestrogen receptor: a stable phenotype in breast cancer. *Br. J Cancer.* 73: 5-12.

Rochefort, H. (1995). Oestrogen- and anti-oestrogen-regulated genes in human breast cancer. *Ciba. Found. Symp.* 191:254-265.

Roger, P., Daures, JP., Maudelonde, T., Pignodel, C., Gleizes, M., Chapelle, J., Marty-Double, C., Baldet, P., Mares, P., Laffargue, F. & Rochefort, H. (2000). Dissociated overexpression of cathepsin D and estrogen receptor alpha in preinvasive mammary tumors. *Hum. Pathol.* 31:593-600.

Roger, P., Sahla, ME, Makela, S., Gustafsson, JA, Baldet, P. & Rochefort, H. (2001). Decreased expression of estrogen receptor beta protein in proliferative preinvasive mammary tumors. *Cancer Res.* 61:2537-2541.

Russell, KS., Haynes, MP., Sinha D., Clerisme, E. & Bender, JR. (2000). Human vascular endothelial cells contain membrane binding sites for estradiol, which mediate rapid intracellular signaling. *Proc Natl Acad Sci U S A.* 97:5930-5935.

Safe, S. (2001). Transcriptional activation of genes by 17 beta-estradiol through estrogen receptor-Sp1 interactions. *Vitam. Horm.* 62:231-252.

Saji,. S, Sakaguchi, H., Andersson, S., Warne,r M. & Gustafsson, J (2001). Quantitative analysis of estrogen receptor proteins in rat mammary gland. *Endocrinology.* 142:3177-3186.

Santen, RJ. (2003). Inhibition of aromatase: insights from recent studies. *Steroids.* 68:559-567.

Segars, JH. & Driggers, PH. (2002). Estrogen action and cytoplasmic signaling cascades. Part I: membrane-associated signaling complexes. *Trends Endocrinol. Metab.* 13:349-354.

Shang, YF. & Brown, M. (2002). Molecular determinants for the tissue specificity of SERMs. *Science.* 295:2465-2468.

Shang, YF., Hu, X., DiRenzo, J., Lazar, MA. & Brown, M. (2000). Cofactor dynamics and sufficiency in estrogen receptor-regulated transcription. *Cell.* 103:843-852.

Sheikh, MS., Garcia, M., Pujol, P., Fontana, JA. & Rochefort, H. (1994). Why are estrogen-receptor-negative breast cancers more aggressive than the estrogen-receptor-positive breast cancers? *Invasion Metastasis.* 14:329-336.

Shi, .L, Dong, B., Li, Z., Lu, Y., Ouyang, T., Li, J., Wang, T., Fan, Z., Fan, T., Lin, B., Wang, ZY. & Xie, YT. (2009). Expression of ER-{alpha}36, a novel variant of estrogen receptor {alpha}, and resistance to tamoxifen treatment in breast cancer. *J Clin. Oncol.* 27:3423-3429.

Shoker, BS., Jarvis, C., Clarke, RB., Anderson, E., Hewlett, J., Davies, MP., Sibson, DR. & Sloane, JP (1999a). Estrogen receptor-positive proliferating cells in the normal and precancerous breast. *Am. J Pathol.* 155:1811-1815.

Shoker, BS., Jarvis, C., Sibson, DR., Walker, C. & Sloane, JP. (1999b). Oestrogen receptor expression in the normal and pre-cancerous breast. *J Pathol.* 188:237-244.

Shupnik, MA. (2004) Crosstalk between steroid receptors and the c-Src-receptor tyrosine kinase pathways: implications for cell proliferation. *Oncogene.* 23:7979-7989.

Sibonga, JD., Dobnig, H., Harden, RM. & Turner, RT. (1998). Effect of the high-affinity estrogen receptor ligand ICI 182,780 on the rat tibia. *Endocrinology.* 139:3736-3742.

Song, RX., McPherson, RA., Adam, L., Bao, Y., Shupnik, MA., Kumar, R. & Santen, RJ. (2002). Linkage of rapid estrogen action to MAPK activation by ERalpha-Shc association and Shc pathway activation. *Mol. Endocrinol.* 16:116-127.

Speir, E., Yu, ZX., Takeda, K., Ferrans, VJ. & Cannon, RO., 3rd. (2000). Competition for p300 regulates transcription by estrogen receptors and nuclear factor-kappaB in human coronary smooth muscle cells. *Circ. Res.* 87:1006-1011.

Speirs, V., Parkes, AT., Kerin, MJ., Walton, DS., Carleton, PJ., Fox, JN. & Atkin, SL. (1999). Coexpression of estrogen receptor alpha and beta: poor prognostic factors in human breast cancer? *Cancer Res.* 59:525-528.

Speirs, V., Skliris, GP., Burdall, SE. & Carder, PJ. (2002). Distinct expression patterns of ER alpha and ER beta in normal human mammary gland. *J Clin. Pathol.* 55:371-374.

Stoner, M., Saville, B., Wormke, M., Dean, D., Burghardt, R. & Safe, S. (2002). Hypoxia induces proteasome-dependent degradation of estrogen receptor alpha in ZR-75 breast cancer cells. *Mol. Endocrinol.* 16:2231-2242.

Sylvia, VL., Walton, J., Lopez, D., Dean, DD., Boyan, BD. & Schwartz, Z. (2001). 17 beta-estradiol-BSA conjugates and 17 beta-estradiol regulate growth plate chondrocytes by common membrane associated mechanisms involving PKC dependent and independent signal transduction. *J Cell Biochem.* 81:413-429.

Tesarik, J. & Mendoza, C. (1997). Direct non-genomic effects of follicular steroids on maturing human oocytes: oestrogen versus androgen antagonism. *Hum. Reprod. Update.* 3:95-100.

Tice, DA., Biscardi, JS., Nickles, AL. & Parsons, SJ. (1999). Mechanism of biological synergy between cellular Src and epidermal growth factor receptor. *Proc Natl Acad Sci U S A.* 96:1415-1420.

Tong, JS., Zhang, QH., Wang, ZB., Li, S., Yang, CR., Fu, XQ., Hou, Y., Wang, ZY., Sheng, J. & Sun, QY. (2010), ER-alpha36, a novel variant of ER-alpha, mediates estrogen-stimulated proliferation of endometrial carcinoma cells via the PKCdelta/ERK pathway. *PLoS One.* 5:e15408.

Toran-Allerand, CD., Guan, X., MacLusky, NJ., Horvath, TL., Diano, S., Singh, M., Connolly, ES., Jr., Nethrapalli, IS. & Tinnikov, A. (2002). ER-X: a novel, plasma membrane-associated, putative estrogen receptor that is regulated during development and after ischemic brain injury. *J Neurosci.* 22:8391-8401.

Touitou, I., Mathieu, M,. & Rochefort, H. (1990). Stable transfection of the estrogen receptor cDNA into Hela cells induces estrogen responsiveness of endogenous cathepsin D gene but not of cell growth. *Biochem. Biophys. Res. Commun.* 169:109-115.

Troyer, KL. & Lee, DC. (2001.) Regulation of mouse mammary gland development and tumorigenesis by the ERBB signaling network. *J Mammary Gland Biol. Neoplasia.* 6:7-21.

Tsai, EM., Wang, SC., Lee, JN. & Hung, MC. (2001). Akt activation by estrogen in estrogen receptor-negative breast cancer cells. *Cancer Res.* 61:8390-8392.

Tzukerman, MT., Esty, A., Santiso-Mere, D., Danielian, P., Parker, MG., Stein, RB., Pike, JW. & McDonnell, DP. (1994). Human estrogen receptor transactivational capacity is determined by both cellular and promoter context and mediated by two functionally distinct intramolecular regions. *Mol. Endocrinol.* 8:21-30.

Vranic, S., Gatalica, Z., Deng, H., Frkovic-Grazio, S., Lee, MJ., Olga Gurjeva, O. & Wang, Z-Y. (2011). ER-α36, a novel isoform of ER-α66, is commonly over-expressed in apocrine and adenoid cystic carcinomas of the breast". *J. of Clinical Pathology.* 64: 54-57.

Wang, ZY., Zhang, XT., Shen, P., Loggie, BW., Chang, Y. & Deuel, TF. (2005). Identification, cloning, and expression of human estrogen receptor-alpha36, a novel variant of human estrogen receptor-alpha66. *Biochem. Biophys. Res. Commun.* 336:1023-1027.

Wang, ZY., Zhang, XT., Shen, P., Loggie, BW., Chang, Y. & Deuel, TF. (2006). A variant of estrogen receptor-{alpha}, hER-{alpha}36: transduction of estrogen- and antiestrogen-dependent membrane-initiated mitogenic signaling. *Proc Natl Acad Sci U S A.* 103:9063-9068.

Warner, M., Saji, S. & Gustafsson, JA. (2000.) The normal and malignant mammary gland: a fresh look with ER-beta onboard. *J Mammary Gland Biol. Neoplasia.* 5:289-294.

Watson, C., Norfleet, A., Pappas, T. & Gametchu, B. (1999). Rapid actions of estrogens in GH3/B6 pituitary tumor cells via a plasma membrane version of estrogen receptor-α. *Steroids.* 64:5–13

Watters, JJ., Campbell, JS., Cunningham, MJ., Krebs, EG. & Dorsa, DM. (1997). Rapid membrane effects of steroids in neuroblastoma cells: effects of estrogen on mitogen activated protein kinase signaling cascade and c-fos immediate early gene transcription. *Endocrinology.* 138:4030-4033.

Xie, H., Sun, M., Liao, XB., Yuan, LQ., Sheng, Z.F, Meng, JC., Wang, D., Yu, ZY., Zhang, LY, Zhou, HD., Luo, XH., Li, H., Wu, XP., Wei, QY., Tang, SY., Wang, ZY. & Liao, EY. (2011). Estrogen receptor alpha36 mediates a bone-sparing effect of 17beta-estrodiol in postmenopausal women. *J Bone Miner. Res.* 26:156-168.

Yamashita, H., Iwase, H., Toyama, T. & Fujii, Y. (2003). Naturally occurring dominant-negative Stat5 suppresses transcriptional activity of estrogen receptors and induces apoptosis in T47D breast cancer cells. *Oncogene.* 22:1638-1652.

Zeps, N., Bentel, JM., Papadimitriou, JM., Dawkins, HJ. (1999). Murine progesterone receptor expression in proliferating mammary epithelial cells during normal pubertal development and adult estrous cycle. Association with eralpha and erbeta status. *J Histochem. Cytochem.* 47:1323-1330.

Zhang, XT., Kang, LG., Ding, L., Vranic, S., Gatalica, Z. & Wang, ZY. (2011). A positive feedback loop of ER-alpha36/EGFR promotes malignant growth of ER-negative breast cancer cells. *Oncogene.* 30:770-780.

Zhao, L., O'Neill, K. & Brinton, RD. (2006). Estrogenic agonist activity of ICI 182,780 (Faslodex) in hippocampal neurons: implications for basic science understanding of estrogen signaling and development of estrogen modulators with a dual therapeutic profile. *J Pharmacol. Exp. Ther.* 319:1124-1132.

Zhao, L., O'Neill, K., Diaz Brinton, R. (2005,) Selective estrogen receptor modulators (SERMs) for the brain: current status and remaining challenges for developing Neuro-SERMs. *Brain Res. Rev.* 49:472-493.

Zheng, WH., Andersson, S., Cheng, G., Simpson, ER., Warner, M. & Gustafsson, JA. (2003). Update on estrogen signaling. *FEBS Lett.* 546:17-24.

Zou, Y., Ding, L., Coleman, M. & Wang, ZY. (2009). Estrogen receptor-alpha (ER-alpha) suppresses expression of its variant ER-alpha 36. *FEBS Lett.* 583:1368-1374.

4

Metabolomics and Transcriptional Responses in Estrogen Receptor Positive Breast Cancer Cells

Soma Mandal, Protiti Khan, Lin Li and James R. Davie
Manitoba Institute of Cell Biology, University of Manitoba, Winnipeg, Manitoba, Canada

1. Introduction

Estrogen exposure is well recognized as a high risk factor of breast cancer, despite the fact that the hormone transcriptionally regulates the expression of tumor suppressor genes, like BRCA1 (Hockings *et al.*, 2008). Estrogen acts through the estrogen receptor α (ERα) in target cells (Ali and Coombes, 2000). ERα overexpression occurs in about 70% of breast cancers, referred as "ER positive" (ER+) (Dickson and Lippman, 1988). ERα is a primary target for chemoprevention as well as other therapeutic interventions for breast cancer with the ER+ phenotype. Clinically, in pathological lesions such as women with benign breast tumors, who underwent surgery, presented with a high proportion of ER positivity than the control group. In such cases, logistic regression yielded an adjusted odds ratio of 6.5 for risk of development of breast cancer compared to 0.3 odds ratio for PR (progesterone receptor); there was an increased proportion of cells expressing ERα by immunohistochemical staining, thereby demonstrating the importance of ERα as a breast cancer risk marker (Khan *et al.*, 1994). Estrogen or E2 mostly exerts its mitogenic effects by the modulation of metabolic responses and through the transcriptional induction of genes regulating crucial cellular processes like the cell cycle (Prall *et al.*, 1998). Microarray and RNA interference studies suggest that the transcriptional regulation of about 60% of estrogen responsive genes (induced or repressed) is dependent upon ERα and Sp1/3 transcription factors (Bazley and Gullick, 2005). The basal expression of ERα, in turn, is regulated by Sp1 in ER+ breast cancer cells (deGraffenried *et al.*, 2002). Sp1 and Sp3 are ubiquitously expressed in mammalian cells and are abnormally expressed in various cancers, including breast (Li and Davie, 2010). Sp1 and Sp3 bind to the same DNA sequence defined as Sp1/3 sites, with similar affinity. Sp1 and Sp3 play important roles in regulating genes critical to the initiation and progression of breast cancers (Hirokawa, 1984; Lu and Archer, 2010). Targeting these proteins is a promising cancer therapeutic approach (Jia *et al.*, 2010).

In most cases, ER+ breast cancers present a better clinical prognosis than the ER- breast cancers. Moreover, it is an encouraging fact that the leading antiestrogenic drugs such as tamoxifen have effectively improved the overall survival of pre and postmenopausal women by the reduction of cancer incidence and formation of new tumors (Ferguson and Davidson, 1997; Muss, 2001). However, a major obstacle to breast cancer treatment is the development of drug resistance. Resistance is commonly associated with an increased expression of Erb proteins including EGFR (epidermal growth factor receptor); in addition, there is evidence of non-hormonal role of ERα in hormone sensitive MCF-7 cells to maintain basal proliferation (Salazar *et al.*, 2011). Interestingly, there was no expression of Erb2 and 3, but ERα supported a population of basal fraction of actively dividing S phase cells which were unaffected by hormone depletion or hydroxy tamoxifen treatment (Salazar *et al.*, 2011). Like breast tumors, breast cancer cell lines can also yield clonal populations of tamoxifen resistant cells that have variable ER dependence (Coser *et al.*, 2009). This *in vitro* evidence supports the fact that the basal population of hormone sensitive cells may be a prerequisite condition for eventual occurrence of hormone insensitive tumors where current therapies such as tamoxifen are no more effective (Salazar *et al.*, 2011). Development of resistance to tamoxifen or aromatase inhibitors (AIs) is a result of adaptive changes which lead to the activation of alternate signaling pathways. ER+ tumors unresponsive to front line therapy drugs such as tamoxifen or AIs will eventually become resistant; as seen in xenograft or cell line models, there is an eventual constitutive activation of the RAS-MAPK (RAS-mitogen activated protein kinase) signaling pathway and dependency on growth factor receptor (EGFR/HER1 and HER2/neu) signaling. Constitutive RAS-MAPK activation by EGFR or HER2 overexpression in ER- breast cancers results in the downstream activation of mitogen and stress activated kinase 1 and 2 (MSK1 and MSK2) as well as several MSK substrates that are implicated in oncogenic programming. Given these detrimental adaptive cellular changes, there is a lot of attention given to breast cancers during the ER+ stage, such that alternative strategies can be used to circumvent the problem of drug resistance. One such approach is the use of synthetic peptides with sequences of natural biological molecules, such as ERα. A peptide analog, ERα17p with a 17 amino acid motif (PLMIKRSKKNSLALSLT; P295-T311 of ERα) was synthesized which contained the third nuclear localization signal of ERα, a proteolysis site, as well as a binding site for calmodulin. This 17 amino acid motif of ERα is responsible for a number of post-transcriptional modifications as well as of the recruitment of co-regulators. It was reported to elicit (pseudo)-estrogenic responses in ER+ MCF-7 cells (Gallo *et al.*, 2007). Further studies showed that the ERα17p peptide induced apoptosis in the ER+ MCF-7 and T47D cells and also in the ER- MDA-MB-231 and SKBr-3 cells through ERα independent mechanisms. This peptide also caused regression of ER- breast cancer tumor xenografts without apparent toxicity. This suggested a potentially new attractive tool for the development of promising therapeutic approaches, and also provided an insight to the cellular fate of ERα (Pelekanou *et al.*, 2011).

The differences of the ER+ or ER- breast cancer not only relate to their morphology, but are also largely due to the differential metabolomics and differences in their transcriptional responses, which overall is a reflection of the selectivity of gene usage. Differences between these two wide phenotypes are reflected in the metabolism of sugars, fatty acids, proteins or even drugs that accelerate or decelerate proliferation. In the ER+ breast cancer cells, E2 is pivotal in controlling diverse energy metabolic pathways such as glucose transport, glycolysis, TCA (tricarboxylic acid) cycle, mitochondrial respiratory chain, adenosine nucleotide translocator and fatty acid β-oxidation and synthesis respectively. Estrogen has positive effects on carbohydrate and lipid metabolism. Absence of ERα causes hyperplasia and hypertrophy of the adipose tissue, insulin resistance, and reduced energy expenditure respectively [(Chen *et al.*, 2009) and references therein]. Hence disturbances in the E2/ER metabolic pathways are likely to cause metabolic diseases such as heart disease, obesity and also cancer. Thus breast cancer progression and unresponsiveness to therapy are interrelated.

MCF-7 is a model cell line of the ER+ phenotype and the highly metastatic MDA-MB-231 is a model cell line of ER- phenotype. Both these cell lines have been widely used for *in vitro* cell culture and *in vivo* xenograft studies. We used microarray expression data obtained from public repositories for MCF-7 (non-stimulated) and MDA-MB-231 to compare interrelated factors that regulate the transition of breast cancer towards the more aggressive phenotype (Mandal *et al.*, 2007b; Mandal and Davie, 2007). In this chapter, we review, discuss, and compare some salient features and experimental findings of major energy metabolic pathways, the importance of pathways that are constitutively activated and transcriptional responses with particular emphasis on ER+ breast cancers.

2. Glucose metabolism

The binding of estrogen to its receptor induces crucial metabolic changes through the activation of various estrogen responsive genes. Estrogen stimulates glucose metabolism, including glycolysis and glycogen synthesis, in target organs such as the uterus, which is a classic estrogen target organ (Shinkarenko *et al.*, 1994; Smith and Gorski, 1968). It has been shown in many studies that estrogen stimulates the incorporation of labeled glucose (^{14}C-labeled glucose) into lipid, RNA, and protein (Bitman *et al.*, 1965; Nicolette and Gorski, 1964; Swigart *et al.*, 1961). The influence of estrogen in glucose metabolism is also well studied in another estrogen target tissue, the breast. Several studies in breast cancer cell lines have that the incorporation of the glucose analogue, [^{18}F]-fluoro-2-deoxy-D-glucose (^{18}F-FDG) varies with the ERα status, the acquisition of drug resistance, or alterations in the expression of ERα. Clinically, ^{18}F-FDG is used for non-invasive detection of breast cancer and staging of axillary lymph node metastases by PET (positron emission tomography) scan (Utech *et al.*, 1996). PET technology utilizes the metabolic characteristic of enhanced glucose utilization by tumor cells (Moreno-Sanchez *et al.*, 2007). Hence this advanced technology can be effectively used to study metabolic characteristics in drug resistance or hormone related metabolic changes.

Tumors refractory to chemotherapy are prone to the acquisition of drug resistance. One of the mechanisms of acquired resistance is through alterations of glucose metabolism and the differential expression of GLUT (glucose transporter) expression. The higher gene and protein expression of GLUTs in tumors is well documented (Macheda *et al.*, 2005; Medina and Owen, 2002; Wood and Trayhurn, 2003). This phenomenon provides an advantage to tumors to harness increased glucose utilization through the glycolysis pathway. Glucose transporters such as GLUT12, initially identified in MCF-7 cells, have been shown to have deregulated and increased expression in breast tumors (Rogers *et al.*, 2003). Facilitated transport of polar glucose molecules across the plasma membrane is dependent on GLUT proteins. GLUT proteins 1-5 have been identified in mammalian cells. These transporter proteins impart unique metabolic properties to cells (Rogers *et al.*, 2003). There is evidence that in both the ER+ MCF-7 cells and the ER- MDA-MB-231 cells, there is an increased expression of GLUT1 under hypoxic conditions (Rivenzon-Segal *et al.*, 2003). MCF-7 cells rendered resistant to the drug 5-fluorouracil by long term exposure (the drug-sensitive parental cell line in medium with increasing concentrations for a period of two years), had a decreased ^{18}F-FDG incorporation. Microarray data showed that the expression of GLUTs 8 and 10 was decreased in resistant cells, while GLUT1 was only increased in cells resistant to the lowest concentration of 5-fluorouracil. There were no alterations in the hexokinase activity, but there was a increase in glucose transport (Smith *et al.*, 2007). On the other hand, estrogen produces an positive increase in the ^{18}F-FDG uptake which has been demonstrated in ER+ cells. A comparative study between the ER+ T47D cells and the ER- cell lines, MDA-MB-231 and MDA-MB-468 demonstrated the dependence of estrogen in mediating the glucose uptake. In the ER- breast cancer cells, the ^{18}F-FDG uptake was totally absent; this correlated positively with the fact that these cells are totally unresponsive to the estrogen dependent effect on glucose uptake. To further demonstrate this estrogen dependence, it was seen that when the ER+ T47D cells were pretreated with the pure antiestrogen ICI182,780 (fulvestrant), the glucose uptake was totally abrogated. Unlike fulvestrant, the partial antiestrogen tamoxifen was incapable of blocking this estrogen response (Ko *et al.*, 2010).

Comparison of metabolic and morphological differences between normal breast and ER+ breast cancer cells gave insights into the adaptive responses adaptive responses which enable cancer cells to better utilize cellular energy resources. Glucose metabolism was studied in the finite lifespan normal human mammary epithelial cell line (HMECs) as well as the classical ER+ the classical ER+ MCF-7 cancer cell line. Cells were induced to grow rapidly under routine tissue culture conditions in nutrient rich media containing ^{13}C-labeled glucose and the isotopic enrichment of cellular metabolites was quantified to calculate metabolic fluxes in key pathways. Cells grown in culture dishes of various sizes (with different surface areas) exhibited very different metabolic and morphological profiles. MCF-7 cells have about an 80% smaller exposed surface area and contain 26% less protein per cell than the HMECs. The per-cell glucose consumption, lactate production, and glutamine consumption rate was 225-250% higher per cell relative to the cancer cells. However, the calculated flux per the exposed area for glucose, lactate, and glutamine was much higher in MCF-7 cells; MCF-7 cells also consumed amino acids at rates much higher than that required for protein synthesis demonstrating a greater efficacy of transport mechanisms (Meadows *et al.*, 2008). In addition, the energy efficiency was much higher in MCF-7 cells which also had a higher dependence on the TCA cycle. These observations form the basis of rational drug design for metabolic drugs (Meadows *et al.*, 2008).

2.1 Glucose metabolism – A comparative analysis in ER+ and ER- breast cancer cells

Glycolysis is the metabolic pathway where glucose is oxidized to pyruvate under aerobic conditions to yield ATP; however, under anaerobic conditions, pyruvate is converted to lactic acid. This biochemical pathway is regulated by the enzymes hexokinase, phosphofructokinase, and pyruvate kinase respectively, which are also potential sites of control and in most organisms these steps are irreversible. The opposite action of glycolysis is gluconeogenesis, which occurs when the blood sugar level falls, thus aiding in the replenishment of blood sugar levels. The gene expression in glycolysis and gluconeogenesis pathways is depicted in Fig. 1A in the ER+ MCF-7 cells and the ER- MDA-MB-231 cells. Some of the key patterns of gene expression are seen between the ER+ and ER- phenotypes:

a. In both cases, the expression of genes and proteins coding for facilitated transmembrane GLUTs (SLCs, solute carrier family of proteins) is either absent or down-regulated. Interestingly, the protein encoded by the gene, *GPI* (phosphoglucose isomerase) catalyzing the irreversible isomerization of G-6-PO_4 (glucose-6-phosphate) to F-6-PO_4 (fructose-6-phosphate), is key in energy pathways and is down-regulated in MDA-MB-231 cells whereas, it is up-regulated in MCF-7 cells. This agrees with our previous studies where we had shown that the more aggressive ER+ cells have a reduced utilization of genes involved in the energy production and expenditure pathways similar to the ER- breast cancer phenotype (Mandal and Davie, 2007).

b. Of the three isozymes of PFK (phosphofructokinase) which catalyze the conversion of fructose 6-phosphate (F-6-PO_4) to the 1, 6-diphosphate form, PFKM is highly expressed in MCF-7 cells and is down-regulated in MDA-MB-231 cells; PFKM is responsible for the phosphorylation of F 6-PO_4 to F 1, 6-bisPO_4. On the other hand, expression of PFKP is quite high in MDA-MB-231 cells and this isoform is responsible for the catalytic conversion of F 6-PO_4 to F 1, 6-bisPO_4 and PFKP is a key regulatory enzyme of glycolysis. Mutations in this key enzyme can cause glycogen storage disease.

c. A crucial difference is the down-regulated expression of the isozymes of lactate dehydrogenase (LDH) in MCF-7 (LDHA, LDHC) versus their up-regulation in MDA-MB-231 cells. The proteins encoded by both these genes catalyze the conversion of L-lactate and NAD to pyruvate and NADH as the final step of anaerobic glycolysis, a feature of the metastatic phenotype.

d. Genes encoding for glycolytic enzymes like phosphoglycerate kinases (*PGK1/2*) are either down-regulated (*PGK1* in MCF-7), or have low expression (*PGK1* in MDA-MB-231), or are absent (*PGK2*, in MCF7 and MDA-MB-231).

e. Aldolases catalyzing the reversible aldol cleavage of fructose 1, 6-biphosphate and fructose 1-phosphate to dihydroxyacetone phosphate and either glyceraldehyde-3-phosphate or glyceraldehyde respectively are either absent (*ALDOA, B*) or are highly expressed in MCF-7 cells, but down-regulated in MDA-MB-231 cells. The same pattern of opposite gene expression is also seen with *TPI1* (triosephosphate isomerase 1), which catalyzes the isomerization of glyceraldehydes 3-phosphate (G3P) and dihydroxy-acetone phosphate (DHAP) in glycolysis and gluconeogenesis.

Glycogenesis is the glycogen synthesis process, in which glucose molecules are added to chains of glycogen for storage. We compared the gene expression analysis between MCF-7 and MDA-MB-231 cells where in general, there was a down-regulation or absence of genes involved in critical steps [such as debranching (AGL), phosphate transfer to glucose molecules (*PGM1*)] within the pathway (Fig. 1B). Notably, mutations of most of the genes involved in the glycogenesis pathway are associated with glycogen storage disease. Interestingly, there was a selective up-regulation of genes *(PPP2R3A, PPP2CA, PPP2R5A, PPP2R5B, PPP2R2C)* in MDA-MB-231 cells encoding for protein phosphatases; the proteins of these genes are involved in the negative control of cell division and growth.

3. Fatty acid (FA) metabolism

The first step to the biosynthesis of fatty acids is the transport of citrate from the mitochondria to the cytoplasm. Lipogenesis is controlled by the enzyme fatty acid synthase or FASN, which is highly expressed in breast carcinomas and is thus an important cancer therapeutic target. The breakdown of fatty acids is regulated by carnitine palmitoyltransferase-1 or CPT-I. The preferential expression of FASN in cancer cells including breast cancer, in particular in ER+ breast cancer cells, is of importance because the production and levels of palmitate substantially differ in cancer cells. Blocking FASN has antiproliferative effects on breast cancer cells. A natural antibiotic, known as cerulenin derived from the fungus, *C. ceruleans*, caused apoptosis in cancer cells; C75 is a natural derivative of cerulenin. C75 has antitumor effects and its action is postulated to be on CPT-1 and production of high levels of malonyl CoA respectively. In a comparative study between C75 and EGCG (epigallocatechin-3-gallate), a main constituent of green tea, it was seen that EGCG caused induction of apoptosis uncoupled to the effects of CPT-1 in breast cancer cells through the targeted inhibition of FASN (Puig *et al.*, 2008). (Information source of individual genes: www.ncbi.nlm.nih.gov).

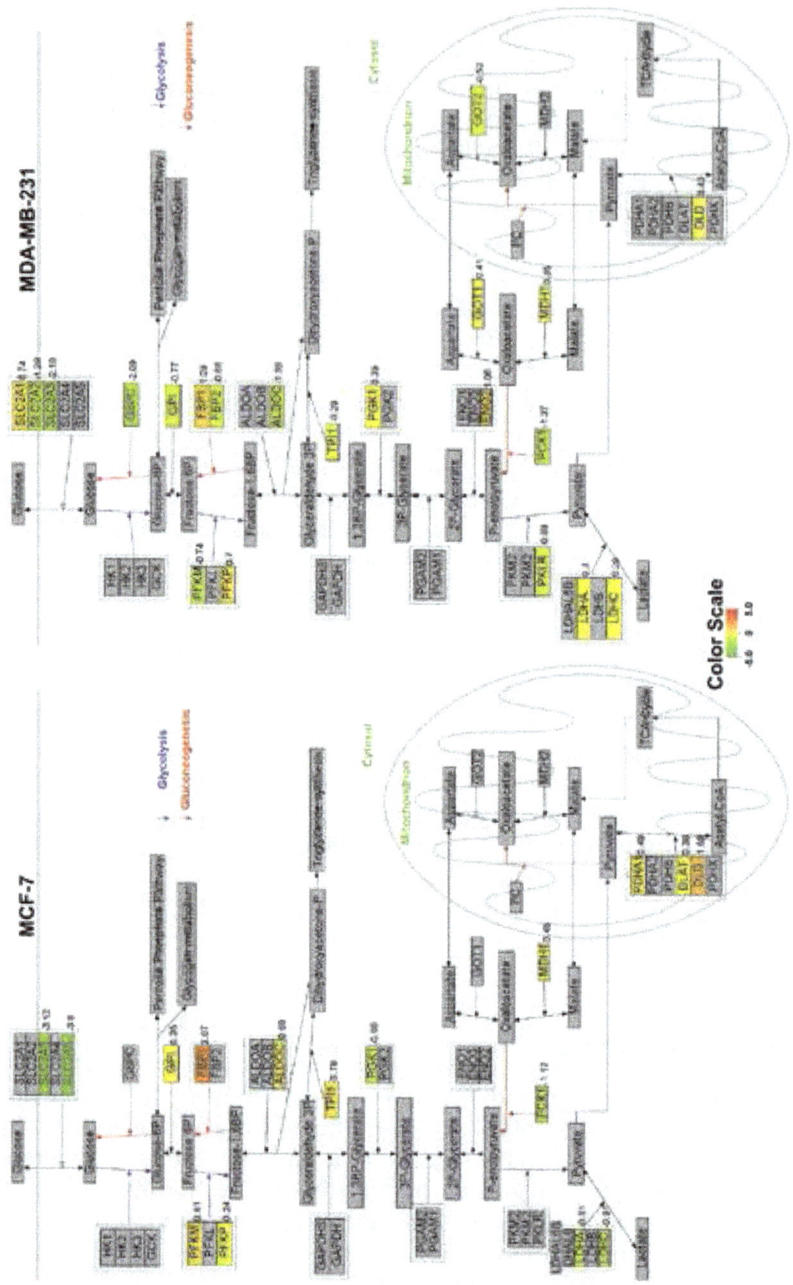

Fig. 1A. A comparative view of the glycolysis and gluconeogenesis pathways operating in the ER+ MCF-7 and ER- MDA-MB-231 cells is shown. The pathway maps were generated using the pathway visualization tool, PathVisio (Version 2). The software generated a color scale for the visualization of expression (red is up-regulation and green is down-regulation of gene expression). Expression values (SLR, signal log ratio) with a cutoff value of ≥ 0.2 or ≤- 0.2 was used and in case of duplicate SLR values, an average SLR was taken. **Note**: Only the controlled irreversible steps of each pathway are colored.

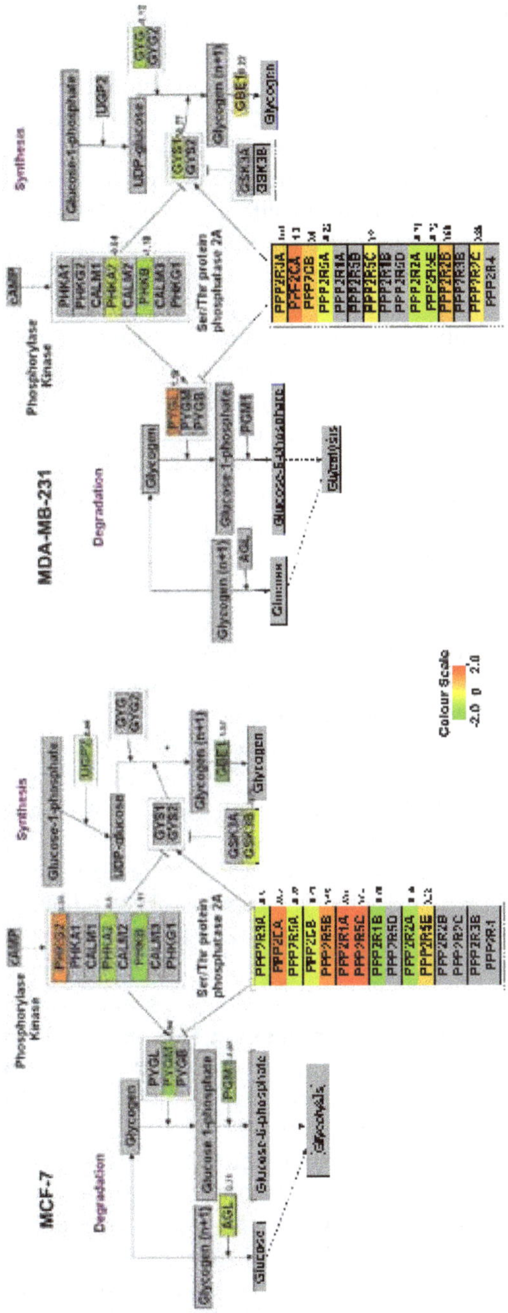

Fig. 1B. A comparative view of the glycogenesis pathway operating in MCF-7 and MDA-MB-231 cells is shown. The pathway maps were generated using the pathway visualization tool, PathVisio (Version 2). The software generated a color scale for the visualization of expression (red is up-regulation and green is down-regulation of gene expression). Expression values (SLR, signal log ratio) with a cutoff value of ≥ 0.2 or ≤- 0.2 was used and in case of duplicate SLR values, an average SLR was taken.

The n-3 PUFAs (n-3 polyunsaturated fatty acids) have beneficial effects as chemopreventive and chemotherapeutic agents in the treatment of cancer. It is of particular interest that in recent years several *in vitro* and *in vivo* xenograft studies and clinical trials have presented evidence that there are beneficial effects of n-3 PUFAs when administered with conventional antineoplastic drugs and radiotherapy against many different types of cancers including breast cancer. Combination of drugs such as doxorubicin/epirubicin/paclitaxel with the n-3 PUFA, DHA (docosahexaenoic acid) had antiproliferative effects such as apoptosis induction, inhibition of neo-angiogenesis, or inhibition of invasiveness in MCF-7 and MDA-MB-231 cells [(Calviello *et al.*, 2009) and references therein]. The cellular antiproliferative actions of n-3 PUFAs include modulation of metabolism, expression of cell cycle and apoptosis factors including caspases, and the ability of fatty acids to sensitize tumor cells to anticancer drugs by increasing membrane permeability. Such beneficial properties have been exploited to develop an interesting strategy of drug delivery, which is the design of liposomes for the targeted delivery of anticancer drugs. This system utilizes the fact that conventional drugs like doxorubicin and cisplatin in liposomal formulations are activated by secretory phospholipase A_2 or $sPLA_2$ which is overexpressed in inflammatory and tumor tissues (Andresen *et al.*, 2005; Laye and Gill, 2003). However, such an approach has not been successful in ER+ (MCF-7) or ER- (MDA-MB-231) cells (Rasmussen *et al.*, 2010). The metabolic modulatory effects of PUFAs leading to antiproliferation include alterations in arachidonic acid (AA) oxidative metabolism and metabolic conversion of n-3 PUFAs to bioactive derivatives. The cellular production of some AA-derived eicosanoids such as prostaglandin E_2 is high in cancer and their formation is inhibited by n-3 PUFAs. Moreover, n-3 PUFAs also competitively inhibit the COX2 enzyme (a very potent oncogene) to produce the less biologically effective n-3 PUFA derived eicosanoids (Chell *et al.*, 2006). A promising finding is the ability of n-3 PUFA to overcome resistance of breast cancer cells treated with tamoxifen. As the n-3 PUFAs are known to inhibit the Akt activity, it was found that EPA (eicosapentaenoic acid) cotreatment of breast cancer cells overexpressing Akt made cells more responsive to tamoxifen. Conjugated preparations of novel anticancer agent, propofol with n-3 PUFAs, DHA and EPA caused significant induction of apoptosis, induction of caspase 3 activity, inhibition of cell adhesion and migration in MDA-MB-231 cells. The drug alone or in combination with the n-3 PUFAs was minimally effective to cause these effects (Siddiqui *et al.*, 2005).

3.1 FA metabolism – A comparative analysis in ER+ and ER- breast cancer cells

In general, the ER+ MCF-7 cells show a greater number of up-regulated genes for proteins catalyzing the FA biosynthesis in comparison to the ER- MDA-MB-231 cells (Fig. 2A). The key features of gene expression are as follows:

a. Notably, the gene expressing the primary enzyme for FA biosynthesis is *FASN*, which is up-regulated in MCF-7 cells in contrast to a down-regulated expression in MDA-MB-231 cells. Genes encoding for enzymes catalyzing the production of FA acetyl Co-A esters from the TCA cycle intermediate, citrate and acetyl CoA (*ACYL, FASN*), or via its intermediate malonyl CoA (ACACB), were up-regulated in MCF-7 cells, but were down-regulated or absent in MDA-MB-231 cells (*ACYL, FASN, ACACA, ACACB*).
b. Interestingly, in both cell types, genes for the enzymes catalyzing the production of triglycerides from FA CoA (*ACSL1, 3, ACAS2*) were down-regulated. These ligases play a key role not only in biosynthesis, but also in FA degradation. Thus, while it is evident that MCF-7 cells differ from ER- cells in the production of palmitate, the synthesis of triglycerides seems to be restricted in both cell types and may be a predominant adaptive response of cancer cells (Fig. 2A).

Similar to FA biosynthesis, genes encoding for enzymes of FA degradation and cholesterol biosynthesis (Fig. 2B) are also mostly up-regulated in MCF-7 cells in contrast to MDA-MB-231 cells.

a. Genes regulating cholesterol biosynthesis may be favored in a hormone responsive environment, cholesterol being the building block of all steroid hormones, including estradiol. Notably among them, is *SQLE* (squalene epoxidase), the protein product of which is a key enzyme in cholesterol key enzyme of cholesterol biosynthesis. MCF-7 cells have an up-regulated expression of the gene, while it is down-regulated in MDA-MB-231 cells. Clinical studies have shown that higher expression of *SQLE* is inversely correlated with distant metastasis-free survival in ER+ stage 1/II breast cancer patients (Helms *et al.*, 2008).
b. Other notable differences include the up-regulated expression of genes of enzymes (*MVK, PMVK*) producing the phosphorylated forms of mevalonic acid, which is a key intermediate of steroid biosynthesis, in MCF-7 cells.
c. Gene of the enzyme catalyzing the dimerization of 2 farnesyl diphosphate molecules to form squalene, is down-regulated, but forms an important step in cholesterol synthesis. It may be assumed that this step of cholesterol biosynthesis, and hence the synthesis of squalene is tightly controlled with respect to the need of steroid hormone synthesis.
d. Notably, in both cell lines, the NAD(P) dependent steroid dehydrogenase-like (NSDHL) enzyme is slightly up-regulated; this may be indicative of an advantage of cancer cells to produce cholesterol depending on its cellular needs.
e. Two other genes whose proteins (*SC4MOL, CYP51A1*) are involved in the synthesis of the cholesterol intermediate, lathosterol are either absent (MDA-MB-231) or down-regulated (MCF-7). Notably, among these, the *CYP51A1* gene encodes for a member of the cytochrome P450 superfamily of monooxygenase enzymes which catalyze many reactions involved in drug metabolism and synthesis of cholesterol, steroids and other lipids. The absence or down-regulation of this enzyme allows cancer cells to metabolize therapeutic drugs aimed to arrest or cause death and thus aid in their overall survival.

4. Retinoic acid (RA) metabolism

The retinoids comprise of RA (vitamin A, all-*trans* retinoic acid) and related signaling molecules which are essential in the differentiation of various types of stem cells. A compromised retinoid signaling is often seen early in carcinogenesis including in breast carcinogenesis, where retinoids interact with the estrogen signaling pathways. These molecules are used for cancer therapeutics because they can induce differentiation and growth arrest. Efficacy of retinoid treatment is often challenged by the fact that these molecules are rapidly metabolized. Moreover, compromised responses, including resistance, to pharmacological doses of retinoids to cancer cells are also the result of epigenetic changes, such as the expression of various transcriptional coactivators and corepressors, the hypermethylation of CpGs in specific promoters in cancer cells, and the activities of other signaling pathways respectively. A combination therapy of retinoids with epigenetic drugs such as histone deacetylase or DNA methytransferase inhibitors or with other classical chemotherapeutic drugs may be a potential alternative route of treatment (Tang and Gudas, 2011). Moreover, another reason limiting the potent anticarcinogenic activities of RA is the fact that it exhibits a paradoxical behavior in that in some cancers it facilitates proliferation rather than inhibition of growth (Schug *et al.*, 2008). (Information source of individual genes: www.ncbi.nlm.nih.gov)

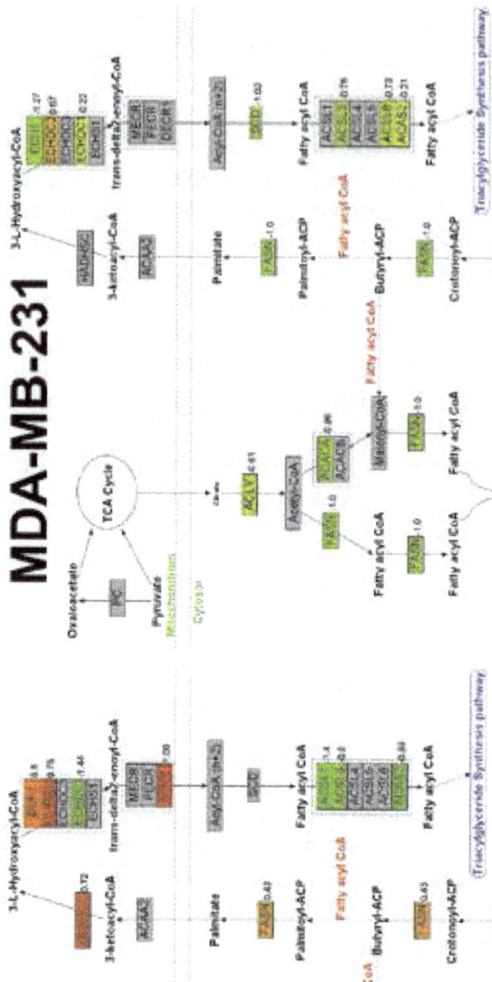

Fig. 2A. A comparative view of fatty acid biosynthesis pathways operating in MCF-7 and MDA-MB-231 cells is shown. The pathway maps were generated using the pathway visualization tool, PathVisio (Version 2). The software generated a color scale for the visualization of expression (red is up-regulation and green is down-regulation of gene expression). Expression values (SLR, signal log ratio) with a cutoff value of ≥ 0.2 or ≤- 0.2 was used and in case of duplicate SLR values, an average SLR was taken.

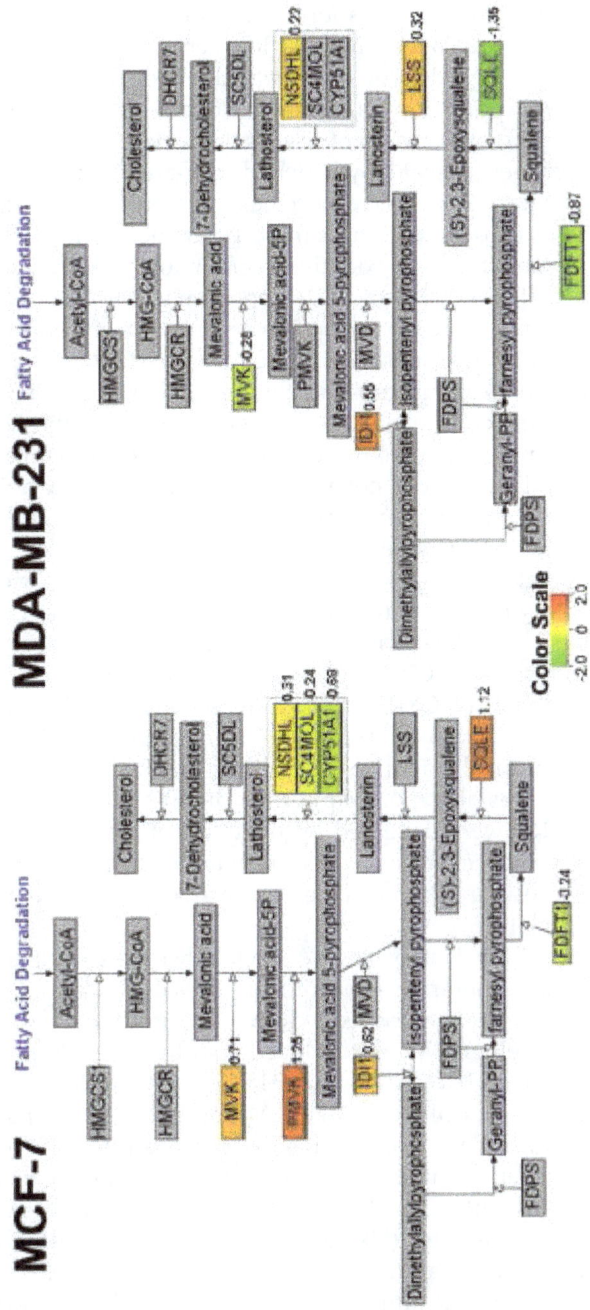

Fig. 2B. A comparative view of fatty acid degradation pathway operating in MCF-7 and MDA-MB-231 cells is shown. The pathway maps were generated using the pathway visualization tool, PathVisio (Version 2). The software generated a color scale for the visualization of expression (red is up-regulation and green is down-regulation of gene expression). Expression values (SLR, signal log ratio) with a cutoff value of ≥ 0.2 or ≤- 0.2 was used and in case of duplicate SLR values, an average SLR was taken.

The intracellular concentrations of various forms of retinoids are under the control of several metabolic enzymes (Duester, 2008). Within the RA generating tissue, retinol or vitamin A (retinol) is first converted to the aldehyde form (retinaldehyde) and then to the carboxylic acid (retinoic acid, RA). The expression of several alcohol and retinol dehydrogenases is widespread and overlapping in a variety of tissues. However, during mouse embryogenesis, the expression of the enzymes (retinaldehyde dehydrogenases) responsible for the second step which leads to RA generation, is tissue specific and non-overlapping (Mic *et al.*, 2002). Oxidation of RA leads to its degradation to more polar metabolites such as 4-oxo-RA (and other more polar RA metabolites); this oxidative degradation is catalyzed by three cytochrome P450 (CYP) enzymes, CYP26A1, B1, and C1 respectively (bu-Abed *et al.*, 1998). Enzymes controlling the synthesis of RA are expressed in very low levels in breast cancers relative to normal breast cells. The ability of normal HMECs from reduction mammoplasty has been shown to be competent in RA synthesis and the ability is still retained by immortal, non-tumorigenic breast epithelial cells, such as MCF10A. However, in the ER+ MCF-7 and T47D cells, the impaired RA activity appeared due to the impaired biosynthesis of RA; treatment with the CYP26 inhibitor, liarozole did not affect the low and undetectable levels of RA (Mira *et al.*, 2000). Likewise, a defect found in human primary breast tumors is the aberrantly high expression of the degradation enzyme, CYP26A1. The ducts and lobules of normal breast tissues demonstrated weak staining which was in contrast to distinct strong cytoplasmic staining in 46% of breast carcinomas (primary and metastatic breast carcinomas) examined within a tissue microarray. Kaplan-Meier analysis of these breast cancer cases suggested an association of high expression of CYP26A1 with a lower disease free and overall survival period. While overexpression of CYP26A1 in transfected AC2M2 (a breast metastatic ER-variant cell line) caused a decreased sensitivity to apoptosis, CYP26A1 siRNA silencing partially abrogated cells from the apoptosis sensitivity. In RA sensitive ER+ T47D cells, the induction of this enzyme was also more rapid than the ER- MDA-MB-231 cells. The growth inhibitory properties of RA were increased by the effect of treatment of an RA metabolism inhibitor, liarozole. Thus both *in vivo* and *in vitro* evidence suggested the potential oncogenic capacity (decreased apoptosis and increased cell survival) of RA degradation enzymes (Osanai *et al.*, 2010; Sonneveld *et al.*, 1998).
Studies show that two critical steps in RA metabolism responsible for synthesis and degradation of RA are sometimes impaired in breast cancers. Thus, defects in RA metabolism influences its effectiveness as a cancer antiproliferative drug in the ER+/ER- breast cells. RA inhibited cell growth and induced apoptosis in ER+ breast cancer cell lines, MCF-7 and T47D, but not in ER- MDA-MB-231 and MDA-MB-453 cells. The differences were due to the ability of ER+ cells to uptake RA rapidly (by hour 2) and by hour 24 there was a disappearance of RA uptake from the medium and cells leaving oxidation products in the culture medium. In sharp contrast, ER- cells showed lower accumulation without any sharp increase and subsequent steep decline; the result was the presence of more RA in these cells and the culture medium (Okamoto *et al.*, 2000). Interestingly, the ER- cell line MDA-MB-468 cells still retain the ability to synthesize RA (Mira *et al.*, 2000). Though a triple negative ER- cell line with EGFR amplification, the MDA-MB-468 cells are responsive to novel drugs along with the nuclear localization of a pseudo wild-type p53 and delocalization of mutant p53 (Mandal *et al.*, 2007a).

4.1 Comparative analysis of RA metabolism between ER+ and ER- cells

RA acts through its binding to the RA receptor (RAR), which in turn is bound to DNA as a heterodimer with the retinoid X receptor (RXR) in the RA response elements (RAREs).

Binding of RA ligand to RAR alters the conformation of the RAR resulting in the transcriptional induction or repression of RA target genes. As discussed in the previous paragraphs, the genes of proteins catalyzing the metabolism of RA has profound effects on breast cancer and hence also on its antiproliferative actions. Here we discuss the pattern of expression of genes encoding for proteins involved in RA metabolism in the ER+ and ER- breast cancer cells (Fig. 3). Essentially, there is a generalized down-regulation of genes encoding proteins involved in the production of various RA metabolites. Major differences are seen in RAR, RA binding proteins, and sulfotransferase enzymes (SULT) respectively. The key differences and similarities are discussed below:

a. The protein encoded by SCARB1 is a plasma membrane receptor for HDL (high density lipoprotein) cholesterol. SCARB1 protein mediates cholesterol transfer to and from HDL. This gene is down-regulated in both cell lines. Among the metabolic genes, there is retinol saturase, (*RETSAT*); the protein of this gene catalyzes the conversion of all-trans retinol to all-trans-13, 14-dihydroretinol, an intermediate of 13, 14-dehydroRA. All-trans-13, 14-dihydroretinol binds to the RARs in the nucleus and it is selectively up-regulated in MCF-7, but is absent in MDA-MB-231 cells. Also, in the ER+ MCF-7 we see a selective up-regulation of CYP2E1, a RA degradation enzyme, which is highly up-regulated in aggressive breast tumors as discussed above. The first step of RAR activation is mediated by the delivery of RA from the cytosol to the receptor in the nucleus, a step which involves the cellular retinoic acid-binding protein 2 (*CRABP2*); this gene is highly up-regulated in MCF-7 cells (Schug *et al.*, 2008).
b. In MCF-7 cells the expression of genes encoding for SULT enzymes, *SULT2A1* and *B1*, are highly up-regulated. These enzymes catalyze the sulfate conjugation of many hormones, neurotransmitters, drugs, and xenobiotic compounds. In particular, the enzyme SULT2B1 sulfates dehydroepiandrosterone, but not 4-nitrophenol, a typical substrate for the phenol and estrogen sulfotransferase subfamilies. MDA-MB-231 cells did not show expression of these genes. In support of this, we found that the GO term molecular functions are associated with sulfotransferase activity within the RA network in E2 stimulated MCF-7 cells; genes of the RA network are associated with biological processes such as the cell cycle and its regulation, protein metabolic processes amino acid methylation and alkylation and sulphur compound biosynthetic process respectively.
c. *RARa/RXRa*-these RARs are selectively up-regulated in MCF-7, but are low in expression and absent in MDA-MB-231 cells. This selective expression can be correlated to the fact that RARa protein is involved with functions such as apoptosis and differentiation and together as hetero/homodimers mediate the biological effects by RA-mediated gene activation.
d. *RARb/RXRb-RARb* binds to RA and mediates cellular signaling in embryonic morphogenesis, cell growth and differentiation. This protein has antiproliferative effects in many cell types. This gene is down-regulated in both cell types; however, its heterodimeric counterpart, RXRb gene lies within the MHC class II region on chromosome 6a, is selectively up-regulated in MDA-MB-231 cells. The significance of this discrepancy is unknown, but may be a feature of de-regulated immune responses present in ER- breast cancer cells (Mandal *et al.*, 2007b).

   RARg/RXRG-these nuclear hormone receptors are ligand-dependent transcriptional regulators. RXRg, the counterpart of RARg, mediates the antiproliferative effects of RA. RXRg is expressed at significantly lower levels in non-small cell lung cancer cells. This receptor pair is down-regulated in MDA-MB-231 cells, but RARg is selectively up-regulated in MCF-7 cells. (Information source of individual genes: www.ncbi.nlm.nih.gov)

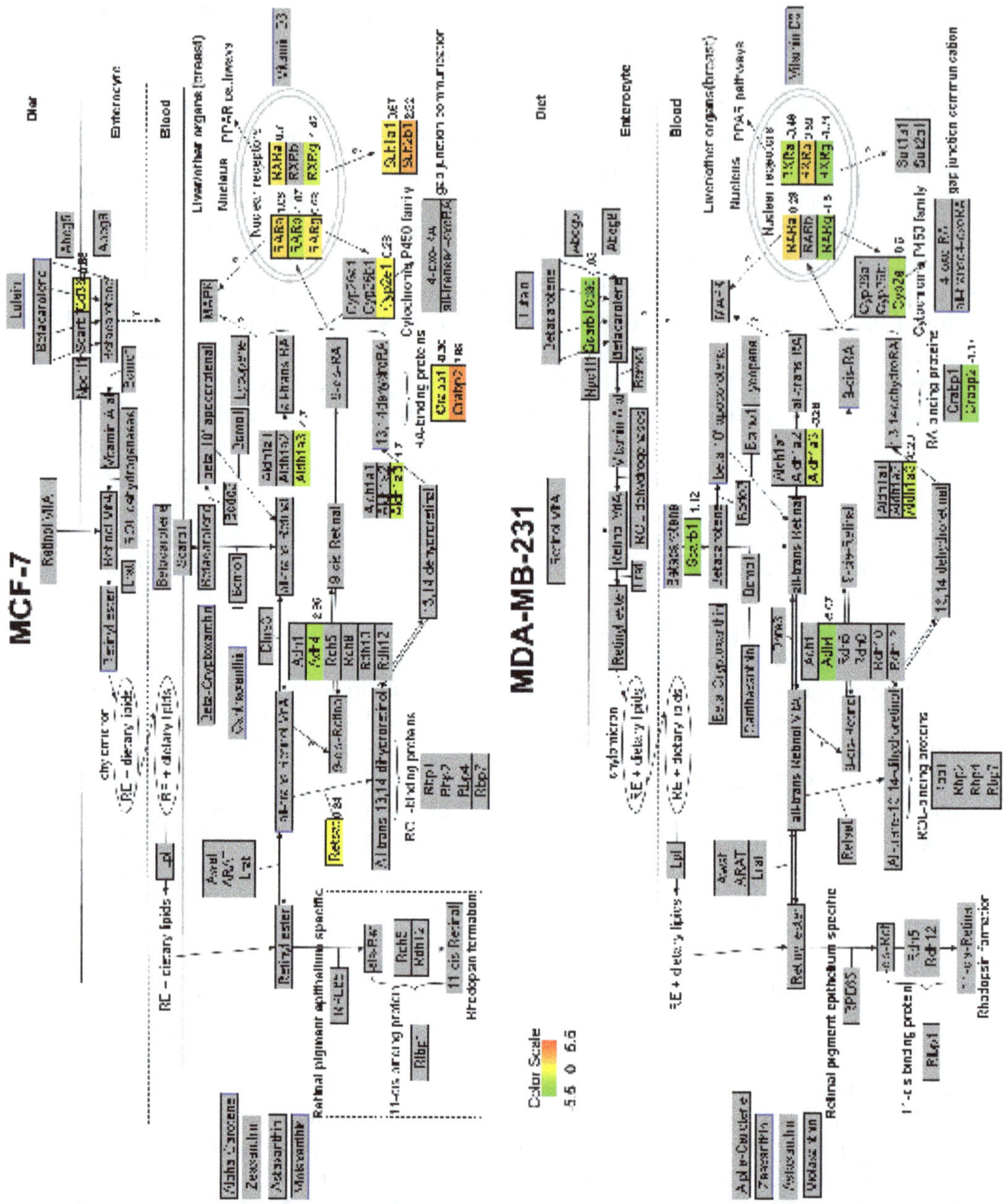

Fig. 3. A comparative view of retinoic acid metabolic pathways operating in MCF-7 and MDA-MB-231 cells is shown. The pathway maps were generated using the pathway visualization tool, PathVisio (Version 2). The software generated a color scale for the visualization of expression (red is up-regulation and green is down-regulation of gene expression). Expression values (SLR, signal log ratio) with a cutoff value of ≥ 0.2 or ≤- 0.2 was used and in case of duplicate SLR values, an average SLR was taken. Abbreviations used: ROL=retinol; RAL=retinaldehyde; RA=retinoic acid; RE=retinyl ester; RPE=retinal pigment epithelium.

5. The role of mitogen and stress activated kinase (MSK) in breast cancer

Mitogen and stress activated kinases 1 and 2 (MSK1/RPS6KA5, MSK2/RPS6KA4) are serine-threonine kinases that are activated by the p38 or RAS-MAPK signaling pathway. In breast cancer, there is overexpression of the growth factor receptors EGFR/HER1 and HER2/neu; in 25-30% of breast tumors HER2 is overexpressed and 45% of breast tumors test positive for EGFR (Klijn *et al.*, 1992; Slamon *et al.*, 1989). The overexpression of these receptors leads to the constitutive activation of the RAS-MAPK signaling pathway and the subsequent phosphorylation and activation of MSK1 and MSK2. Once activated, MSK1 and 2 can act on several substrates that are relevant to cancer signaling pathways. Importantly, MSKs can phosphorylate the serine residues S10 and S28 on the N-terminal tail of the histone protein H3 (Soloaga *et al.*, 2003). MSK1/2 mediated H3 modification is an event that can lead to chromatin remodeling and the expression of immediate-early (IE) genes such as *FOS*, *COX2*, and *JUN*, which are often up-regulated during oncogenesis (Drobic *et al.*, 2010; Dunn *et al.*, 2005). MSK proteins can also phosphorylate and activate various transcription factors such as CREB, ATF1, ER81, and the p65 subunit of NFκB, which activate the transcription of genes involved in tumorigenic and metastatic progression (Arthur and Cohen, 2000; Vermeulen *et al.*, 2003; Wiggin *et al.*, 2002).

The role of MSKs in cancer progression spans from their contribution to the process of anchorage-independent growth to a potential role in epithelial mesenchymal transition (EMT). MSK has been implied in the anchorage independent growth of mouse epidermal cells, *H-ras* transformed mouse fibroblasts and v-Src transformed mouse Balb3T3 cells (Kim *et al.*, 2008; Perez-Cadahia *et al.*, 2011; Tange *et al.*, 2009). Inhibition of MSK by the small molecule inhibitor H89 implicates MSK in the EMT process in *H-RAS* overexpressing Caco-H human colon cancer cells (Pelaez *et al.*, 2010). In the ER+ breast cancer cell line MCF-7, stimulation with the phorbol ester 12-O-tetradecanoylphorbol-13-acetate (TPA) causes the activation of the RAS-MAPK pathway and hence H3S10 phosphorylation and the induction of the E2 response gene, *TFF1* (trefoil factor 1), which has been implicated in breast cancer progression (Espino *et al.*, 2006). Interestingly, MSK activation by TPA in MCF-7 cells induces H3S10 phosphorylation but not H3S28 phosphorylation by an unknown mechanism (Espino *et al.*, 2006). However, a recent study has called into question the value of using *TFF1* as a prognostic marker in breast cancer, as it demonstrates that knockdown of *TFF1* in MCF-7 cells leads to enhanced colony formation in soft agar, and that *TFF1* knock-out mice have a higher tumor incidence in mammary glands (Buache *et al.*, 2011).

In the ER- MDA-MB-231 and SKBR-3 cells, MSK is implicated in the expression of the pro-inflammatory cytokine IL-6, whereby IL-6 is constitutively expressed and MSK is recruited to the IL-6 promoter following TNF-α signaling. The MSK-mediated expression of IL-6 involves MSK-mediated phosphorylation of NFκBp65^{S276}, recruitment of MSK and phosphorylation of H3S10 on the IL-6 promoter, followed by subsequent chromatin remodeling of the promoter via the recruitment of the BRG1 subunit of the SWI/SNF chromatin remodeling complex (Ndlovu *et al.*, 2009). Similarly, MSK mediated H3S10 phosphorylation can induce the chromatin remodeling of the mouse mammary tumor virus (MMTV) promoter in MTVL breast cancer cells that have a stably integrated luciferase reporter gene driven by the MMTV promoter (Vicent *et al.*, 2008). In this system, progestin treatment leads to the formation of a ternary complex comprised of the PR and phosphorylated ERK (pERK) and MSK1 (pMSK1). The PR/pERK/pMSK1 complex is recruited to the MMTV promoter followed by phosphorylation of H3S10 by pMSK, leading to the displacement of the HP1γ repressor complex and the subsequent activation of gene transcription in these cells (Vicent *et al.*, 2008; Vicent *et al.*, 2009). In the ER- cells (eg., MDA-MB-231) MSK has been implicated in the migration and invasion of cells to lymphatic endothelial cells *in vitro* as well as in *in vivo* mouse xenograft model through the possible NFκB binding to the chemokine receptor CCR7 (Pan *et al.*, 2009). MSK has also been implicated in cancer-related inflammation through *COX2* expression. It has been observed that MSK-mediated *COX2* expression in mouse epidermal cells induces neoplastic transformation (Yan *et al.*, 2006). MSK recruitment and H3S10 and H3S28 phosphorylation occur at the upstream regulatory promoter region of *COX2* in mouse fibroblasts in addition to the recruitment of chromatin remodeling factors and transcriptional activation histone marks at these sites (Drobic *et al.*, 2010). In MCF-7, TPA selectively induces *COX2* expression (Degner *et al.*, 2006). From these data it can be speculated that MSK may be involved in *COX2* expression/regulation in breast cancer cells, although this has yet to be experimentally reported. MSKs contribute to breast cancer progression through a variety of mechanisms including the induction of genes involved in transformation or inflammation, and priming gene promoters for chromatin remodeling and activation.

5.1 A comparative analysis of the MAPK pathway in ER+ and ER- breast cancer

As discussed in the previous paragraphs, genes of the MAPK pathway have profound effects on the progression of breast cancer. An overall comparison between MCF-7 and MDA-MB-231 shows that all the caspases are either absent or down-regulated in both cell lines, *EGFR* is up-regulated in the MDA-MB-231. cells, and the early responsive genes, *FOS* and *JUN* are oppositely expressed, and the p50/p105 (NFκB1) subunit of NFκB is up-regulated. *BDNF* (brain-derived neurotrophic factor) is highly expressed in MDA-MB-231 cells, but is totally absent in MCF-7 cells. The high expression of *BDNF* is of speculative importance because the gene encoding for this protein of the nerve growth factor family is responsible for the survival of striatal neurons and also responds to stress. Different members of MAP kinases are differntially up/down-regulated in the two cell lines, which may be a reflection of aggressiveness. The key differences and similarities are discussed below (Fig. 4):

a. *DUSP*- dual specificity protein phosphatase enzymes play important roles in regulating cellular response to environmental stress are also negative regulators of cell proliferation. They negatively regulate members of the mitogen-activated protein (MAP) kinase superfamily, which are associated with cellular proliferation and differentiation. Different members of this family of phosphatases have distinct substrate specificities for various MAP kinases, different tissue distribution and subcellular localization, and different modes of inducibility of their expression by extracellular stimuli. Interestingly, genes encoding for these phosphatases are down-regulated in MCF-7 and are up-regulated in MDA-MB-231 cells.
b. *PRKC (B, Z, H, G, D)*-Protein kinase C (PKC) is a family of serine- and threonine-specific protein kinases that can be activated by calcium and second messenger DAG (diacylglycerol). PKC family members phosphorylate a wide variety of protein targets and participate in diverse cellular signaling pathways. PKCs are major receptors for phorbol esters; in the comparative gene analysis, we find that most of the PKCs are down-regulated or absent with the exception of a few, but we have shown that the ER+ MCF-7 cells activate the MAPK pathway in response to TPA (Espino *et al.*, 2006). (Information source of individual genes: www.ncbi.nlm.nih.gov)

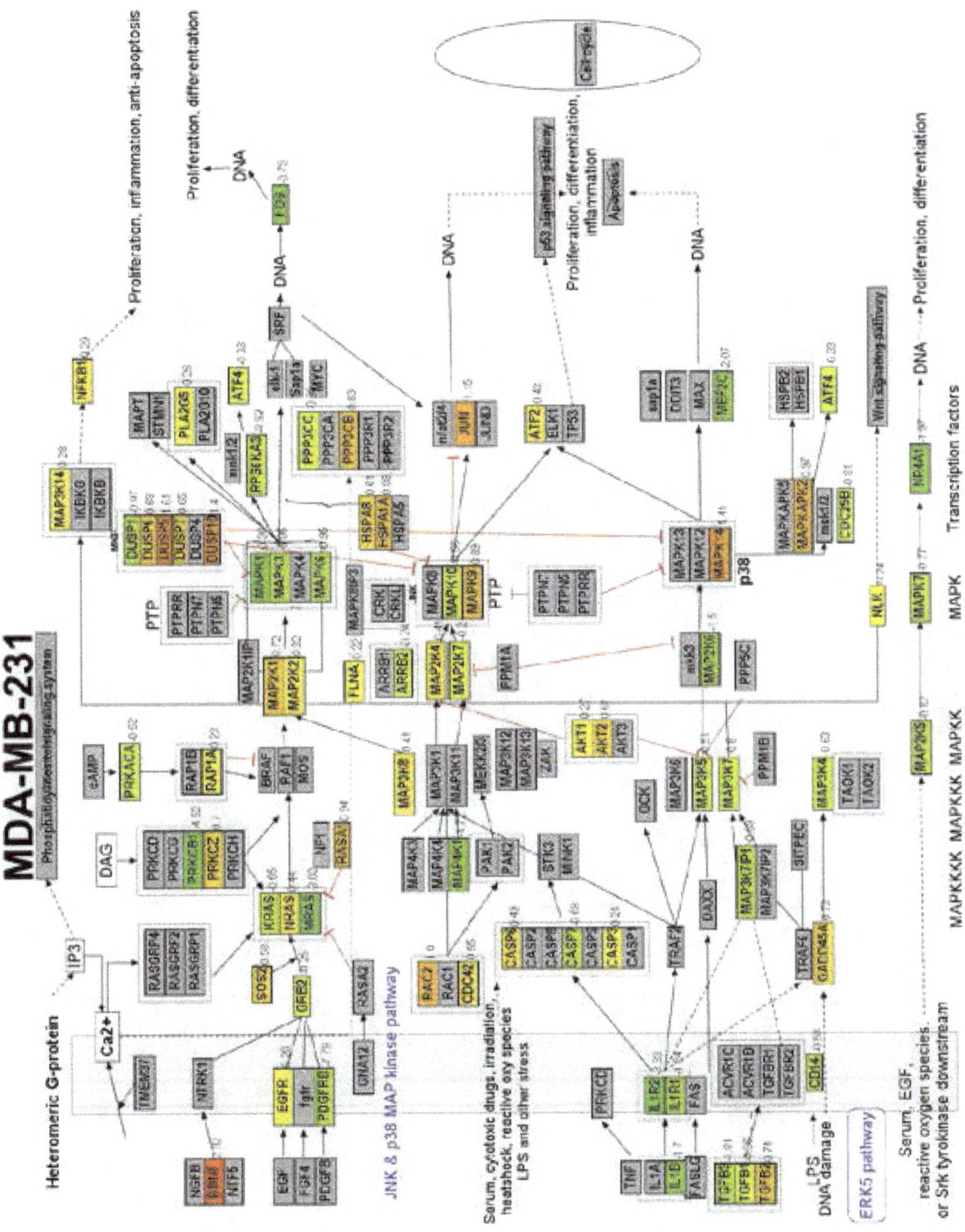

Fig. 4. (Continued)

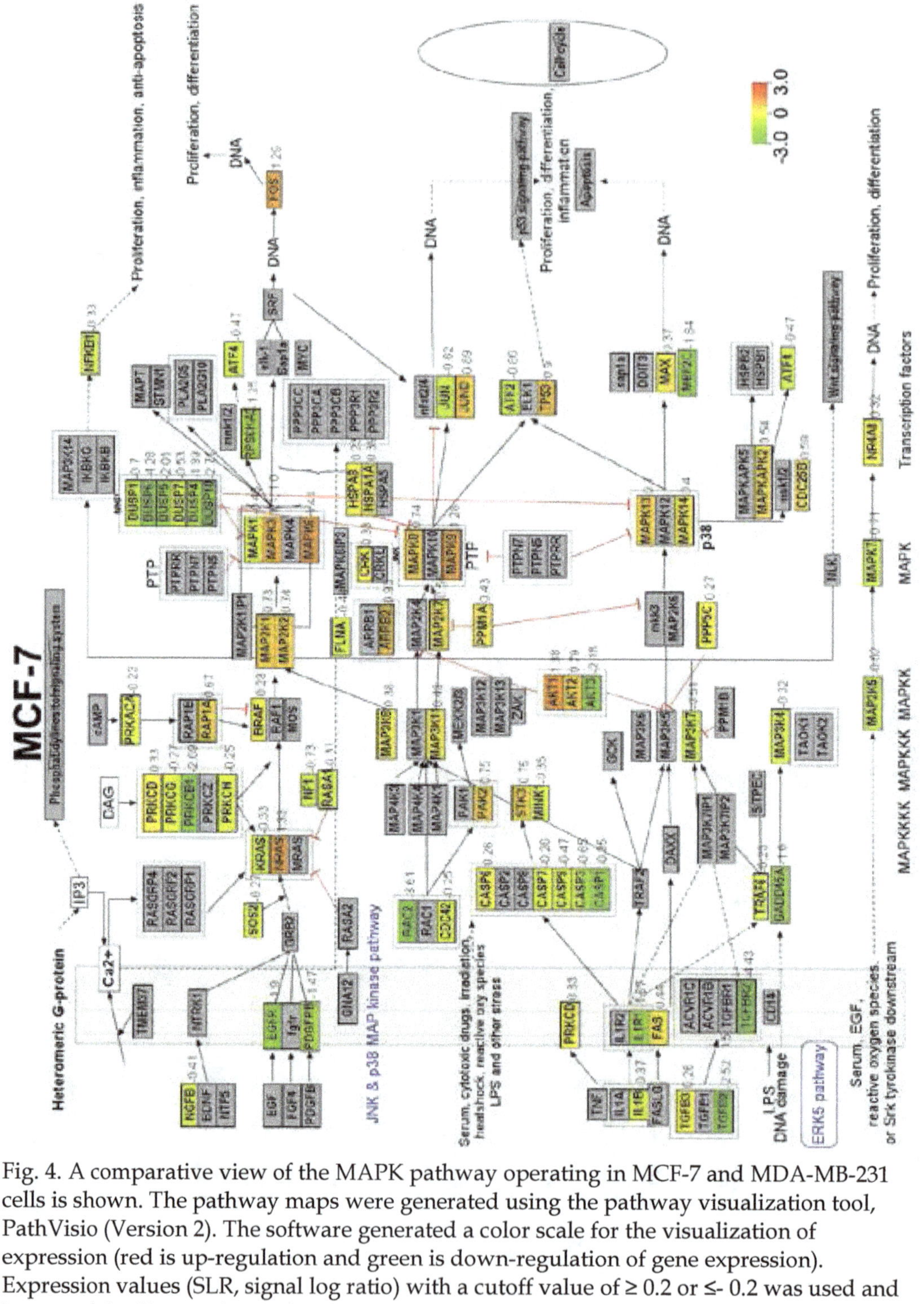

Fig. 4. A comparative view of the MAPK pathway operating in MCF-7 and MDA-MB-231 cells is shown. The pathway maps were generated using the pathway visualization tool, PathVisio (Version 2). The software generated a color scale for the visualization of expression (red is up-regulation and green is down-regulation of gene expression). Expression values (SLR, signal log ratio) with a cutoff value of ≥ 0.2 or ≤- 0.2 was used and in case of duplicate values, an average SLR was taken.

6. Role of transcription factors, Sp1 and Sp3 in breast cancer

Sp1 and Sp3 proteins are overexpressed in breast tumors and contribute to the proliferative and angiogenic phenotype, characteristics which correlate to poor prognosis (Li *et al.*, 2004; Mertens-Talcott *et al.*, 2007). There are an estimated 12000 Sp1 and Sp3 binding sites in human genome (Cawley *et al.*, 2004). Inhibition of Sp1 binding to DNA by mithramycin A or knocking down Sp1 to the normal expression level, decreased tumor formation, growth and metastasis (Lou *et al.*, 2005; Yuan *et al.*, 2007). Likewise, antiproliferative agents such as, betulinic acid and curcumin reduced the expression of Sp1 and Sp3 and their target genes (*EGFR, CCND1, VEGF, SREBF2, CD151*), which have roles in metastasis (Chadalapaka *et al.*, 2010; Kang and Chen, 2009). Knocking out Sp1/Sp3 was lethal and caused the death of knockout mice at different developmental stages. Compounded Sp1 and Sp3 knockout mice were not viable suggesting that both these transcription factors are required to maintain appropriate gene expression programs (Bouwman *et al.*, 2000; Kruger *et al.*, 2007; Marin *et al.*, 1997; Van Loo *et al.*, 2003). This agrees with the fact that Sp1 and Sp3 are autoregulated genes with Sp1 and Sp3 binding sites in their proximal promoter regions (Nicolas *et al.*, 2001).

In the estrogen and breast cancer context, it is known that many estrogen responsive genes have Sp1/3(s) sites in the estrogen response elements of their promoters (Castro-Rivera *et al.*, 2001; Higgins *et al.*, 2006; Mandal and Davie, 2010; Sun *et al.*, 2002; Sun *et al.*, 2005). *TFF1* is a highly expressed estrogen responsive gene in malignant breast epithelial cells but not normal mammary cells (Rio *et al.*, 1987). In our studies, we predicted and validated a Sp1/3 site 6 bp upstream of the imperfect ERE site and the dynamic association of ERα, Sp protein, KATs and HDACs on the *TFF1* proximal promoter in response to E2 using TFSEARCH, ChIP (chromatin immunoprecipitation) assay and promoter analysis. We found Sp3, but not Sp1, to be the major Sp protein activating the *TFF1* upstream promoter region in response to E2 (Sun *et al.*, 2005). This was supported by other studies where it was shown that Sp3 plays a major role in ERα/Sp-mediated gene expression in MCF-7 cells (Khan *et al.*, 2007). In general, Sp1 usually activates transcription and Sp3 represses or most weakly activates transcription (Higgins *et al.*, 2006; Jaiswal *et al.*, 2006; Noe *et al.*, 2001). Though in some studies it was shown that Sp1 and Sp3 synergistically enhanced gene promoter function, we have shown that Sp1 and Sp3 did not exist in the same protein complexes in the *TFF1* promoter in MCF-7 cells (Hantusch *et al.*, 2007; He *et al.*, 2005; Lee *et al.*, 2009; Li and Davie, 2008).

6.1 Regulation of transcriptional responses of Sp1 and Sp3

Sp1 and Sp3 have multiple isoforms, of which Sp1 has two and Sp3 has four isoforms (Li and Davie, 2010). Four Sp3 isoforms have been reported. The two long forms of Sp3 and Sp1 contain two trans-activation domains A and B, one serine /threonine rich domain for post-translational modifications (PTMs) and the DNA binding domain C. Sp1 has domain D at the C-terminus which is critical for its synergistic activation. As the Sp family signature, the DNA binding domain C features the three Cys2His2 zinc 'fingers' required for sequence-specific DNA association. The consensus Sp1 and Sp3 binding DNA sequence is GGGGCGGGG. Although recognizing the same DNA binding sequence, Sp1 and Sp3 differ structurally in the location of their inhibitory domains; it is at the N-terminus for Sp1 and for Sp3 this domain lies immediately in front of the DNA binding domain (Suske, 1999).

PTMs such as sumoylation and acetylation of Sp1 and Sp3 regulate their functional roles (Li *et al.*, 2004; Li and Davie, 2010). Sumoylated Sp1 was deficient in proteolytic processing; it was proposed that Sp1 sumoylation preserves the integrity of a negative regulatory domain and inhibits the Sp1-dependent transcription (Spengler and Brattain, 2006). In another study however, sumoylation was found to aid in Sp1 interaction with the proteosome (Wang *et al.*, 2008). The major sumoylation of Sp3 long and short forms occurs at K551, which is a single lysine in its inhibitory domain and a minor sumoylation site (K120) is in the long form. The K551 modification silenced or significantly decreased Sp3 activity and mutation of this site converted the short Sp3 isoforms into potent transactivators of the SRC 1A gene promoter, but did not affect the transcriptional properties of Sp3 long forms (Ellis *et al.*, 2006; Ross *et al.*, 2002; Sapetschnig *et al.*, 2002; Spengler *et al.*, 2008). Interestingly, acetylation of K551 by KAT p300 converts Sp3 to a transcriptional activator; thus the activity of Sp3 can be repressing or activating depending on PTM of K551 (Ammanamanchi *et al.*, 2003). Sp1 can also be acetylated by p300, but the exact role of acetylation is unclear (Song *et al.*, 2003). Another PTM is methylation within or around Sp1/3 site(s), which regulates Sp1 and Sp3 association with DNA to regulate gene expression (Mudduluru and Allgayer, 2008). Whereas methylation within the consensus Sp1/3 site did not influence binding of Sp1/Sp3 to the $p21^{Waf1/Cip1}$ promoter, this modification outside the GC boxes reduced Sp1/Sp3 binding to $p21^{Waf1/Cip1}$ and mouse *Abcc6* promoter with repression of gene expression (Zhu *et al.*, 2003). Thus these Sp1/Sp3 PTMs likely influence the functional roles of these transcription factors for gene activation and repression.

6.2 A comparative analysis of Sp1-Sp3 interactions in ER+ and ER- breast cancer – The Sp1 and Sp3 target genes

Sp1 and Sp3 participate in the regulation of tissue-specific, viral, and inducible genes (Davie *et al.*, 2008; Lu and Archer, 2010). Genes include regulators of cell cycle progression and arrest (eg. cyclins), pro- and anti-angiogenic factors involved in invasion and metastasis, pro- and anti-apoptotic factors involved in genomic stability, proto-oncogenes (eg. *MYC*), tumor suppressors (eg. *p53*), enhancers of cell proliferation and oncogenesis (Abdelrahim *et al.*, 2002; DesJardins and Hay, 1993; Feng *et al.*, 2000; Kavurma *et al.*, 2001; Lagger *et al.*, 2003; Olofsson *et al.*, 2007; Yuan *et al.*, 2007). Analysis by Ingenuity Pathway Analysis (IPA) tool showed that in MCF-7 and MDA-MB-231 cells, Sp1 and Sp3 share a network of interconnected genes inclusive of all categories discussed above (Fig. 5A, 5B). Fig. 5C is a snapshot cluster view of the Sp1-Sp3 gene network. Comparison showed that in the ER+ MCF-7 cells Sp1 was up-regulated and Sp3 was expressed at lower levels, while Sp3 was highly expressed in the MDA-MB-231 cells. In case of the $p21^{Waf1/Cip1}$ promoter, we also observed a lower Sp3 association in response to estrogen stimulation in MCF-7 cells (Mandal and Davie, 2007). We demonstrated that both Sp1 and Sp3 associated with *TFF1*, but Sp3, not Sp1, plays a major role in the estrogen activated ERα/Sp-mediated gene expression in MCF-7 cells (Khan *et al.*, 2007; Li and Davie, 2008). Therefore, in the context of estrogen stimulation, Sp1 and Sp3 play dual roles in regulating gene expression.

7. Conclusions

The evidence presented here show that metabolic patterns, transcriptional responses and gene expression in pathways in ER+ cells considerably differ from the ER- breast cancer counterpart. Generally, gene expression of energy metabolic pathways is low to absent for the more metastatic ER- cancer cells. Estrogen is a major mitogen which drives metabolic processes related to glucose and fatty acid metabolism and the hormone is also responsible

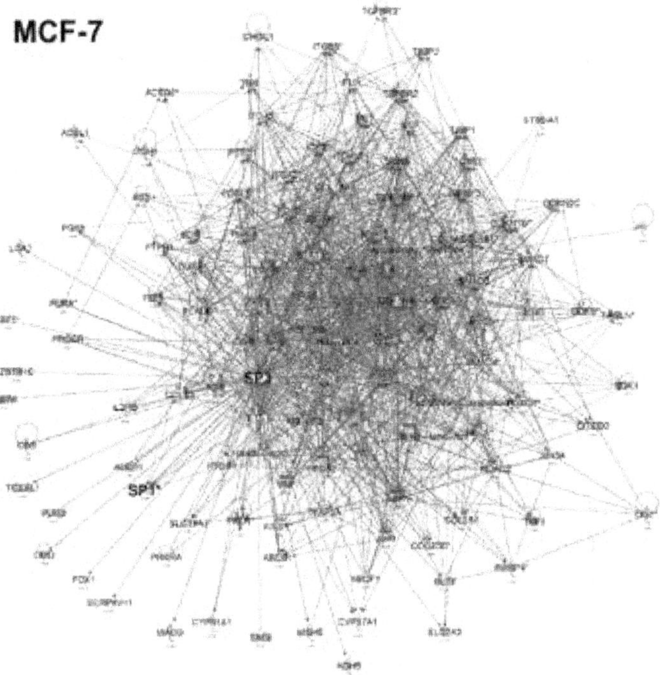

5A

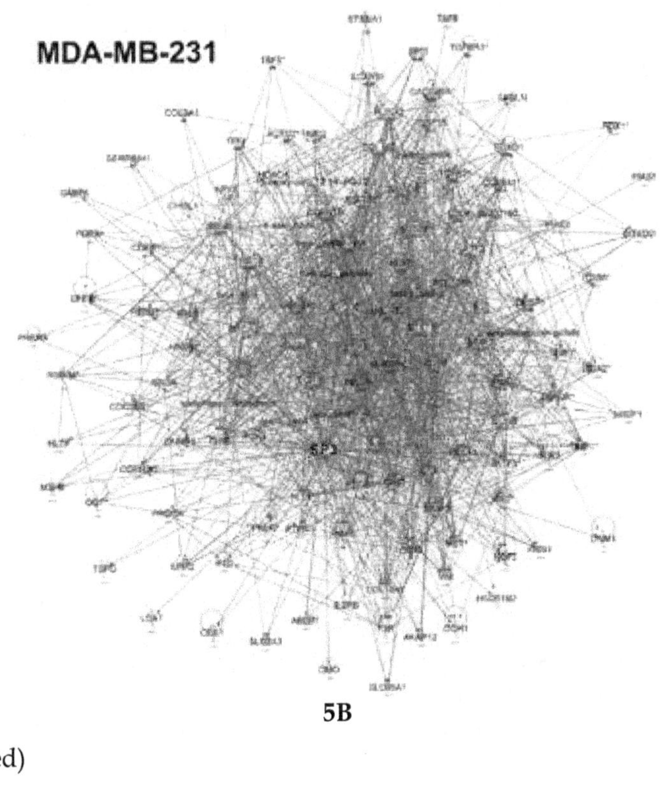

5B

Fig. 5. (Continued)

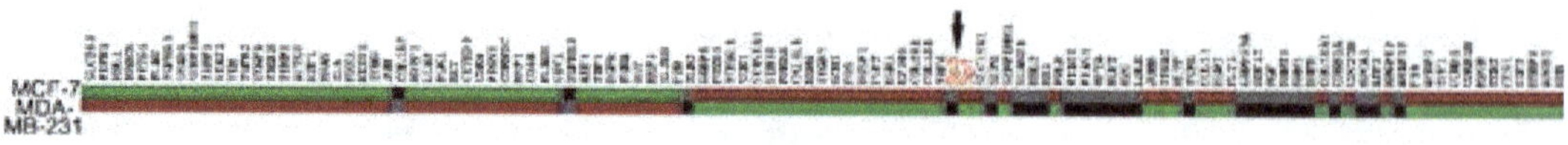

5C

Fig. 5. A network of genes connected to the transcription factors Sp1 and Sp3 in (A) in the ER+ MCF-7 and the (B) ER- MDA-MB-231 cells. This network was generated using IPA (Ingenuity Pathway Analysis) tool. Red indicates positive and green indicates negative expression. (C) A cluster view of the genes in the network (Cluster Tree view; red is positive, green is negative, grey is total absence of expression); cluster analysis was done as described previously (Eisen *et al.*, 1998). Expression values (SLR, signal log ratio) with a cutoff value of ≥ 0.2 or ≤- 0.2 was used and in case of duplicate values, an average SLR was taken.

for the Sp1 and Sp3 transcriptionally driven expression of many estrogen responsive genes. The functional role of Sp1 and Sp3 in estrogen stimulated breast cancer cells is determined by the type of PTM, protein interaction, promoter context, collectively all of which contribute to the progression of the disease. The contribution of MSK to breast cancer progression is manifold. Importantly, MSK proteins can be inhibited by small molecules (e.g. H89) which reverse the epigenetic effects of MSK on gene transcription, and thereby make MSK an attractive target for cancer therapy. Moreover, it has been shown that treatment with MEK1/2 inhibitors such as PD98059, can cause radio-sensitization of MCF-7 cells in clonogenic survival assay. The MAPK pathway can also be proapoptotic in breast cancer cells. In the ER+ T47D cells, p38 kinase inhibitors (SB202190, SB203580, PD169316) abolished activin-mediated growth arrest, suggesting that this pathway can be utilized by a growth factor for growth inhibitory effects (Cocolakis *et al.*, 2001). Further studies are required to determine the mechanisms by which MEK1/2 inhibitors commit cells to killing via apoptotic and non-apoptotic mechanisms (Qiao *et al.*, 2002). On the other hand, targeting these major transcription factors is also a promising therapeutic approach. Most of the current studies have focused on Sp1 mRNA/protein expression and more studies on Sp3 isoforms are required to develop better Sp protein targeting cancer therapies. Several approaches to the development and delivery of metabolic drugs also hold promise to the treatment of hormone responsive tumors.

8. Acknowledgments

Research support has been provided by a grant from the Canadian Breast Cancer Foundation to JRD and a Canada Research Chair to JRD. Lin Li was a recipient of the U.S. Army Medical and Materiel Command Breast Cancer Research Program Foundation Studentship grant W81XWH-05-1-0284.

9. References

Abdelrahim, M. *et al.* (2002). Small inhibitory RNA duplexes for Sp1 mRNA block basal and estrogen-induced gene expression and cell cycle progression in MCF-7 breast cancer cells. *J Biol Chem* 277, 28815-28822.

Ali, S., Coombes, R. C. (2000). Estrogen receptor alpha in human breast cancer: occurrence and significance. *J Mammary Gland Biol Neoplasia* 5, 271-281.

Ammanamanchi, S. *et al.* (2003). Acetylated sp3 is a transcriptional activator. *J Biol Chem* 278, 35775-35780.

Andresen, T. L. *et al.* (2005). Advanced strategies in liposomal cancer therapy: problems and prospects of active and tumor specific drug release. *Prog Lipid Res* 44, 68-97.

Arthur, J. S., Cohen, P. (2000). MSK1 is required for CREB phosphorylation in response to mitogens in mouse embryonic stem cells. *FEBS Lett* 482, 44-48.

Bazley, L. A., Gullick, W. J. (2005). The epidermal growth factor receptor family. *Endocr Relat Cancer* 12 Suppl 1, S17-S27.

Bitman, J. *et al.* (1965). Kinetics of in vivo glycogen synthesis in the estrogen-stimulated rat uterus. *Endocrinology* 76, 63-69.

Bouwman, P. *et al.* (2000). Transcription factor Sp3 is essential for post-natal survival and late tooth development. *EMBO J* 19, 655-661.

bu-Abed, S. S. *et al.* (1998). Mouse P450RAI (CYP26) expression and retinoic acid-inducible retinoic acid metabolism in F9 cells are regulated by retinoic acid receptor gamma and retinoid X receptor alpha. *J Biol Chem* 273, 2409-2415.

Buache, E. *et al.* (2011). Deficiency in trefoil factor 1 (TFF1) increases tumorigenicity of human breast cancer cells and mammary tumor development in TFF1-knockout mice. *Oncogene.*

Calviello, G. *et al.* (2009). Antineoplastic effects of n-3 polyunsaturated fatty acids in combination with drugs and radiotherapy: preventive and therapeutic strategies. *Nutr Cancer* 61, 287-301.

Castro-Rivera, E. *et al.* (2001). Estrogen regulation of cyclin D1 gene expression in ZR-75 breast cancer cells involves multiple enhancer elements. *J Biol Chem* 276, 30853-30861.

Cawley, S. *et al.* (2004). Unbiased mapping of transcription factor binding sites along human chromosomes 21 and 22 points to widespread regulation of noncoding RNAs. *Cell* 116, 499-509.

Chadalapaka, G. *et al.* (2010). Drugs that target specificity proteins downregulate epidermal growth factor receptor in bladder cancer cells. *Mol Cancer Res* 8, 739-750.

Chell, S. *et al.* (2006). Mediators of PGE2 synthesis and signalling downstream of COX-2 represent potential targets for the prevention/treatment of colorectal cancer. *Biochim Biophys Acta* 1766, 104-119.

Chen, J. Q. *et al.* (2009). Regulation of energy metabolism pathways by estrogens and estrogenic chemicals and potential implications in obesity associated with increased exposure to endocrine disruptors. *Biochim Biophys Acta* 1793, 1128-1143.

Cocolakis, E. *et al.* (2001). The p38 MAPK pathway is required for cell growth inhibition of human breast cancer cells in response to activin. *J Biol Chem* 276, 18430-18436.

Coser, K. R. *et al.* (2009). Antiestrogen-resistant subclones of MCF-7 human breast cancer cells are derived from a common monoclonal drug-resistant progenitor. *Proc Natl Acad Sci U S A* 106, 14536-14541.

Davie, J. R. *et al.* (2008). Nuclear organization and chromatin dynamics--Sp1, Sp3 and histone deacetylases. *Adv Enzyme Regul* 48, 189-208.

Degner, S. C. *et al.* (2006). Conjugated linoleic acid attenuates cyclooxygenase-2 transcriptional activity via an anti-AP-1 mechanism in MCF-7 breast cancer cells. *J Nutr* 136, 421-427.

deGraffenried, L. A. *et al.* (2002). Sp1 is essential for estrogen receptor alpha gene transcription. *J Steroid Biochem Mol Biol* 82, 7-18.

DesJardins, E., Hay, N. (1993). Repeated CT elements bound by zinc finger proteins control the absolute and relative activities of the two principal human c-myc promoters. *Mol Cell Biol* 13, 5710-5724.

Dickson, R. B., Lippman, M. E. (1988). Control of human breast cancer by estrogen, growth factors, and oncogenes. *Cancer Treat Res* 40, 119-165.

Drobic, B. *et al.* (2010). Promoter chromatin remodeling of immediate-early genes is mediated through H3 phosphorylation at either serine 28 or 10 by the MSK1 multi-protein complex. *Nucleic Acids Res* 38, 3196-3208.

Duester, G. (2008). Retinoic acid synthesis and signaling during early organogenesis. *Cell* 134, 921-931.

Dunn, K. L. *et al.* (2005). The Ras-MAPK signal transduction pathway, cancer and chromatin remodeling. *Biochem Cell Biol* 83, 1-14.

Eisen, M. B. *et al.* (1998). Cluster analysis and display of genome-wide expression patterns. *Proc Natl Acad Sci U S A* 95, 14863-14868.

Ellis, D. J. *et al.* (2006). The modification of Sp3 isoforms by Sumoylation has differential effects on the SRC1A promoter. *Gene* 379, 68-78.

Espino, P. S. *et al.* (2006). Chromatin modification of the trefoil factor 1 gene in human breast cancer cells by the Ras/mitogen-activated protein kinase pathway. *Cancer Res* 66, 4610-4616.

Feng, X. H. *et al.* (2000). Smad2, Smad3 and Smad4 cooperate with Sp1 to induce p15(Ink4B) transcription in response to TGF-beta. *EMBO J* 19, 5178-5193.

Ferguson, A. T., Davidson, N. E. (1997). Regulation of estrogen receptor alpha function in breast cancer. *Crit Rev Oncog* 8, 29-46.

Gallo, D. *et al.* (2007). Calmodulin-independent, agonistic properties of a peptide containing the calmodulin binding site of estrogen receptor alpha. *Mol Cell Endocrinol* 268, 37-49.

Hantusch, B. *et al.* (2007). Sp1/Sp3 and DNA-methylation contribute to basal transcriptional activation of human podoplanin in MG63 versus Saos-2 osteoblastic cells. *BMC Mol Biol* 8, 20.

He, S. *et al.* (2005). Differential intranuclear organization of transcription factors Sp1 and Sp3. *Mol Biol Cell* 16, 4073-4083.

Helms, M. W. *et al.* (2008). Squalene epoxidase, located on chromosome 8q24.1, is upregulated in 8q+ breast cancer and indicates poor clinical outcome in stage I and II disease. *Br J Cancer* 99, 774-780.

Higgins, K. J. *et al.* (2006). Vascular endothelial growth factor receptor-2 expression is induced by 17beta-estradiol in ZR-75 breast cancer cells by estrogen receptor alpha/Sp proteins. *Endocrinology* 147, 3285-3295.

Hirokawa, T. (1984). [Experimental chemotherapy using a transplanted head and neck cancer model in athymic nude mice]. *Nippon Jibiinkoka Gakkai Kaiho* 87, 182-194.

Hockings, J. K. *et al.* (2008). Involvement of a specificity proteins-binding element in regulation of basal and estrogen-induced transcription activity of the BRCA1 gene. *Breast Cancer Res* 10, R29.

Jaiswal, A. S. *et al.* (2006). 7,12-Dimethylbenzanthracene-dependent transcriptional regulation of adenomatous polyposis coli (APC) gene expression in normal breast epithelial cells is mediated by GC-box binding protein Sp3. *Carcinogenesis* 27, 252-261.

Jia, Z. *et al.* (2010). Combined treatment of pancreatic cancer with mithramycin A and tolfenamic acid promotes Sp1 degradation and synergistic antitumor activity. *Cancer Res* 70, 1111-1119.

Kang, Q., Chen, A. (2009). Curcumin inhibits srebp-2 expression in activated hepatic stellate cells in vitro by reducing the activity of specificity protein-1. *Endocrinology* 150, 5384-5394.

Kavurma, M. M. *et al.* (2001). Sp1 phosphorylation regulates apoptosis via extracellular FasL-Fas engagement. *J Biol Chem* 276, 4964-4971.

Khan, S. *et al.* (2007). Role of specificity protein transcription factors in estrogen-induced gene expression in MCF-7 breast cancer cells. *J Mol Endocrinol* 39, 289-304.

Khan, S. A. *et al.* (1994). Estrogen receptor expression of benign breast epithelium and its association with breast cancer. *Cancer Res* 54, 993-997.

Kim, H. G. *et al.* (2008). Mitogen- and stress-activated kinase 1-mediated histone H3 phosphorylation is crucial for cell transformation. *Cancer Res* 68, 2538-2547.

Klijn, J. G. *et al.* (1992). The clinical significance of epidermal growth factor receptor (EGF-R) in human breast cancer: a review on 5232 patients. *Endocr Rev* 13, 3-17.

Ko, B. H. *et al.* (2010). 17beta-estradiol augments 18F-FDG uptake and glycolysis of T47D breast cancer cells via membrane-initiated rapid PI3K-Akt activation. *J Nucl Med* 51, 1740-1747.

Kruger, I. *et al.* (2007). Sp1/Sp3 compound heterozygous mice are not viable: impaired erythropoiesis and severe placental defects. *Dev Dyn* 236, 2235-2244.

Lagger, G. *et al.* (2003). The tumor suppressor p53 and histone deacetylase 1 are antagonistic regulators of the cyclin-dependent kinase inhibitor p21/WAF1/CIP1 gene. *Mol Cell Biol* 23, 2669-2679.

Laye, J. P., Gill, J. H. (2003). Phospholipase A2 expression in tumours: a target for therapeutic intervention? *Drug Discov Today* 8, 710-716.

Lee, V. H. *et al.* (2009). Regulation of RASSF1A in nasopharyngeal cells and its response to UV irradiation. *Gene* 443, 55-63.

Li, L., Davie, J. R. (2008). Association of Sp3 and estrogen receptor alpha with the transcriptionally active trefoil factor 1 promoter in MCF-7 breast cancer cells. *J Cell Biochem* 105, 365-369.

Li, L., Davie, J. R. (2010). The role of Sp1 and Sp3 in normal and cancer cell biology. *Ann Anat* 192, 275-283.

Li, L. *et al.* (2004). Gene regulation by Sp1 and Sp3. *Biochem Cell Biol* 82, 460-471.

Li, Y. *et al.* (2011). The histone modifications governing TFF1 transcription mediated by estrogen receptor. *J Biol Chem.*

Lou, Z. *et al.* (2005). Down-regulation of overexpressed sp1 protein in human fibrosarcoma cell lines inhibits tumor formation. *Cancer Res* 65, 1007-1017.

Lu, S., Archer, M. C. (2010). Sp1 coordinately regulates de novo lipogenesis and proliferation in cancer cells. *Int J Cancer* 126, 416-425.

Macheda, M. L. *et al.* (2005). Molecular and cellular regulation of glucose transporter (GLUT) proteins in cancer. *J Cell Physiol* 202, 654-662.

Mandal, S. *et al.* (2007a). A novel series of potent cytotoxic agents targeting G2/M phase of the cell cycle and demonstrating cell killing by apoptosis in human breast cancer cells. *Bioorg Med Chem Lett* 17, 4955-4960.

Mandal, S. *et al.* (2007b). S100A7 (psoriasin) influences immune response genes in human breast cancer. *Exp Cell Res* 313, 3016-3025.

Mandal, S., Davie, J. R. (2007). An integrated analysis of genes and pathways exhibiting metabolic differences between estrogen receptor positive breast cancer cells. *BMC Cancer* 7, 181.

Mandal, S., Davie, J. R. (2010). Estrogen regulated expression of the p21(Waf1/Cip1) gene in estrogen receptor positive human breast cancer cells. *J Cell Physiol* 224, 28-32.

Marin, M. *et al.* (1997). Transcription factor Sp1 is essential for early embryonic development but dispensable for cell growth and differentiation. *Cell* 89, 619-628.

Meadows, A. L. *et al.* (2008). Metabolic and morphological differences between rapidly proliferating cancerous and normal breast epithelial cells. *Biotechnol Prog* 24, 334-341.

Medina, R. A., Owen, G. I. (2002). Glucose transporters: expression, regulation and cancer. *Biol Res* 35, 9-26.

Mertens-Talcott, S. U. *et al.* (2007). The oncogenic microRNA-27a targets genes that regulate specificity protein transcription factors and the G2-M checkpoint in MDA-MB-231 breast cancer cells. *Cancer Res* 67, 11001-11011.

Mic, F. A. *et al.* (2002). Novel retinoic acid generating activities in the neural tube and heart identified by conditional rescue of Raldh2 null mutant mice. *Development* 129, 2271-2282.

Mira, Y. L. *et al.* (2000). Retinol conversion to retinoic acid is impaired in breast cancer cell lines relative to normal cells. *J Cell Physiol* 185, 302-309.

Moreno-Sanchez, R. *et al.* (2007). Energy metabolism in tumor cells. *FEBS J* 274, 1393-1418.

Mudduluru, G., Allgayer, H. (2008). The human receptor tyrosine kinase Axl gene--promoter characterization and regulation of constitutive expression by Sp1, Sp3 and CpG methylation. *Biosci Rep* 28, 161-176.

Muss, H. B. (2001). Role of adjuvant endocrine therapy in early-stage breast cancer. *Semin Oncol* 28, 313-321.

Ndlovu, N. *et al.* (2009). Hyperactivated NF-{kappa}B and AP-1 transcription factors promote highly accessible chromatin and constitutive transcription across the interleukin-6 gene promoter in metastatic breast cancer cells. *Mol Cell Biol* 29, 5488-5504.

Nicolas, M. *et al.* (2001). Cloning and characterization of the 5'-flanking region of the human transcription factor Sp1 gene. *J Biol Chem* 276, 22126-22132.

Nicolette, J. A., Gorski, J. (1964). Effect of estradiol on glucose-u-c-14 metabolism in the rat uterus. *Arch Biochem Biophys* 107, 279-283.

Noe, V. *et al.* (2001). Sp1 involvement in the 4beta-phorbol 12-myristate 13-acetate (TPA)-mediated increase in resistance to methotrexate in Chinese hamster ovary cells. *Eur J Biochem* 268, 3163-3173.

Okamoto, K. *et al.* (2000). Differences in uptake and metabolism of retinoic acid between estrogen receptor-positive and -negative human breast cancer cells. *Cancer Chemother Pharmacol* 46, 128-134.

Olofsson, B. A. *et al.* (2007). Phosphorylation of Sp1 in response to DNA damage by ataxia telangiectasia-mutated kinase. *Mol Cancer Res* 5, 1319-1330.

Osanai, M. *et al.* (2010). Oncogenic and cell survival properties of the retinoic acid metabolizing enzyme, CYP26A1. *Oncogene* 29, 1135-1144.

Pan, M. R. *et al.* (2009). Tubocapsanolide A inhibits transforming growth factor-beta-activating kinase 1 to suppress NF-kappaB-induced CCR7. *J Biol Chem* 284, 2746-2754.

Pelaez, I. M. *et al.* (2010). Oncogenic RAS alters the global and gene-specific histone modification pattern during epithelial-mesenchymal transition in colorectal carcinoma cells. *Int J Biochem Cell Biol* 42, 911-920.

Pelekanou, V. *et al.* (2011). The estrogen receptor alpha-derived peptide ERalpha17p (P(295)-T(311)) exerts pro-apoptotic actions in breast cancer cells in vitro and in vivo, independently from their ERalpha status. *Mol Oncol* 5, 36-47.

Perez-Cadahia, B. *et al.* (2011). Role of MSK1 in the malignant phenotype of Ras-transformed mouse fibroblasts. *J Biol Chem* 286, 42-49.

Prall, O. W. *et al.* (1998). Estrogen regulation of cell cycle progression in breast cancer cells. *J Steroid Biochem Mol Biol* 65, 169-174.

Puig, T. *et al.* (2008). Fatty acid metabolism in breast cancer cells: differential inhibitory effects of epigallocatechin gallate (EGCG) and C75. *Breast Cancer Res Treat* 109, 471-479.

Qiao, L. *et al.* (2002). Pharmocologic inhibitors of the mitogen activated protein kinase cascade have the potential to interact with ionizing radiation exposure to induce cell death in carcinoma cells by multiple mechanisms. *Cancer Biol Ther* 1, 168-176.

Rasmussen, N. *et al.* (2010). Effect of free fatty acids and lysolipids on cellular uptake of doxorubicin in human breast cancer cell lines. *Anticancer Drugs* 21, 674-677.

Rio, M. C. *et al.* (1987). Specific expression of the pS2 gene in subclasses of breast cancers in comparison with expression of the estrogen and progesterone receptors and the oncogene ERBB2. *Proc Natl Acad Sci U S A* 84, 9243-9247.

Rivenzon-Segal, D. *et al.* (2003). Glycolysis and glucose transporter 1 as markers of response to hormonal therapy in breast cancer. *Int J Cancer* 107, 177-182.

Rogers, S. *et al.* (2003). Differential expression of GLUT12 in breast cancer and normal breast tissue. *Cancer Lett* 193, 225-233.

Ross, S. *et al.* (2002). SUMO-1 modification represses Sp3 transcriptional activation and modulates its subnuclear localization. *Mol Cell* 10, 831-842.

Salazar, M. D. *et al.* (2011). During hormone depletion or tamoxifen treatment of breast cancer cells the estrogen receptor apoprotein supports cell cycling through the retinoic acid receptor alpha1 apoprotein. *Breast Cancer Res* 13, R18.

Sapetschnig, A. *et al.* (2002). Transcription factor Sp3 is silenced through SUMO modification by PIAS1. *EMBO J* 21, 5206-5215.

Schug, T. T. *et al.* (2008). Overcoming retinoic acid-resistance of mammary carcinomas by diverting retinoic acid from PPARbeta/delta to RAR. *Proc Natl Acad Sci U S A* 105, 7546-7551.

Shinkarenko, L. *et al.* (1994). 13C NMR kinetic studies of the rapid stimulation of glucose metabolism by estrogen in immature rat uterus. *NMR Biomed* 7, 209-217.

Siddiqui, R. A. *et al.* (2005). Anticancer properties of propofol-docosahexaenoate and propofol-eicosapentaenoate on breast cancer cells. *Breast Cancer Res* 7, R645-R654.

Slamon, D. J. *et al.* (1989). Studies of the HER-2/neu proto-oncogene in human breast and ovarian cancer. *Science* 244, 707-712.

Smith, D. E., Gorski, J. (1968). Extrogen control of uterine glucose metabolism. An analysis based on the transport and phosphorylation of 2-deoxyglucose. *J Biol Chem* 243, 4169-4174.

Smith, T. A. *et al.* (2007). Decreased [18F]fluoro-2-deoxy-d-glucose incorporation and increased glucose transport are associated with resistance to 5FU in MCF7 cells in vitro. *Nucl Med Biol* 34, 955-960.

Soloaga, A. *et al.* (2003). MSK2 and MSK1 mediate the mitogen- and stress-induced phosphorylation of histone H3 and HMG-14. *EMBO J* 22, 2788-2797.

Song, C. Z. *et al.* (2003). Functional interplay between CBP and PCAF in acetylation and regulation of transcription factor KLF13 activity. *J Mol Biol* 329, 207-215.

Sonneveld, E. *et al.* (1998). Human retinoic acid (RA) 4-hydroxylase (CYP26) is highly specific for all-trans-RA and can be induced through RA receptors in human breast and colon carcinoma cells. *Cell Growth Differ* 9, 629-637.

Spengler, M. L., Brattain, M. G. (2006). Sumoylation inhibits cleavage of Sp1 N-terminal negative regulatory domain and inhibits Sp1-dependent transcription. *J Biol Chem* 281, 5567-5574.

Spengler, M. L. *et al.* (2008). Phosphorylation mediates Sp1 coupled activities of proteolytic processing, desumoylation and degradation. *Cell Cycle* 7, 623-630.

Sun, J. M. *et al.* (2002). The transcriptional repressor Sp3 is associated with CK2-phosphorylated histone deacetylase 2. *J Biol Chem* 277, 35783-35786.

Sun, J. M. *et al.* (2005). Estrogen regulation of trefoil factor 1 expression by estrogen receptor alpha and Sp proteins. *Exp Cell Res* 302, 96-107.

Suske, G. (1999). The Sp-family of transcription factors. *Gene* 238, 291-300.

Swigart, R. H. *et al.* (1961). Glycogen in the uterus of alloxan-diabetic rats. *Endocrinology* 68, 643-646.

Tang, X. H., Gudas, L. J. (2011). Retinoids, retinoic acid receptors, and cancer. *Annu Rev Pathol* 6, 345-364.

Tange, S. *et al.* (2009). Phosphorylation of histone H3 at Ser10: its role in cell transformation by v-Src. *Biochem Biophys Res Commun* 386, 588-592.

Utech, C. I. *et al.* (1996). Prospective evaluation of fluorine-18 fluorodeoxyclucose positron emission tomography in breast cancer for staging of the axilla related to surgery and immunocytochemistry. *Eur J Nucl Med* 23, 1588-1593.

Van Loo, P. F. *et al.* (2003). Impaired hematopoiesis in mice lacking the transcription factor Sp3. *Blood* 102, 858-866.

Vermeulen, L. *et al.* (2003). Transcriptional activation of the NF-kappaB p65 subunit by mitogen- and stress-activated protein kinase-1 (MSK1). *EMBO J* 22, 1313-1324.

Vicent, G. P. *et al.* (2008). Convergence on chromatin of non-genomic and genomic pathways of hormone signaling. *J Steroid Biochem Mol Biol* 109, 344-349.

Vicent, G. P. *et al.* (2009). Erk signaling and chromatin remodeling in MMTV promoter activation by progestins. *Nucl Recept Signal* 7, e008.

Wang, Y. T. *et al.* (2008). Sumoylation of specificity protein 1 augments its degradation by changing the localization and increasing the specificity protein 1 proteolytic process. *J Mol Biol* 380, 869-885.

Wiggin, G. R. *et al.* (2002). MSK1 and MSK2 are required for the mitogen- and stress-induced phosphorylation of CREB and ATF1 in fibroblasts. *Mol Cell Biol* 22, 2871-2881.

Wood, I. S., Trayhurn, P. (2003). Glucose transporters (GLUT and SGLT): expanded families of sugar transport proteins. *Br J Nutr* 89, 3-9.

Yan, Y. *et al.* (2006). NFAT3 is specifically required for TNF-alpha-induced cyclooxygenase-2 (COX-2) expression and transformation of Cl41 cells. *J Cell Sci* 119, 2985-2994.

Yuan, P. *et al.* (2007). Therapeutic inhibition of Sp1 expression in growing tumors by mithramycin a correlates directly with potent antiangiogenic effects on human pancreatic cancer. *Cancer* 110, 2682-2690.

Zhu, W. G. *et al.* (2003). Methylation of adjacent CpG sites affects Sp1/Sp3 binding and activity in the p21(Cip1) promoter. *Mol Cell Biol* 23, 4056-4065.

5

Targeting HER-2 Signaling Network: Implication in Radiation Response

In Ah Kim
Department of Radiation Oncology, Seoul National University, Republic of Korea

1. Introduction

The Human Epidermal Growth Factor Receptor 2 (HER2) oncogene encodes a 185 kDa type I tyrosine kinase receptor that is a member of the epidermal growth factor receptor (EGFR) family including HER1, HER2, HER3 and HER4 (Yarden & Sliwkowski, 2001). Overexpression of HER2 is observed in 25-30% of human breast cancers and is associated with poor prognosis (Slamon et al., 1989; Cooke et al., 2001).

HER2 overexpression activates multiple signaling pathways and promotes tumor growth, proliferation, and survival. The underlying mechanism for this action was elucidated by several studies involving critical components of the HER2 regulated pathway including phosphatidylinositol 3-kinase (PI3K) and mitogen-activated protein kinase (MAPK) cascades (Huang & Lau, 1999). The most widely used anti-HER2 therapy is the recombinant humanized antibody trastuzumab, which represented the proof of principle for the targeting of tyrosine kinase receptors in breast cancer. Trastuzumab exerts its antitumor activity by induction of receptor degradation (Klapper et al., 2000), prevention of HER2 ectodomain cleavage (Molina et al., 2001), inhibition of HER2 kinase signal transduction via antibody-dependent cellular cytotoxicity (Clynes et al., 2000) and inhibition of angiogenesis (Izumi et al., 2002). Trastuzumab has been approved as a front-line therapy for HER2-positive breast cancer patients in both adjuvant and metastatic settings (Hudis, 2007), however, trastuzumab fails in 50-70% of HER2-positive patients (Vogel et al., 2002; Slamon et al., 2001).

Radiotherapy is employed as an integral part of the current comprehensive breast cancer treatment regimen, and may be used to eradicate remaining cancer cells in the breast, chest wall, or axilla after surgery or to reduce the size of an advanced tumor before surgery. A series of studies have shown the evidences regarding the potential value of targeting HER-2 signaling to enhance the anti-tumor activity of ionizing radiation. However, therapeutic resistance, resulting from several factors including activation of downstream pathway or alternative survival pathways, as well as molecular resistance mechanisms, has been emerged as an important issue in clinic.

We have been trying to identify the component(s) implicated in radiation response in HER-2 signaling network and also screening the useful approaches to overcome therapeutic resistance such as targeting downstream effectors, ligand-independent modulation via heat shock protein 90 (HSP90) inhibition and epigenetic modulation of HER-2 signaling via inhibition of histone deacetylases (HDACs). The efficacy and clinical relevance of each strategy and the diverse mechanisms of radiosensitization will be discussed.

2. Targeting downstream signaling

Overamplification of the HER2 gene results in formation of a ligand-independent HER2 homodimer that is able to initiate downstream signaling cascades such as the PI3K and MAPK pathways (Pinkas-Kramarski et al., 1996). While the inhibition of MEK-ERK signaling did not increase the radiosensitivity of SKBR3 breast cancer cells exhibiting over-amplification of HER2, selective inhibition of PI3K-Akt-mTOR pathway components radiosensitized SKBR3 cells (No et al., 2009). Loss of PTEN (phosphatase and tensin homolog deleted one chromosome ten) expression results in trastuzumab resistance, and PI3K inhibitors restore trastuzumab sensitivity in PTEN-deficient cells (Nagata et al., 2004). Berns et al. recently provided strong confirmatory evidence that activation of the PI3K pathway through loss of the tumor suppressor PTEN or through oncogenic stimulation of PI3K can mediate trastuzumab resistance (Berns et al., 2007).

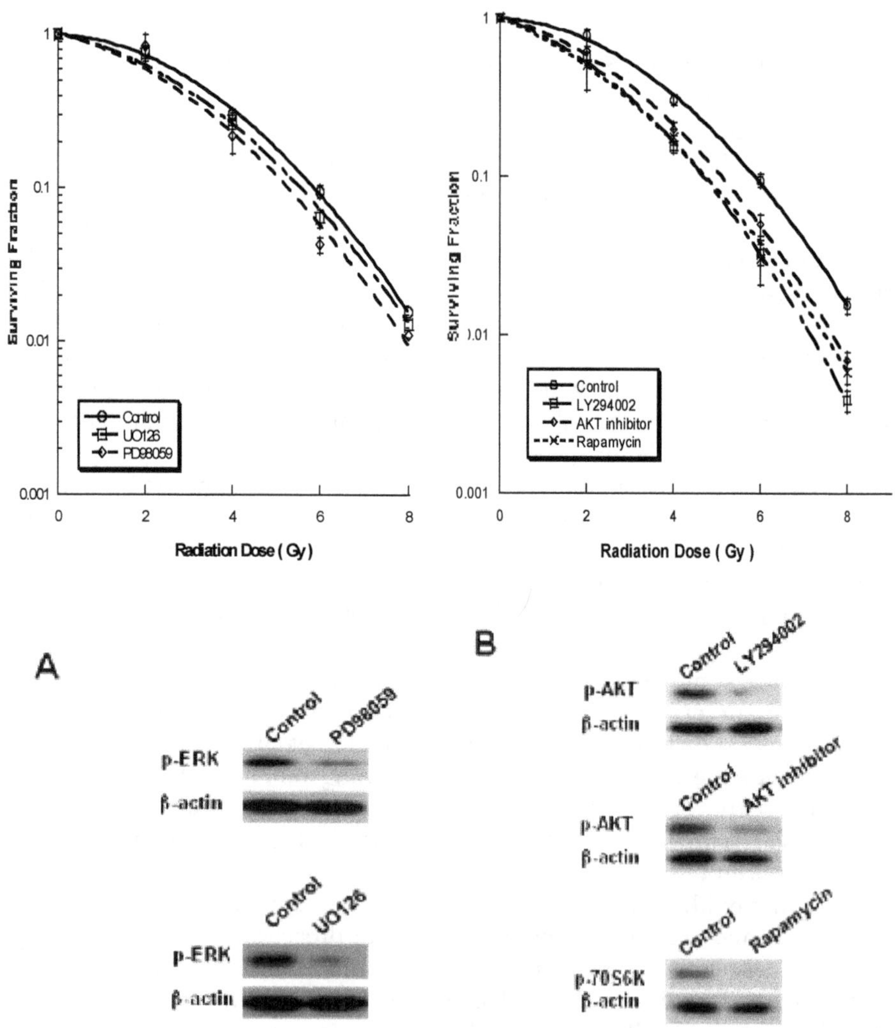

Fig. 1. Targeting downstream of HER-2 signaling (No et al, 2009).

2.1 Targeting PI3K-AKT-mTOR pathway

2.1.1 Targeting PI3K

PI3K, a heterodimer consisting of p85 regulatory subunit and a 110 catalytic subunit, plays a central role in growth regulation and tumorigenesis. It generates specific inositol lipids (PIP2, PIP3) that have been implicated in the regulation of cell proliferation, differentiation, survival, and angiogenesis (Engelman et al., 2006). Recently, several groups reported that 18-40% of human breast cancers harbor somatic mutations of PI3K (Levin et al, 2005), resulting in constitutive activation of PI3K signaling. PTEN inhibits PI3K by dephosphorylation of the second messenger PIP3. PTEN appears to be controlled by down-regulation of gene expression and genetic alterations of this tumor suppressor are found in a moderate proportion of breast cancers.

2.1.2 Targeting AKT

AKT/PKB is a serine/threonine kinase that plays an important role in cancer progression and cell survival and is activated in a PI3K-dependent manner by a variety of stimuli through growth factor receptors. Among the specific AKT family members, increased AKT1 activity was reported in 40% of breast cancers (Manning et al., 2007). We previously showed that inhibition of AKT1 using RNAi increased radiosensitivity of EGFR- or Ras-activated cell lines (Kim et al., 2005) and the other study showed that AKT inhibitor (API) or AKT1 siRNA inhibited repair of DNA double strand breaks (DSBs) in EGFR-activated lung cancer cell lines as measured by the γH2AX foci assay (Toulany et al., 2008). SKBR3 breast cancer cells having activated HER-2 signaling also showed similar findings (Figure 3, No et al., 2009).

2.1.3 Targeting m-TOR

The mammalian target of rapamycin (mTOR) is an important downstream component of the PI3K-AKT signaling pathway. mTOR inhibitors can effectively block the pro-growth, pro-proliferative, and pro-survival actions of mTOR by inactivating its downstream effectors such as p70S6 kinase and 4E-binding protein1 and decreasing protein synthesis (Shaw et al., 2006; Guertin & Sabatini, 2007). mTOR presents an attractive target in the pathway because its inhibition could avoid possible side effects associated with inhibition of upstream PI3K/AKT signaling molecules with broader function. We previously showed that the radiosensitizing effect of Rapamycin is related to inhibition of DNA damage repair, as demonstrated by the γH2AX foci assay using SKBR3 cells (Fig. 2, No et al., 2009). Recent report showed that RAD001 attenuated prosurvival AKT/mTOR signaling and increased radiation sensitivity of MDA-MB-231 breast cancer cells (Albert et al., 2006).

2.1.4 Targeting class I PI3K and m-TOR

One of the reasonable approaches would be the targeting more than one component of tumor specific signaling that less affect normal cell survival. Inhibition of PI3K using LY294002 lacks specificity and has shown unacceptable toxicities in preclinical studies. Previous study showed that specific inhibition of class I PI3K using RNAi enhanced the radiosensitivity of tumor cells having activated PI3K signaling resulting from overexpression of EGFR or mutation of RAS oncogene (Kim et al., 2005). The PI103 is known as a dual inhibitor which targets class I PI3K and mTOR signaling which reduce radiation survival of tumor cells with AKT activation. (Prevo et al., 2008). PI103 effectively radiosensitized SKBR3 cells with activated HER2 signaling and this sensitizing effect

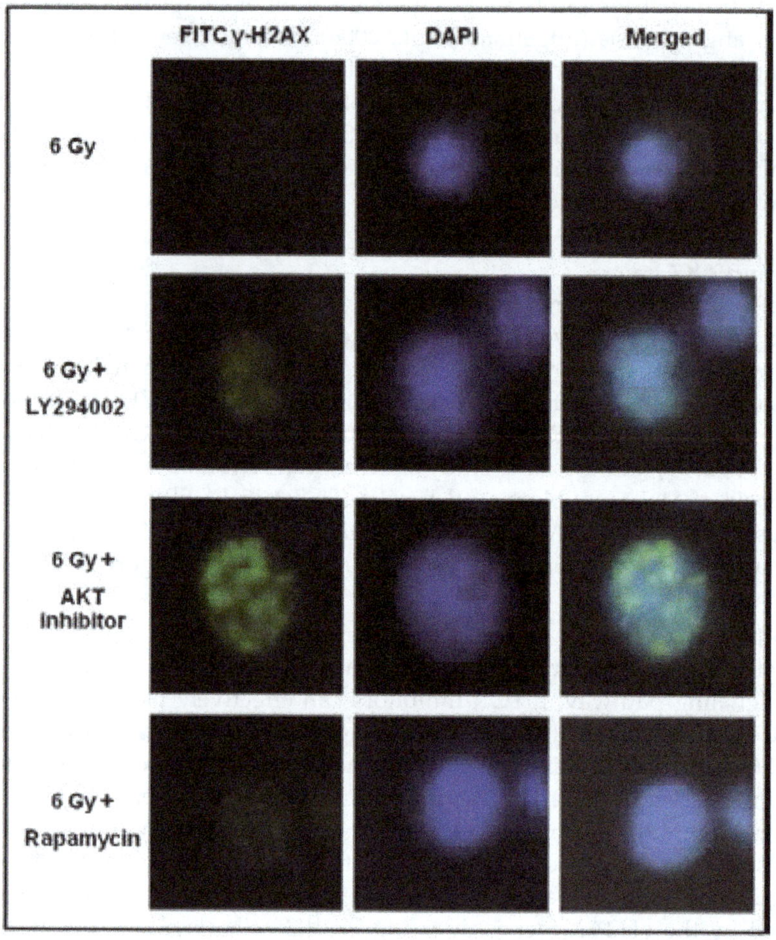

Fig. 2. Persistent γH2AX foci following orradiation by selective inhibition of PI3K-AKT-mTOR signalling (No et al., 2009).

was associated with prolongation of γH2AX foci following irradiation. Decreased phosphorylation of DNA-PKs by pretreatment of inhibitors targeting PI3K-AKT indicated that the functional requirement of PI3K-AKT pathway in regulation of DNA repair following radiation (Fig.3 & 4, No et al., 2009). While apoptosis was the major mode of cell death when the cells were pretreated with LY294002 or AKT inhibitor VIII, cells were pretreated by Rapamycin or PI103 showed the mixed mode of cell death including autophagy (Fig. 5, No et al., 2009).

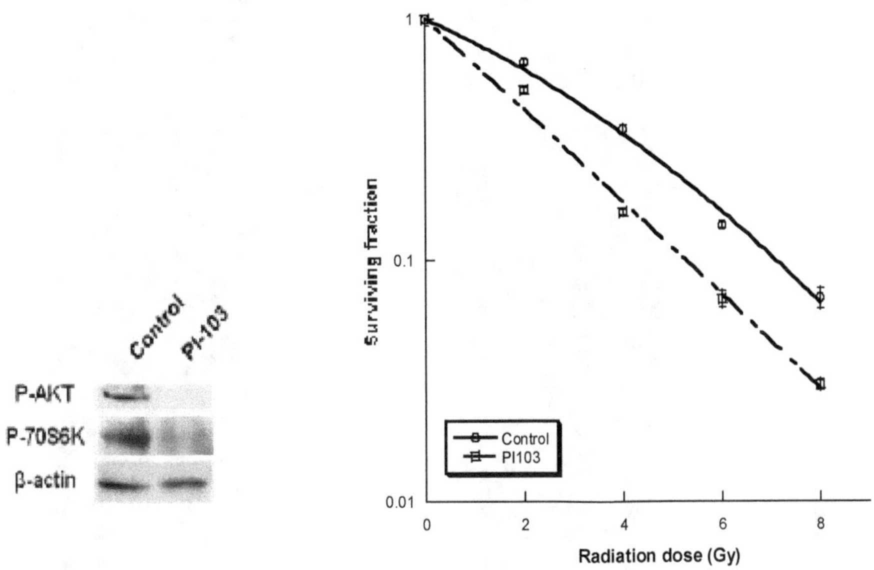

Fig. 3. Targeting Class I PI3K and m-TOR using dual inhibitor (No et al., 2009).

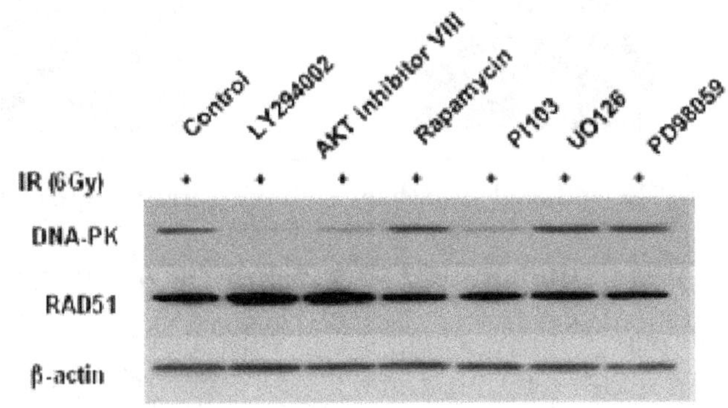

Fig. 4. Targeting Class I PI3K-Akt down-regulated DNA-PK expression (No et al., 2009).

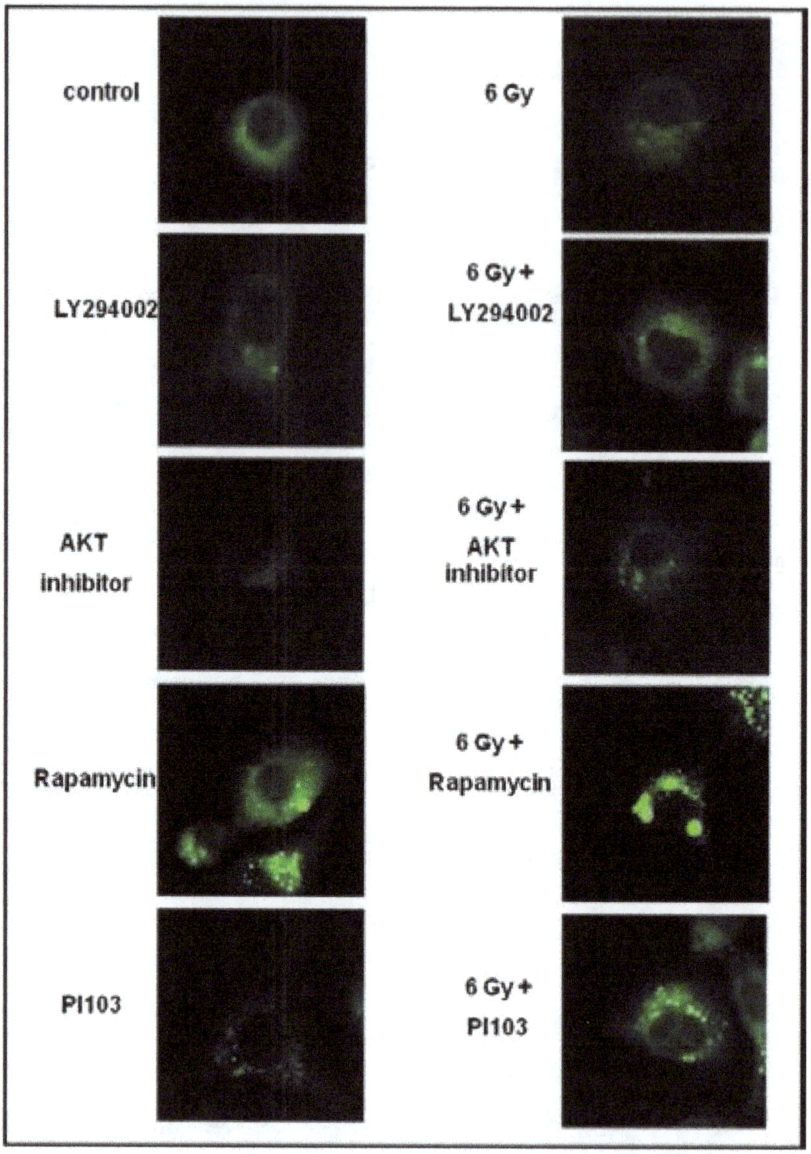

Fig. 5. Rapamycin and PI103 induced autophagy following irradiation. (No et al., 2009).

3. Ligand-independent modulation of HER-2 signaling: HSP90 inhibition

The majority of breast cancers involve multiple molecular abnormalities that are likely to be involved in malignant progression. It is possible that several different molecules from diverse pathways have synergistic properties that promote malignant relapse or metastasis. In that situation, HSP90 could be a pivotal key molecule, as its chaperone function ensures the correct conformation, activity, intracellular localization, and proteolytic turnover of a range of proteins involved in cell growth, differentiation, and survival (Neckers et al., 2003). This molecular chaperon is essential for the stability and function of many oncogenic client proteins, which contributes to the hallmark trait of cancers such as ER, HER-2, and AKT (Powers & Workman, 2006). The inhibition of multiple targets through the abrogation of HSP90 could be more effective in the management of breast cancers, since its inhibition counteracts multiple oncogenic molecules and prosurvival signaling pathways at the same time.

Additional data supports the identification of HSP90 as an important molecular target relevant to breast cancers. HER2, which is associated with poor prognosis in breast cancer, is one of the most important client proteins of HSP90, and HSP90 inhibitors have shown antitumor activity in a HER2-driven xenograft model (Kamal et al, 2003). Additionally, HSP90 inhibitors bind selectively to HSP90 in cancerous cells versus normal cells (Munster et al, 2001). Breast cancer cells resistant to conventional chemotherapy, radiation therapy, and trastuzumab, are known to involve the PI3K signaling pathway. The key molecule of this pathway, AKT, is also an important client protein of HSP90.

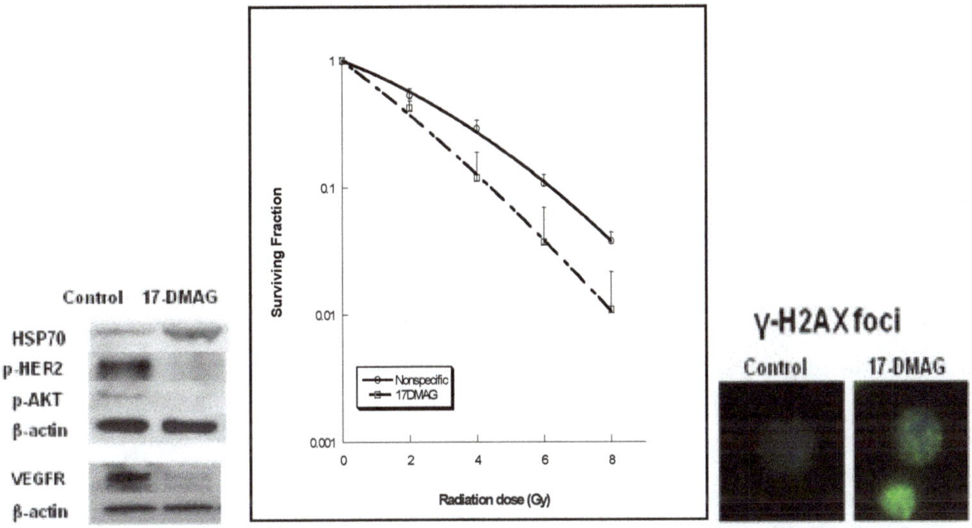

Fig. 6. 17-DMAG, a HSP90 inhibitor radiosensitized SKBR-3 cells with HER-2 overexpression.

A HSP90 inhibitor, 17-(allylamino)-17-demethoxy-geldanamycin (17-AAG) downregulated HER2 in trastuzumab-resistant breast cancer cells (Zsebik et al., 2006). We also have observed that 17-DMAG, led to downregulation of HER-2 and p-AKT, and radiosensitized HER-2 activated breast cancer cells. This radiosensitizing effect was associated with persistence of γH2AX foci following irradiation (Figure 6, unpublished data).

Our previous immunihistochemical study using tissue samples from 212 patients who underwent surgical resection for primary invasive breast cancer, have shown that expression of HSP90 from invasive breast cancer was associated with an increased risk of early recurrence (Fig. 7, Song et al., 2010). Co-expression of HSP90 and PI3K or expression of HSP90 in combination with the loss of PTEN was significantly associated with RFS especially in the patient group having HER-2 overexpression (Fig.8, Song et al., 2010). This study provides direct evidence that the expression of HSP90 predicts early relapse in patients with invasive breast cancers and validates the significance of HSP90 as a clinically significant therapeutic target.

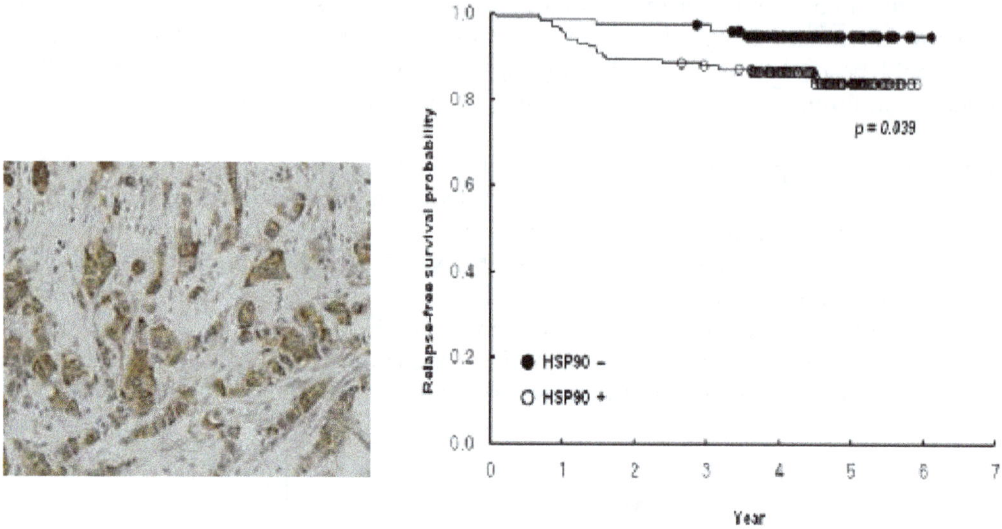

Fig. 7. Relapse free survival of patients according to HSP90 overexpression (Song et al., 2010).

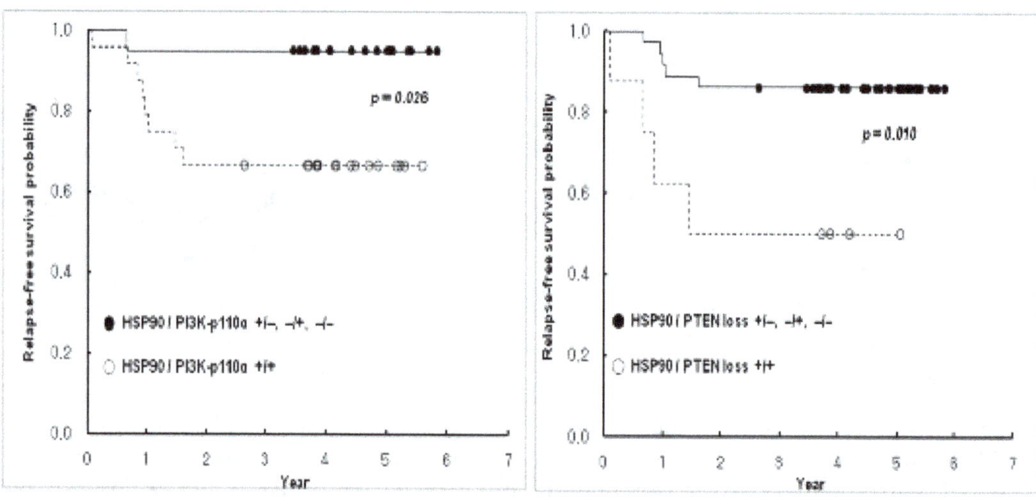

Fig. 8. Relapse free survival of patients with HER-2 overexpression (Song et al., 2010).

4. Epigenetic modulation of HER-2 signlaing: Histone deacetylase inhibition

Histone deacetylase inhibitiors (HDIs) are capable of modifying gene expression without directly interacting with DNA by affecting the acetylation state of DNA-associated proteins, as well as other proteins.

We previously reported that HER-2 activated cells were preferentially radiosensitized by LBH589, the cinnamyl hydroxamic acid analogue panHDAC inhibitor compared to the effect of TSA or SK7041 at iso-effective concentrations and that this was associated with down-regulation of HER-2 signaling of SKBR-3 cells (Fig.9, Kim et al., 2009).

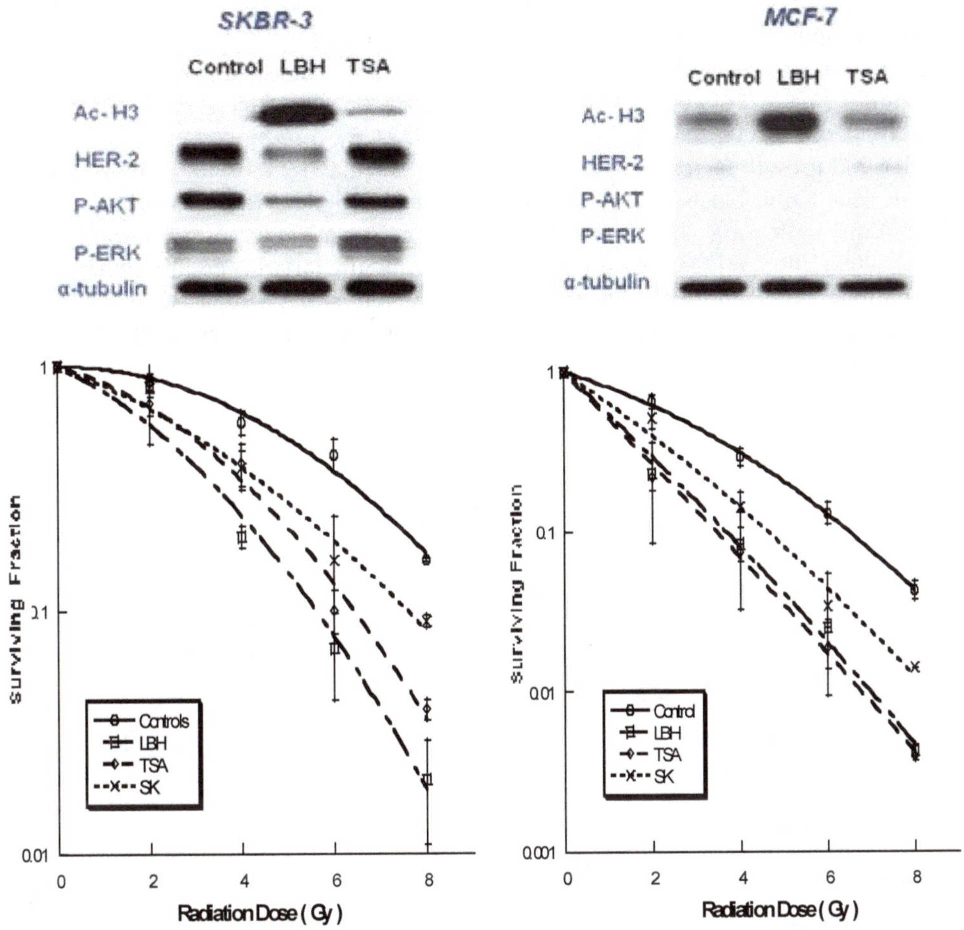

Fig. 9. LBH589 preferentially radiosensitizes breast cancer cells with HER-2 amplification (Kim et al., 2009).

The acetylation level of HSP90 and the relative inhibition of HDAC6 by the three different HDIs at iso-effective concentrations provided a mechanistic clue to explain this preferential radiosensitization by LBH589. Selective inhibition of HDAC6 led to acetylation of HSP90 resulting in ubiquitination and depletion of pro-survival client proteins including HER-2 and its downstream effectors. Specific inhibition of HDAC6 using RNAi increased acetylation of HSP 90 and attenuated the expression level of its client proteins such as p-AKT and p-ERK. This was associated with increased radiosensitivity of SKBR-3 cells (Fig.10, unpublished data).

The first evidence of non-nuclear and non-histone associated activity for a HDAC member came from the characterization of HDAC 6, one of the class IIB members. It possesses two deacetylase domains and zinc finger motif. The central part of this motif is similar to region found in BRAP (BRCA1-associated protein 2) and several ubiquitin-specific proteases. This motif is also known as PAZ (polyubiquitin-associated zinc finger) due to its ubiquitin-binding ability. It has been implicated as a critical link between proteasome degradation and autophagy (Kawaguchi et al., 2003; Boyault et al., 200; Pandei et al., 2007). HDAC6 has been implicated in modulating receptor tyrosine kinase signaling. Increased acetylation of heat shock protein such as HSP90 by HDAC 6 inhibition may lead to mis-folding and degradation of survival associated client proteins such as oncogenic tyrosine kinases, RAF, and AKT (Bali et al., 2005). Stable knockdown of HDAC6 expression also causes a decrease platelet-derived growth factor receptor α (Kamera et al., 2008). Lee et al. recently found that HDAC6 deficient fibroblasts were more resistant to oncogenic Ras and HER2-dependent transformation, indicating a critical role of HDAC6 in oncogene-induced transformation (Lee et al., 2008). Thus, HDAC6 could be a good therapeutic target regulating critical cancer-relevant biologic functions. These reports and the current study suggest that HDAC 6 may be a useful target for overcoming therapeutic resistance to available HER2 inhibitors combined with radiation.

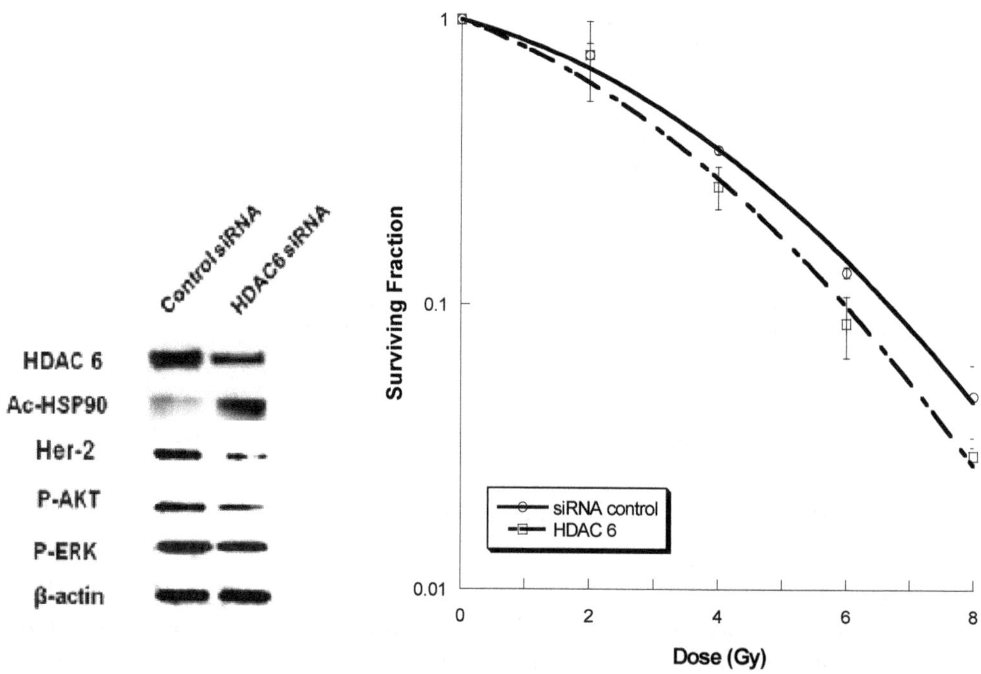

Fig. 10. Selective inhibition of HDAC6 radiosensitized SKBR-3 cells.

5. Conclusion

Identification of the prognostic significance of HER2 and its targeted therapy are the best examples of proof of concept (Hassa et al., 2005). A series of studies have shown solid preclinical and clinical evidences regarding the potential value of targeting HER-2 signaling to enhance the anti-tumor activity of ionizing radiation (Sartor et al., 2003; Sambade et al.,

2010). However, therapeutic resistance resulting from several factors including activation of downstream pathway or alternative survival pathways, as well as molecular resistance mechanisms, have emerged as an important issue in the clinic. Based on previous studies and our data, we propose that targeting downstream, ligand-inependent modulation via HSP90 inhibitor, and epigentic modulation via HDAC inhibiton could be an alternative approaches to tackle factors such as these that limit the therapeutic benefit of HER-2 targeted therapy combined with radiation.

6. Acknowledgment

This work was supported by the National Research Foundation grants (Nuclear R&D Program, BAERI #2007-2001193, #313-2007-2-E00381 and #531-2006-1-E00061) from Korean Ministry of Education, Science & Technology to Kim IA and Cancer Control Program(#0820010) from Korean Ministry of Health & Welfare

7. References

Yarden Y, Sliwkowski M. (2001) Untangling the ErbB signalling network. *Nature Rev Mol Cell Biol* 2:127-37.

Slamon DJ, Godolphin W, Jones LA, Holt JA, Wong SG, Keith DE, et al. (1989). Studies of HER2/neu proto-oncogene in human breast and ovarian cancer. *Science*; 244: 707-712.

Cooke T, Reeves J, Lanigan A, Stanton P. (2001). HER2 as a prognostic and predictive marker for breast cancer. *Ann Oncol*; 12: S23-S28.

Huang MC, Lau YK: Basic science of HER2/neu. a review (1999). *Semin Oncol* 26:51-59.

Klapper L, Waterman H, Sela M, Yarden Y. (2000) Tumor-inhibitory antibodies to HER2/ErbB2 may act by recruiting c-Cbl and enhancing ubiquitination of HER2. *Cancer Res* 60:3384-8.

Molina MA, Codony-Servat J, Albanell J, Rojo F, Arribas J, Balselga J. (2001). Trastuzumab, a humanized anti-her2 receptor monoclonal antibody inhibits basal and activated HER2 ectodomain cleavage in breast cancer cells. *Cancer Res* 61: 4744-9.

Clynes RA, Towers TL, Presta LG, Ravetch JV. (2000). Inhibitory Fc receptors modulate in vivo cytotoxicity against tumor targets. *Nat Med* 6: 443-6.

Izumi Y, Xu L, di Tomaso E, Fukumura D, Jain RK. (2002) Tumour biology: Herceptin acts as an anti-angiogenic cocktail. *Nature* 416:279-80.

Hudis CA. Trastuzumab - mechanism of action and use in clinical practice. (2007) *N Engl J Med* 357:39-51.

Vogel CL, Cobleigh MA, Tripathy D, Gutheil JC, Harris LN, Fehrenbacher L,et al. (2002). Efficacy and safety of trastuzumab as a single agent in first-line treatment of HER2 overexpressing metastatic breast cancer. *J Clin Oncol* 20:719-26.

Slamon DJ, Leyland-Jones B, Shak S, Fuchs H, Paton V, Bajamonde A, et al. (2001). Use of chemotherapy plus monoclonal antibody against HER2 for metastatic breast cancer that overexpress HER2. *N Engl J Med* 344:783-792.

Kim IA, Bae SS, Fernandes A, Wu J, Muschel RJ, McKenna WG, et al. (2005). Selective inhibition of Ras, Phosphoinositide 3 kinase, and Akt isoforms increases the radiosensitivity of human carcinoma cell lines. *Cancer Res* 1: 65(17):7902-10.

Berns K, Horlings HM, Hennessy BT, Madiredjo M, Hijmans EM, Beelen K, et al. (2007). A functional Genetic Approach identifies the PI3K pathway as a major determinant of tratuzumab resistance in breast cancer. *Cancer Cell* 12: 395-402.

Nagata Y, Lan KH, Zhou X, Tan M, Esteva FJ, Sahin AA, et al. (2004). PTEN activation contributes to tumor inhibition by tratuzumab, and loss of PTEN predicts trastuzumab resistance in patients. *Cancer Cell* 6:117-27.

Pinkas-Kramarski R, Soussan L, Waterman H, Levkowitz G, Alroy I, Klapper L, Lavi S, et al. (1996). Diversification of Neu differentiation factor and epidermal growth factor signaling by combinatorial receptor interactions. *EMBO J* 15:2452-67.

Engelman JA, Luo J, Catley LC. (2006). The evolution of phosphatidylinositol 3-kinases as regulators of growth and metabolism. *Nat Rev Genetics* 7: 606-619.

Lee JY, Engelman JA, Catley LC. (2007). PI3K charges ahead. *Science* 317: 206-207.

Levine DA, Bogomolniy F, Yee CJ, Lash A, Barakat RR, Borgen PI et al. (2005). Frequent mutation of PI3KA gene in ovarian and breast cancers. *Clin Can Res* 11:2875-8.

Manning BD, Catley LC. AKT/PKB Signaling: Navigating Downstream. (2007). *Cell* 129:1261-1274.

Toulany M, Kehlbach R, Florczak U, Sak A, Wang S, Chen J, et al. (2008). Targeting of AKT1 enhances radiation toxicity of human tumor cells by inhibiting DNA-PKs-dependent DNA double-strand break repair. *Mol Can Ther* 7(7):1772-1781.

Bozulic L, Surucu B, Hynx D, Hemmings BA. (2008). PKBα/AKT1 acts downstream of DNA-PK in DNA double-stand break response and promotes survival. *Mol Cell* 30:203-213

Shaw RJ, Cantley LC. (2006). Ras, PI3K and mTOR signalling controls tumour cell growth. *Nature* 441:424-430.

Guertin DA, Sabatini DM (2007). Defining the role of mTOR in Cancer. *Cancer Cell* 12:9-22.

Albert JM, Kim KW, Cao C, Lu B. (2006). Targeting the Akt/mammalian target of rapamycin pathway for radiosensitization of breast cancer. *Mol Cancer Ther* 5: 1183-42.

Prevo R, Deutsch E, Sampson O, Diplexcito J, Cengel K, Harper J, et al. (2008). Class I PI3 kinase inhibition by the pyridinylfuranopyrimidine inhibitor PI-103 enhances tumor radiosensitivity. *Cancer Res* 15:68(14):5915-23.

Neckers L, Ivy SP. (2003). Heat shock protein 90. *Curr Opin Oncol* 15:419-424.

Powers M, Workman P. Targeting multiple signalling pathways by heat shock protein 90 molecular chaperone inhibiotrs. *Endocrine -Related Cancer* 2006, 13:S125-35

Kamal A, Thao L, Sensintaffar J, Zhang L, Boehm MF, Fritz LC, Burrows FJ. (2003). A high-affinity conformation of HSP90 confers tumour selectivity on HSP90 inhibitors. *Nature* 425:407-410.

Munster PN, Basso A, Solit D, Norton L, Rosen N. Modulation of HSP90 function by ansamycin sensitize breast cancer cells to chemotherapy-induced apoptosis in a RB- and schedule-dependent manner. *Clin Cancer Res* 2001, 7:2228-36

Zsebik B, Citri A, Isola J, Yarden Y, Szöllosi J, Vereb G. HSP90 inhibitor 17-AAG reduces ErbB2 levels and inhibits proliferation of the trastuzumab resistant breast tumor cell line JIMT-1. *Immunol Lett* 2006, 104:146-155.

McKee JA, Yao TP. Histone deacetylases in the response to misfolded proteins p167-169 in *Histone Deacetylases: transcriptional regulation and other cellular functions.* edited by Verdin E. Humania pres. 2006

Kawaguchi Y, Kovacs JJ, McLaurin A, Vance JM, Ito A, Yao P. The Deacetylase HDAC6 regulates aggresome formation and cell viability in response to misfolded protein stress. *Cell* 2003;115:727-738

Boyault C, Sadoul K, Pabion M, Khochbin S. (2007). HDAC6, at the crossroad between cytoskelecton and cell signaling by acetylation and ubiquitination. *Oncogene* 26:5468-5476

Pandey UB, Nie Z, Batlevi Y, McCray BA, Ritson GP, Nedelsky NB, Schwartz SL, DiProspero NA, Knight MA, Schuldiner O, Padmanabhan R, Hild M, Berry DL, Garza D, Hubbert CC, Yao TP, Baehrecke EH, Taylor JP. (2007). HDAC6 rescues neurodegeneration and provides an essential link between autophagy and the UPS. *Nature* 14:447(7146):859-63.

Bali P, Pranpat M, Bradner J, Balasis M, Fiskus W, Guo F, Bhalla K. (2005). Inhibition of Histone Deacetylase 6 acetylates and disrupts the chaperone function of Heat Shock Protein 90. *J Biol Chem* 29:26729-26734

Kamemura K, Ito A, Shimazu T, Matsuyama A, Maeda S, Yao TP, Horinouchi S, Khochbin S, Yoshida M. (2008). Effects of downregulated HDAC6 expression on the proliferation of lung cancer cells. *Biochem Biophys Res Commun* 12:374 (1):84-89

Lee YS, Lim KH, Guo X, Kawaguchi Y, Gao Y, Barrientos T, Ordentlich P, *et al.* (2008). The cytoplasmic deacetylase HDAC6 is required for efficient oncogenic tumorigenesis. *Can Res* 68:7561- 7569

Huang SM, Bock JM, Harari PM. (1999). Epidermal growth factor recetor blockade with C225 modulates proliferation, apoptosis and radiosensitivity in squmous cell carcinomas of head and neck. *Cancer Res* 59:1935-1940

Bonner JA, Harari PM, Giralt J, Azarnia N, ShinDM, Cohen RB, Jones CU, *et al.* (2006). Radiotherapy plus Cetuximab for squamous-cell carcinoma of head and neck. *N Engl J Med* 9: 354 (6):567-78

Sartor CI. Epidermal growth factor family receptors and inhibitors: radiation response modulators.(2003). *Semin Radiat Oncol* 13(1): 22-30

Sambade MJ, Kimple RJ, Camp JT, *et al.* (2010). Lapatinib in combination with radiation diminishes tumor regrowth in HER2+ and basal-like/EGFR+ breast tumor xenografts. *Int J Radiat Oncol Biol Phys* 77:575-581.

No M, Choi EJ, Kim IA. (2009). Targeting HER2 signaling pathway for radiosensitization: Alternative strategy for therapeutic resistance. *Cancer Biology & Therapy* 8(24):2351-2361

Kim IA, No M, Lee JM *et al.* (2009). Epigenetic modulation of radiation response in human cancer cells with activated EGFR or HER-2 signaling: Potential role of histone deacetylase 6. *Radiotherapy & Oncology*: 92:125-132

Song CH, Park SY, Eom KY, Kim JH, Kim SW, Kim JS, Kim IA. (2010). Potential prognostic value of heat-shock protein 90 in the presence of phosphatidylinositol-3-kinase overexpression or loss of PTEN, in invasive breast cancers. *Breast Cancer Res.* 12(2):R20.

6

Brain Metastases Progression of Breast Cancer

Ala-Eddin Al Moustafa[1,2,3], Amber Yasmeen[2], Lina Ghabreau[4], Ali H. Mohamed[4] and Amal Achkhar[1,5]

[1]*Syrian Research Cancer Centre of the Syrian Society against Cancer, Aleppo*
[2]*Oncology Department, Faculty of Medicine, McGill University, Montréal*
[3]*Department of Mechanical Engineering, Concordia University, Montréal*
[4]*Deaptement of Pathology, Faculty of Medicine/University of Aleppo, Aleppo*
[5]*Faculty of Pharmacy, University of Aleppo, Aleppo*
[1,4,5]*Syria*
[2,3]*Canada*

1. Introduction

The development of brain metastases is one of the complications of breast cancer most feared by patients, having connotations of loss of identity and independence (Mayer, 2007). Clinically evident brain metastases occur in 20-30% of patients with metastatic breast cancer (Landis et al., 1999; Lin et al., 2004) and median survival of patients who develop breast cancer brain metastases (BCBMs) is generally poor, ranging from 2 to 9 months (Altundag et al., 2007; Lee et al., 2008; Ogawa et al., 2008). The treatment of metastasis to the brain is complicated by the unique characteristics of the brain. The blood-brain barrier (BBB), with its tight junctions and lack of lymphatic drainage, makes the delivery of chemotherapeutic agents difficult and represents a therapeutic haven from chemotherapy (Patchell, 2003; Ballabh et al., 2004; Nathoo et al., 2005). In addition, brain metastatic disease is the most poorly understood aspect of cancer progression. The potential of malignant cells to spread to distant organs including lung, bone and brain is the leading cause of death from breast cancer. Some breast cancer metastases display tissue-specific patterns to distant organs, such as the brain (Palmieri et al., 2006-2007; Sanna et al., 2007) and bone (Yang et al., 2007; Wang et al., 2007). The metastatic process is a complex phenomenon, and involves several genes. Recent studies recognize cell adhesion proteins especially E-cadherin and matrix metalloproteinases (MMPs), growth factor receptors such as EGF-R, ErbB-2, VEGF, and contributions from signal transduction pathways in addition to the activation of specific chemokines/cytokines, as major regulators of the metastatic process (Zeljko et al., 2011; Klein et al., 2009; Bos et al., 2009; Kennecke et al., 2010; Carotenuto et al., 2010; Hinton et al., 2010). Contrary to non-invasive breast cancer cells, malignant cells must display enhanced migratory behaviour and the ability to breach blood vessel walls and the dense collagenous matrix surrounding tumours. Additionally, metastatic cells must overcome the dynamics of a foreign microenvironment, to colonize and survive at a distant target site. Once metastasis has occurred, tumour growth is highly dependent on the ability of tumours to induce their own vascularization (Harlozinska, 2005; Hinton et al., 2008). There are key events to which malignant cells must adhere to complete their migration and angiogenesis: invasion of the surrounding stromal tissue, intravasation, evasion of programmed cell death and growth within a new microenvironment (Kaplan et al., 2006). These events are governed by several important genes that can regulate cell cancer invasion to a specific organ such as lung, bone and brain. In this chapter, we will discuss the contributions of E-cadherin, MMPs EGF-R, ErbB-2, VEGF and chemokine genes, to the induction and progression of metastasis of breast cancer especially to the brain.

2. MMPs and E-cadherin in brain metastasis

Ecadherin and MMPs family proteins are heavily involved in the metastases of the brain (VanMeter et al., 2001; Lewis-Tuffin et al., 2010). MMPs are a broad family of zinc-dependent proteinases that play a key role in extracellular matrix (ECM) degradation in metastasis (Kessenbrock et al., 2010); their expression is regulated via cytokines, and the ECM metalloprotease inducer is found on the surface of tumour cells. MMP activity is known to correlate with invasiveness, metastasis, and poor prognosis (Murphy, 2008; Kessenbrock et al., 2010). Earlier study found that MMP-2 is present in all metastatic brain tumours tested regardless of the site of origin and that the level of activity inversely correlated with survival (Jäälinojä et al., 2000; Deryugina and Quigley, 2006). Meanwhile, although MMP-9 was found to be up-regulated in all brain metastases and primary brain tumours, there was an inability to correlate up-regulation with survival (Arnold et al., 1999). Furthermore, previous studies showed that MMPs might be involved in the metastases of breast cancer to the brain (Cheng and Hung, 2007). A breast cancer brain metastases rat model was derived from injection of a carcinogen-induced mammary adenocarcinoma cell line in the left ventricle of rat (Mendes et al., 2005). The micro-metastasis in the brain showed a significantly higher expression of MMP-2, -3 and -9 and an increase in MMP-2 and MMP-3 activity compared to the normal brain tissue (Deryugina and Quigley, 2006). Furthermore, the development of brain metastasis was significantly decreased by the treatment with a selective synthetic MMP inhibitor (Mendes et al., 2005). This phenomenon was confirmed by another study in which human breast cancer cells over-expressed with MMP2 were inoculated into the left ventricle, a higher incidence of metastasis to brain was observed (Tester et al., 2004). Another study also showed that brain seeking breast cancer cells have a higher total and active amount MMP-1 and MMP-9 with higher migration and invasion capacity, which could be decreased by the application of MMP-1 and/or MMP-9 inhibitor (Stark et al., 2007).

On the other hand, E-cadherin/catenin complex is vital for the maintenance of both normal and tumour cytoarchitecture as well as a necessary mediator of cell-cell adhesion. β-catenin, as well as plakoglobin (γ-catenin), associate directly with the highly conserved cytoplasmic domain of E-cadherin in a mutually exclusive manner (Yasmeen et al., 2006; Al Moustafa et al., 2008). The E-cadherin/β-catenin complex is linked via α-catenin either directly or indirectly to the actin filament network via the actin-binding proteins α-actinin or vinculin (Yasmeen et al., 2006; Al Moustafa et al., 2008). The association of the E-cadherin/catenin complex with the cytoskeleton is essential for tight cell-cell adhesions. In the metastatic escape of a tumour, clone cells reduced intercellular adhesion and disrupted cytoarchitecture, and are thus prone to separation from the primary tumour mass (Al Moustafa et al., 2011). These clones are then free to invade both locally as well as to continue on to intravasation and further progress in the cascade (Nathoo et al., 2005).

Decreased expression of the E-cadherin/catenin complex has been correlated with invasion, metastasis, and unfavorable prognosis (Bremnes et al., 2002). Shabani et al. (2003) established a correlation between E-cadherin/catenin complex expression and an increased mindbomb homolog 1 (MIB1) index in metastatic adenocarcinomas. Further, E-cadherin is expressed in most meningiomas (Tohma et al., 1992; Figarella-Branger et al., 1994; Howng et al., 2002), and its loss may be associated with tumour progression (Schwechheimer et al., 1998). E-cadherin expression in glioblastoma multiforme or glioblastomas appears to be an exception to the epithelial-mesenchymal transition (EMT) rule, which is an important event in the progression cancer and metastasis (Lewis-Tuffin et al., 2010; Al Moustafa et al., 2011) (Figure 1). The molecular mechanisms underlying the contribution of E-cadherin to growth and/or invasiveness in glioblastomas are currently unknown. Although, the two main sources of brain metastasis - adenocarcinomas of the lung or the breast represent different models of the course of the disease (Bos et al., 2009); Zeljko et al. (2011) have showed that E-cadherin changes were frequent in metastases from both those malignancies. Moreover, Saad et al. (2008) demonstrated that loss of E-cadherin in patients with adenocarcinomas and squamous cell carcinomas of the lung is significantly associated to the increased risk of developing brain metastases. The results of other authors investigating E-cadherin involvement in brain metastasis (Arnold et al., 1999; Shabani et al., 2003; Prudkin et al., 2009) collectively demonstrate that Ecadherin is constantly expressed in metastatic deposits. Furthermore, our recent studies also demonstrated that E-cadherin-catenin complex is involved in cell migration and metastasis *in vivo* and *in vitro* (Yasmeen et al., 2007). In order to investigate the cooperation effect between ErbB-2 receptor and high-risk human papillomavirus (HPV) in breast carcinogenesis and metastasis, we generated double transgenic mice carrying ErbB-2 and E6/E7 of HPV type 16 under mouse mammary tumour virus (MMTV) and human keratin 14 (K14) promoters, respectively. Within six months, these double transgenic mice developed large and extensive invasive breast cancers to several vital organs including lung, bone and brain. Histological analysis of ErbB-2/E6/E7 transgenic mouse tumours revealed the presence of invasive breast carcinomas. However, breast tissues from ErbB-2 and E6/E7 singly transgenic mice showed only *in-situ* cancer and normal mammary phenotype, respectively (Yasmeen et al., 2007). In parallel, to assess the outcome of ErbB-2/E6/E7 cooperation in human breast carcinogenesis, we examined the effect of ErbB-2 and E6/E7 of HPV type 16 on the BT20 breast cancer cell lines. We found that ErbB-2/E6/E7 cooperate in the BT20 cell line to induce large colony formation and cell migration using soft agar and wound healing assays, respectively, in comparison with ErbB-2, E6/E7 and wild type cells. Moreover, we demonstrated that ErbB-2/E6/E7 cooperation induces a nuclear translocation of β-catenin in BT20 cells; regarding the mechanism of this translocation, we reported that ErbB-2/E6/E7 cooperation provokes a dissociation of E-cadherin/catenin complex by tyrosine phosphorylation of β-catenin through pp60(c-Src) kinase phosphorylation. Subsequently, the free β-catenin enters to the nucleus and modulates cell transcription via its association with the Tcf/Lef transcription factors (Yasmeen et al., 2007; Al Moustafa et al., 2008) (Figure 2). In conclusion, our *in vitro* and *in vivo* models demonstrated that the ErbB-2 tyrosine kinase receptor cooperates with E6/E7 of high-risk HPVs in breast tumorigenesis and metastasis via E-cadherin/catenin complex (Yasmeen et al., 2007; Al Moustafa et al., 2008). These studies provide evidence that MMPs and E-cadherin play an important role in brain metastases of breast cancer.

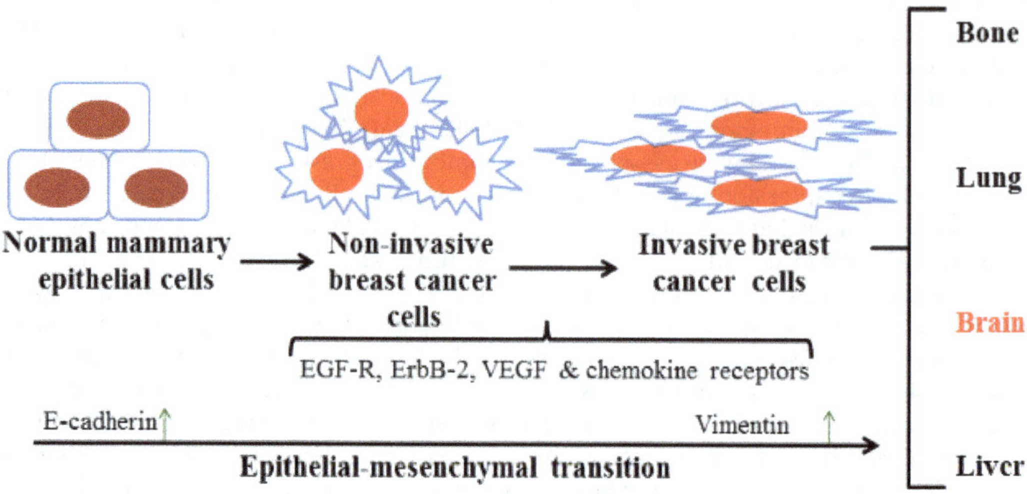

Fig. 1. Transformation of normal mammary epithelial to non-invasive and invasive cancer cells. Several oncogenes can transform normal epithelial cells to cancer ones; meanwhile, other genes such as, EGF-R, ErbB-2, VEGFs and chemokines, convert non-invasive cancer cells to invasive ones which can invade several vital organs including bone, lung, brain and liver. Invasion is a multi-step process which allows cell migration and invasion through dysfunctional cell–cell adhesive interactions, loss of cell–cell junctions and reorganization of the cytoskeleton; these procedures result in the loss of apical polarity and the acquisition of a more spindle-shaped morphology; this process is identified as the epithelial-mesenchymal transition (EMT). This event is accompanied by inhibition of epithelial markers such as E-cadherin and over-expression of mesenchymal markers such as vimentin.

3. EGF-R and ErbB-2 in brain metastasis

The epidermal growth factor receptor (EGFR) is a member of the ErbB family of receptor tyrosine kinases. This family includes four receptors: EGF-R/ErbB-1/HER-1, ErbB-2/HER-2/Neu, ErbB-3/HER-3, and ErbB-4/HER-4 (Carney et al., 2007; Lee-Hoeflich et al., 2008) that are structurally related. All HER members except HER-3 contain intracellular tyrosine kinase domain and all except HER-2, bind to extracellular ligands (Carpenter et al., 1990). Certain discrete genes, with several alternative splice variants, encode either the "Epidermal Growth Factor (EGF) receptor ligands" or the Neuregulins that bind to different ErbB receptors as a co-receptor. Different ligands bind to more than one receptor with high affinity; consequently ErbB-2 ligands readily activate ErbB-2 in combination with the appropriate high affinity co-receptor. The biological activity and affinity is often higher with the presence of ErbB2 complex than without it. The mammalian ligands that bind to the ErbB family include EGF, Transforming growth factor-α (TGF-α), heparin-binding EGF-like growth factor (HB-EGF), amphiregulin (AR), betacellulin (BTC), epiregulin (EPR), epigen, tomoregulin and neuregulins (NRG-1, NRG-2, NRG-3 and NRG-4) (Chang et al., 1997; Bublil and Yarden, 2007). The architecture of ErbB kinases, like most receptor tyrosine kinases (RTKs), is characterized by an extracellular ligand-binding domain, a transmembrane domain, a juxtamembrane (JM) segment, a kinase domain, and a COOH

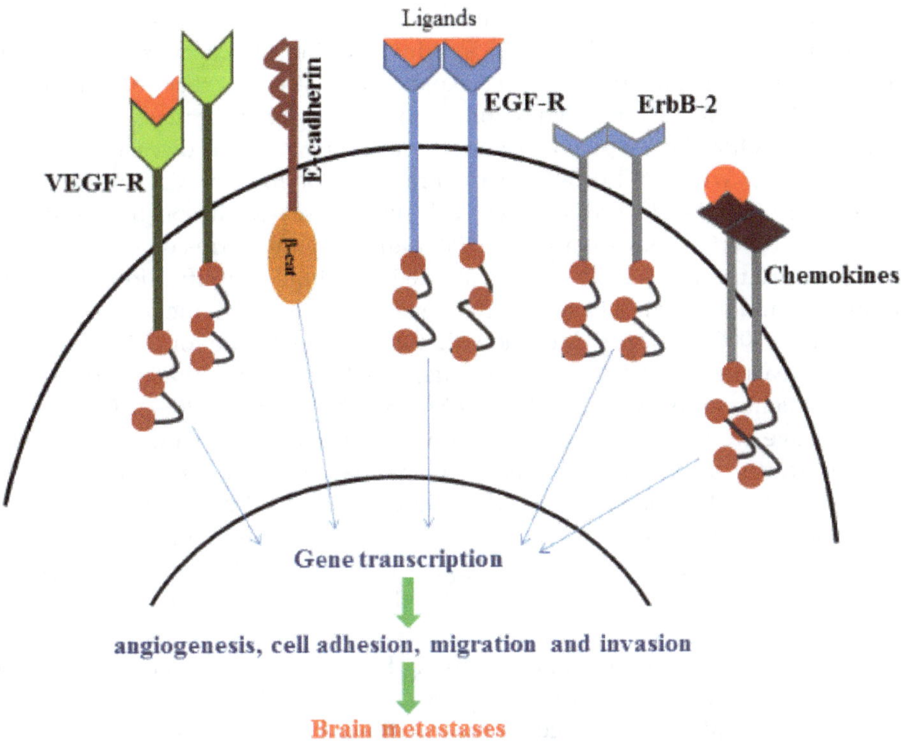

Fig. 2. VEGF-R, EGF-R, ErbB-2 and chemokines receptor signaling pathways in cancer cells. Ligands can activate downstream-signaling pathways of these receptors which also can interact with other protein complexes such E-cadherin/catenins. Therefore, these pathways alter the activity of multiple nuclear transcription factors which in turn can activate several genes implicated in diverse cellular procedures such as angiogenesis, cell adhesion, migration and invasion; after which cancer cells can migrate to several organs including brain.

terminal tail (C-terminal tail). The EGF-R is involved in many cellular processes including cell proliferation, motility, adhesion and angiogenesis via the activation of primarily two pathways: Phosphatidylinositol-3 Kinase (PI3K)/Akt pathway, and the External signal-Regulated Kinase (ERK) pathway (Yasmeen et al., 2006; Bublil and Yarden, 2007) (Figure 2). EGF-R is widely expressed in a variety of human cancers including non-small-cell lung cancer NSCLC, colorectal, pancreatic, breast, ovarian, prostate and gastric cancers (Raymond et al., 2000). It is thought that EGF-R plays an important role in the tumour development and progression (Grandis et al., 2004). In addition to their well established contributions to cell proliferation and survival, EGF-R and ErbB-2 are also linked with other characteristics of aggressive tumours such as local invasion and intravasation (Figure 2), independently of their effects on growth (Xue et al., 2006; Zhan et al., 2006). Gene expression profiling and immunohistochemical studies have indicated that 50–70% of basal-type breast tumours, which are ErbB-2 "triple-negative" carcinomas, exhibit EGF-R expression (Burness et al., 2010). This type of breast cancers is associated with large size, high tumour grade, increased frequency of distant metastases to several vital organs including brain (Da Silva et al., 2007).

ErbB-2/HER-2/Neu oncogene, located on the long arm of chromosome 17 (17q12-q21), is over-expressed or amplified in 18–35% of invasive breast cancers and in 60% of intraductal breast carcinomas but are not over-expressed relative to the normal breast epithelium (Pawlowski et al., 2000). Over-expression of ErbB-2 in breast carcinoma patients is associated with a shorter survival period and more frequent disease recurrence compared with patients without ErbB-2 over-expression (Slamon et al., 1987). Moreover, over-expression of ErbB-2 in breast cancer cell lines increases the portion of cells that present stem-like properties (Korkaya et al., 2008) and display intrinsic resistance to antiestrogen therapy (Jordan et al., 2007; Fan et al., 2009). ErbB-2 amplification/over-expression is a prognostic and predictive factor for the development of CNS metastases (Evans et al., 2004; Gabos et al., 2006). Autopsy data show that the incidence rate for CNS metastases in ErbB-2-positive breast cancer patients is higher (ie, 30% to 50%) than that in ErbB-2-negative breast cancer patients (approximately 30%) (Aragon-Ching et al., 2007). On the other hand, a retrospective study on 9524 women with early stage breast cancer identified ErbB-2 as a clear risk factor for the development of CNS relapse (Pestalozzi et al., 2006). However, the precise biological explanation for the tendency of ErbB-2-positive breast cancer cells to metastasize to CNS has not been completely elucidated; although it has been suggested that it may occur as a result of both the aggressiveness of this breast cancer subtype and of a particular affinity for CNS. Interestingly, the survival time after the diagnosis of brain metastasis is longer for patients with ErbB-2-positive disease than ErbB-2-negative. It is estimated that one-third of women receiving Herceptin for metastatic ErbB-2-positive breast cancer develop CNS metastases during the course of their illness (Bendell et al., 2003; Lai et al., 2004). Herceptin levels in cerebrospinal fluid are 300-fold lower than those in plasma (Pestalozzi et al., 2000; Rusnak et al., 2001), indicating that Herceptin cannot cross the BBB due to its large molecular weight. The inability of Herceptin to cross the BBB may also contribute to the increased incidence of brain metastases in patients with ErbB-2-over-expressing breast cancer. This is most likely because of the inherent aggressiveness of ErbB-2-positive disease, as well as the prolongation in survival and control of extracranial disease attributable to Herceptin therapy (Clayton et al., 2004). Interestingly, ErbB-3 expression was increased in breast cancer cells residing in the brain. Neuregulin-1, the ligand for this receptor, is abundantly expressed in the brain (Law et al., 2004; Da Silva et al., 2010). These findings suggest that neuregulin/ErbB-3 activation is an important mechanism for breast cancer cell colonization of the brain and imply that the inhibition of ErbB family receptors especially EGF-R and/or ErbB-2 may play a significant role in the treatment of patients with brain metastases from breast cancer.

4. VEGFs in brain metastasis

Vascular endothelial growth factor (VEGF) belongs to VEGF family that consists of five members: VEGF (or VEGF-A), VEGF-B, VEGF-C, VEGF-D, and placental growth factor (PlGF) (Li et al., 2001; Nagy et al., 2003; Yamazaki et al., 2003). There are three receptor protein-tyrosine kinases for the VEGF family ligands (VEGFR-1, VEGFR-2, and VEGFR-3), which are primarily expressed by the endothelium and are required for normal vascular development (Millauer et al., 1993; Peters et al., 1993; Terman et al., 1994). Each of these receptors consists of seven immunoglobulin-like loops in the extracellular domain, a single transmembrane domain, and an intracellular protein-tyrosine kinase segment that contains a kinase insert, and a carboxy-terminal tail (Fantl et al., 1993) (Figure 2). Several ligands of

VEGF family bind to two non-enzymatic receptors (neuropilin-1 and -2), and heparan sulfate proteoglycans that are found on the plasma membrane and in the extracellular matrix (Dougher et al., 1997; Gluzman-Poltorak et al., 2000). Binding of VEGF to its receptors induces proliferation and migration of cancer cells (Figure 1 and 2).

Although VEGF is considered potent mitogen for vascular endothehal cells, it is also considerably involved in the mitogenic activity of other cells. VEGF mRNA and protein are found in several tissues and organs (Berse et al., 1992; Ng et al., 2001; Maharaj et al., 2006). Also, VEGF gene expression and protein are found in many of human malignancies such as breast, non-small cell lung, colorectal, neuroblastoma, and prostate carcinomas (Fukuzawa et al., 2002; Hoeben et al., 2004; Xu et al., 2004). On the contrary, VEGF receptors are generally limited to endothelial cells in the cardiovascular and lymphatic systems (Kukk et al., 1996; Lymboussaki et al., 1999).

In the nervous tissue, VEGF is crucial for vascular growth during brain development (Breier et al., 1992; Ogunshola et al., 2000; Vates et al., 2005). However, in the intact adult CNS, the expression of VEGF becomes restricted to the choroid plexus, area postrema cerebellar granule cells (Monacci et al., 1993), and VEGF receptor expression becomes extremely low (Kremer et al., 1997; Soker et al., 1998). VEGF expression was demonstrated to be up-regulated in neurons and astroglia during pathological processes in the CNS that are associated with angiogenesis and increased BBB permeability, including tumours and ischemia (Pietsch et al., 1997; Issa et al., 1999; Lee et al., 1999; Plate et al., 1999; Jin et al., 2000; Graumann et al, 2003). VEGF direct application to fetal cortical and ventral mescencephalic explants has been shown to induce significant angiogenesis and astroglial proliferation (Silverman et al., 1999; Mani et al., 2005; Krum et al., 2008). Furthermore, continuous interstitial infusion of recombinant human VEGF165 protein administered to the cerebrum produced significant increases in the activity and, unexpectedly, in the astroglial proliferation within the adult CNS (Krum et al., 2002). VEGF, thus, was considered a direct astroglial mitogen (Krum et al., 2002).

It was postulated, forty years ago, by Folkman that tumours require to be vascularized to grow (Folkman, 1971). Tumour cells enter the vascular system after switching on the angiogenic process, and forming new ascites, leading to the initiation of metastasis. VEGF, among other various angiogenic factors, plays an essential role in tumour angiogenesis. VEGF is expressed and secreted by most solid tumours, but little occurs in endothelial cells (Ribatti et al., 1998; Shemirani and Crowe, 2000). In contrast, VEGF receptors (VEGFR-1 and VEGFR-2 mRNAs and proteins) are largely expressed in vessels lining and penetrating the tumours; where they are exclusively expressed in endothelial cells (Brown et al., 1995; Mentzel et al., 2001). These observations are consistent with the notion that VEGF acts in a paracrine manner, in which VEGF that is secreted from tumour cells influences nearby endothelial cells.

The finding that VEGF is highly expressed in metastatic cerebral tumours originating from angiosarcoma, renal cell carcinomas, melanomas, and adenocarcinomas provide further evidence that supports the significant role for VEGF in human metastases (Strugar et al., 1994). VEGF expression was associated with considerable staining of microvascular and the formation of vasogenic brain edema, revealing both the angiogenic and permeability properties of VEGF (Strugar et al., 1994). On the other hand, VEGF- mRNA is significantly correlated with vascularisation in both gliomas and meningiomas, indicating a pivotal role for VEGF in the vascularization of primary brain tumours (Samoto et al., 1995). It is currently well established that the formation of metastases correlates with the number of microvessels (the amount of vascularisation) that can be detected in a primary tumour.

A number of mechanisms account for tumour vascularisation, including sprouting angiogenesis, intussusceptions, recruitment of circulating endothelial precursors, cooption, mosaic vessels, and vascular mimicry. VEGF family members are considered the major players that control these mechanisms. Sprouting angiogenesis has been suggested as the mechanism that is used by the brain for vasculrization. In sprouting angiogenesis, VEGF-A produces vasodilatation of preexisting capillaries and increases permeability (Auguste et al., 2005). VEGF-A also induces endothelial cell proliferation (Auguste et al., 2005) and an increase in metalloproteases and plasminogen activators, which lead to the degradation of the extracellular matrix permitting endothelial cell migration (Pepper et al., 1991; Vu et al., 1998; Bergers et al., 2000). Vessel guidance mechanisms that direct host vessels into the tumour have been identified in the brain. VEGF and its receptors have been postulated as important guidance signal. It seems that cells located at the invading front of the blood vessels, huddle VEGFR-2 and follow a VEGF gradient (Gerhardt et al., 2003). Tumour cells injected into the brain were found to develop vascularization immediately by angiogenic sprouting with loss of the BBB. Tumour cells are speculated to be organized in cuffs of pseudopalisading cells around VEGFR-2 positive vessels, and to use these vessels to invade other brain areas. Vessels supply tumour cells with oxygen and nutriments.

A different mechanism of brain tumour vascularization that is distinct from the sprouting mechanism has been described. Accordingly, tumours in the brain can use a cooption mechanism for vascularization (Holash et al., 1999; Fischer et al., 2005). Vessels are surrounded by tumour cells, and cooped endothelial cells are induced to express angiopoietin-2. Binding of angiopoietin-2 to its receptors located at the endothelial cell surface leads to the dissociation of the mural cells from endothelial cells, and an increase in apoptosis. Angiopoietin-2 activity causes a significant decrease in tumour vessel number and an increase in vessel diameter. Accordingly, the scarcity of vessels leads to hypoxia which upregulates VEGF-A expression in tumour cells. As a consequence, strong angiogenesis develops mainly at the tumour periphery (Holash et al., 1999; Zagzag et al., 2000; Fischer et al, 2005). Rat mammary carcinomas was shown to be vascularized by cooption when cells are injected inside the brain. Metastases of Lewis lung carcinoma and melanoma cells into brain have been demonstrated to be partially vascularized by cooption (Holash et al., 1999; Kusters et al., 2002). Decreasing VEGF production, by antisense transfection, to 20–50% of original cell level was shown to be associated with inhibition of both angiogenesis and brain metastasis formation (Yano et al., 2000). In conclusion, VEGF is a key factor in the vascularization and metastasis of primary tumours into brain.

5. Chemokines and chemokine receptors

Chemotactic cytokines, or *chemo-kines*, are a large subfamily of cytokines that coordinate leukocyte recruitment and activation, two crucial elements in the pathogenesis of several immuno-mediated human diseases. Chemokines have been recognized in the last few years as important mediators in the pathogenesis of many human diseases and have assumed growing relevance in clinical pathology as markers of disease onset, progression, and remission (Hinton et al., 2010). Since the description of the first chemokine in 1977, over 40 related molecules have been discovered in humans and chemokines have been recognized as a family of functionally related small secreted molecules named "chemo-kine" because of leukocyte chemoattractant and cytokine-like activities (Luster, 1998; Locati and Murphy,

1999). Human chemokine family is currently known to include more than 40 chemokines and 20 chemokine receptors (Bonecchi et al., 2009). These receptors are defined by their ability to induce directional migration of cells toward a gradient of a chemotactic cytokine (a process known as chemotaxis) (Figure 2). Chemokine receptors are a family of seven transmembrane G protein-coupled cell surface receptors (GPCR) that are classified into four groups (CXC, CC, C, and CX3C) based on the position of the first two cysteines (Murphy et al., 2000; Zlotnik and Yoshie, 2000). While chemokine receptors have been found in many different cell types, these receptors were initially identified on leukocytes and were found to play an important role in the homing of such cells to sites of inflammation (Loetscher et al., 2000).

During the past several years, other types of non-hematopoietic cells have been found to express receptors for various chemokines found in their distinct tissue microenvironments. The interactions between such receptors and their respective chemokines are thought to help coordinate the trafficking and organization of cells within various tissue compartments (Baggiolini, 1998; Moser and Loetscher, 2001). CXCR4 is one of the best studied chemokine receptors, primarily due to its role as a co-receptor for HIV entry (Feng et al., 1996) and its ability to mediate the metastasis of a variety of cancers, including prostate cancer (Zlotnik, 2006a and b; Burger and Kipps, 2006; Sun et al., 2003). CXCR4 is a 352-amino acid rhodopsin-like GPCR that selectively binds the CXC chemokine stromal cell-derived factor 1 (SDF-1), also known as CXCL12 (Fredriksson et al., 2003; Burger and Kipps, 2006). On the other hand, lack of either SDF-1 or CXCR4 resulted in a phenotype almost identical to that of late gestational lethality with defects in B cell lymphopoiesis, bone marrow colonization, and cardiac septal formation (Nagasawa et al., 1996; Zou et al., 1998). These studies indicate that CXCR4 is essential for development, hematopoiesis, organogenesis, as well as vascularization (Tachibana et al., 1998; McGrath et al., 1999) and that it functions as a classical chemokine receptor in adults (Murphy, 1994; Baggiolini, 1998). A growing body of evidence now shows that CXCR4 has a role in both cancer metastasis and in cancer stem cells. The physiological mechanism of tissue-specific recruitment (i.e. a homing system for normal tissue replacement) also seems to be functional for cancer stem cells. The CXCR4-SDF-1 axis seems to have a large influence on the biology of tumours. High levels of SDF-1 in organs and tissue structures such as the lymph nodes, lungs, liver, brain and bones are believed to direct the metastasis of CXCR4-expressing tumour cells. In support of this hypothesis, several researchers have shown that multiple cancers expressing CXCR4 (e.g. breast, ovarian, and prostate cancers, as well as rhabdomyosarcomas and neuroblastomas) metastasize to the bones and the brain through the bloodstream in an SDF-1 (CXCL12)-dependent manner (Dontu et al., 3003; Porcile et al., 2004; Sun et al., 2003; Geminder et al., 2001; Hinton et al., 2010). The CXCR4-SDF-1-mediated trafficking/homing of tumour cells during metastasis seems to share some molecular mechanisms with normal stem cell processes. Additionally, the mobilization, trafficking and homing of both cancer and normal stem cells seem to be multistep processes, as described in several studies (Hattori et al., 2001; Lapidot et al., 2002; Hinton et al., 2010). Previous study by Muller et al. (2001) reported in breast cancer that CXCR4 and CXCL12 are central players in regulating metastasis by showing that normal breast tissues express little CXCR4, whereas breast neoplasms express high levels of CXCR4; CXCR4 signaling in response to CXCL12 mediates actin polymerization and pseudopodia formation, and subsequently induces chemotactic and invasive responses (Muller et al., 2001). These data formed the basis of the hypothesis that malignant cells may employ chemokine receptors to migrate toward chemokine ligands expressed at common metastatic sites, such as the lungs, bone marrow, brain and lymph nodes. Indeed, CXCR4 appears to be one of a limited number of genes that are enriched in a subpopulation of metastatic breast cancer cells, as over-expression of CXCR4 alone significantly increased the number of bone and brain metastases *in vivo* (Kang et al., 2003). Supporting evidence for the hypothesis was demonstrated by Liang et al. (2005) as blocking CXCR4 expression by siRNAs decreased breast cancer cell invasion *in vitro* and inhibited metastasis in animal models. Interestingly, the CXCR4 carboxy-terminal domain appears to play a major role in regulating receptor desensitization and down-regulation, whereas deletion of the C-terminal domain of CXCR4 leads to the down-regulation of cell-to-cell contact, enhanced motility, and proliferation in breast carcinoma cells (Ueda et al., 2006). Elucidation of the underlying mechanisms of breast cancer invasion and metastasis focusing on CXCR4 has resulted in several important observations. Ligand-binding studies indicate that the number and affinity of CXCR4 receptors are similar in nonmetastatic cells versus highly metastatic cells. In metastatic cells, CXCL12 binding to the Gαβγ/GDP protein complex leads to a GTP-for-GDP exchange, allowing Gαi to dissociate from the Gβγ subunit, leading to activation of ERK1/2, IκBα, JNK, Akt, p38 MAPK, and GSK-3αβ. In nonmetastatic cells, CXCR4 is able to independently form a complex with Gαi or Gβ subunits, but no Gαβγ heterotrimer could be associated with CXCR4 and, ultimately, Gβγ-dependent downstream signaling did not occur (Holland et al., 2006). Although the molecular basis for the difference in G-protein signaling in metastatic versus nonmetastatic cells remains to be elucidated, these studies have implications for clinical studies that are examining CXCR4 protein expression but not receptor function. As observed in breast cancer cell lines, detection of CXCR4 protein does not necessarily indicate CXCR4-mediated signaling (Fulton, 2009).

There is increasing evidence that CXCR4 interacts with several growth factor receptor tyrosine kinases. Upon activating IGF-1R, IGF-1 was shown to transactivate CXCR4 signal transduction in metastatic MDA-MB-231 cells but not in nonmetastatic MCF-7 cells, even though both cell lines are positive for IGF-1R and CXCR4 (Akekawatchai et al., 2005). Myofibroblasts associated with breast cancer, but not those in normal breast tissue, produce CXCL12 and enhance growth of tumours through mechanisms that include proliferation and survival of malignant cells and angiogenesis (Allinen et al., 2004; Orimo et al., 2005). Specific alleles of CXCL12 are associated with an increased risk of breast cancer (Razmkhah et al., 2005), and CXCL12 has been shown to transactivate ErbB-2 (Cabioglu et al., 2005). CXCR4 expression was also identified as a predictive factor of worse outcome in some metastatic tumours and in malignant gliomas (Scala et al., 2005; Ottaiano et al., 2006; Bian et al., 2007). CXCL12/CXCR4 axis is supposed to be crucial in brain metastases formation from breast cancer (Hinton et al., 2008). Recently, another CXCL12 receptor has been identified: the orphan G protein-coupled receptor (GPCR) RDC1, now called CXCR7 (Balabanian et al., 2005; Burns et al., 2006). This receptor does not mediate typical GPCR signaling through Gi or Ca2+ mobilization. Recent findings in zebrafish primordial germ cells showed a scavenger activity of CXCR7 generating a CXCL12 gradient that would lead to the formation of a guidance cue for CXCR4-positive cells (Thelen and Thelen, 2008). On the other hand, formation of CXCR4/CXCR7 heterodimers enhancing CXCL12 signaling in embryonic cells was observed, suggesting a potential interaction between the two receptors (Sierro et al., 2007). Nevertheless, CXCL12/CXCR4 relevance in brain metastasis establishment/progression needs more investigation especially on the molecular level.

6. Conclusions/Perspectives

Cancer cell migration and invasion are critical processes in the metastatic cascade. They can be induced and executed by various signalling pathways and regulatory networks. Many of these pathways seem to overlap with developmental processes and are being abused by invasive carcinomas cells and their microenvironment. Although we have made substantial progress in understanding the molecular mechanisms underlying cancer cell migration and invasion in experimental systems, we still lack sufficient insights into the actual processes at work in metastatic cancer patients especially brain metastatic disease. This divergence between clinicopathologic and experimental observations is mainly based on the lack of appropriate surrogate markers and the lack of complex *in vivo* models that appropriately recapitulate human stochastic carcinogenesis. However, it is expected that the ongoing cellular and molecular research on cell migration will provide the urgently needed tools for the development of improved diagnosis, prognosis and eventually for the design of innovative therapies.

There are few therapeutic approaches that are currently under development or in clinical trials specifically targeting metastatic breast cancer of the brain, such as interfering with specific pathways of some regulator genes of invasive cancer cells. However, by interfering with important signaling pathways that are known to modulate cell proliferation, survival, and differentiation, they may also affect cell migration and invasion. Examples are inhibitors against the activities of different receptor tyrosine kinases, such as EGF-R, ErbB-2, VEGF-Rs, fibroblast growth factor receptors, chemokine receptors, and c-Met, as well as various anti-angiogenesis regimen or even in combinations. Altogether, such multifaceted inhibitory approaches may provide efficient therapeutic measures that repress not only primary tumour outgrowth but also metastasis formation by interfering with cancer cell migration and invasion to the brain and other organs. However, the cellular and molecular variations to cancer cell migration discussed above raise the caveat that this endeavour will not be easy. We believe that using microarray technology and new *in vitro* and *in vivo* cancer metastatic models, including brain, should help us to understand the mechanism of cancer metastasis and consequently facilitate the design of more successful, personalized cancer therapies.

7. Acknowledgments

We are grateful to Mrs. A. Kassab and Mr. E Segal for their critical reading of the manuscript. The research works from Dr. Al Moustafa's laboratory has been supported by the Canadian Institutes for Health Research, the Cancer Research Society Inc. of Canada, the National Colorectal Cancer Campaign and the Fonds de la Recherche en Santé du Québec (FRSQ- Réseau du Cancer).

8. References

Akekawatchai C, Holland JD, Kochetkova M, Wallace JC, McColl SR. Transactivation of CXCR4 by the insulin-like growth factor-1 receptor (IGF-1R) in human MDA-MB-231 breast cancer epithelial cells. J Biol Chem. 2005 Dec 2;280(48):39701-8.

Al Moustafa A-E, Achkhar A, Yasmeen A. EGF-receptor signaling and epithelial-mesenchymal transition in human carcinomas. Frontiers in Bioscience journal, in press.

Al Moustafa AE, Kassab A, Darnel A, Yasmeen A. High-risk HPV/ErbB-2 interaction on E-cadherin/catenin regulation in human carcinogenesis. Curr Pharm Des. 2008;14(22):2159-72.

Allinen M, Beroukhim R, Cai L, Brennan C, Lahti-Domenici J, Huang H, Porter D, Hu M, Chin L, Richardson A, Schnitt S, Sellers WR, Polyak K. Molecular characterization of the tumor microenvironment in breast cancer. Cancer Cell. 2004 Jul;6(1):17-32.

Altundag K, Bondy ML, Mirza NQ, Kau SW, Broglio K, Hortobagyi GN, Rivera E. Clinicopathologic characteristics and prognostic factors in 420 metastatic breast cancer patients with central nervous system metastasis. Cancer. 2007 Dec 15;110(12):2640-7.

Aragon-Ching JB, Zujewski JA. (2007). CNS metastasis: an old problem in a new guise. Clin Cancer Res, vol.13, no.6, (mar 2007), pp. 1644-1647.

Arnold SM, Young AB, Munn RK, Patchell RA, Nanayakkara N, Markesbery WR. Expression of p53, bcl-2, E-cadherin, matrix metalloproteinase-9, and tissue inhibitor of metalloproteinases-1 in paired primary tumors and brain metastasis. Clin Cancer Res. 1999 Dec;5(12):4028-33.

Auguste P, Lemiere S, Larrieu-Lahargue F, Bikfalvi A. Molecular mechanisms of tumor vascularization. Crit Rev Oncol Hematol 2005;54:53–61.

Baggiolini M. Chemokines and leukocyte traffic. Nature 1998; 392: 565–8.

Balabanian K, Lagane B, Infantino S, Chow KY, Harriague J, Moepps B, Arenzana-Seisdedos F, Thelen M, Bachelerie F. The chemokine SDF-1/CXCL12 binds to and signals through the orphan receptor RDC1 in T lymphocytes. J Biol Chem. 2005 Oct 21;280(42):35760-6.

Ballabh P, Braun A, Nedergaard M.The blood-brain barrier: an overview: structure, regulation, and clinical implications. Neurobiol Dis. 2004 Jun;16(1):1-13.

Bartholdi, D., Rubin, B.P., Schwab, M.E., 1997. VEGF mRNA induction correlates with changes in the vascular architecture upon spinal cord damage in the rat. Eur. J. Neurosci. 9, 2549–2560.

Bendell JC, Domchek SM, Burstein HJ, et al. 2003. Central nervous system metastases in women who receive trastuzumab-based therapy for metastatic breast carcinoma. Cancer, vol. 97, no. 12, pp. 2972–2977.

Bergers G, Brekken R, McMahon G, et al. Matrix metalloproteinase- 9 triggers the angiogenic switch during carcinogenesis. Nat Cell Biol 2000;2:737–44.

Berse B, Brown LF, Van de Water L, Dvorak HF, Senger DR. Vascular permeability factor (vascular endothelial growth factor) gene is expressed differentially in normal tissues, macrophages, and tumors. Mol Biol Cell 1992;3:211–20.

Bian XW, Yang SX, Chen JH, Ping YF, Zhou XD, Wang QL, Jiang XF, Gong W, Xiao HL, Du LL, Chen ZQ, Zhao W, Shi JQ, Wang JM. Preferential expression of chemokine receptor CXCR4 by highly malignant human gliomas and its association with poor patient survival. Neurosurgery. 2007 Sep;61(3):570-8; discussion 578-9.

Bonecchi R, Galliera E, Borroni EM, Corsi MM, Locati M, Mantovani A. Chemokines and chemokine receptors: an overview. Front Biosci. 2009 Jan 1;14:540-51

Bos PD, Zhang XH, Nadal C, Shu W, Gomis RR, Nguyen DX, Minn AJ, van de Vijver MJ, Gerald WL, Foekens JA, Massagué J. Genes that mediate breast cancer metastasis to the brain. Nature. 2009 Jun 18;459(7249):1005-9.

Breier G, Albrecht U, Sterrer S, Risau W. Expression of vascular endothelial growth factor during embryonic angiogenesis and endothelial cell differentiation. Development 1992;114:521–32.

Bremnes RM, Veve R, Hirsch FR, Franklin WA. The E-cadherin cell-cell adhesion complex and lung cancer invasion, metastasis, and prognosis. Lung Cancer. 2002 May;36(2):115-24.

Brown, L. F., Berse, B., Jackman, R. W. Tognazzi, K. Guidi, A. J. Dvorak, H. F. Senger, D. R. Connolly, J. L. Schnitt, S. J. 1995. "Expression of vascular permeability factor (vascular endothelial growth factor) and its receptors in breast cancer." Hum Pathol 26(1): 86-91.

Bublil EM, Yarden Y. The EGF receptor family: spearheading a merger of signaling and therapeutics. Current opinion in cell biology 2007; 19:124-34.

Burger JA, Kipps TJ. CXCR4: A key receptor in the crosstalk between tumor cells and their microenvironment. Blood 2006; 107: 1761–7.

Burns JM, Summers BC, Wang Y, Melikian A, Berahovich R, Miao Z, Penfold ME, Sunshine MJ, Littman DR, Kuo CJ, Wei K, McMaster BE, Wright K, Howard MC, Schall TJ. A novel chemokine receptor for SDF-1 and I-TAC involved in cell survival, cell adhesion, and tumor development. J Exp Med. 2006 Sep 4;203(9):2201-13.

Burness ML, Grushko TA, Olopade OI. 2010. Epidermal growth factor receptor in triple-negative and basal-like breast cancer: promising clinical target or only a marker?. Cancer J, vol. 16, pp.23–32.

Cabioglu N, Summy J, Miller C, Parikh NU, Sahin AA, Tuzlali S, Pumiglia K, Gallick GE, Price JE. CXCL-12/stromal cell-derived factor-1alpha transactivates HER2-neu in breast cancer cells by a novel pathway involving Src kinase activation. Cancer Res. 2005 Aug 1;65(15):6493-7.

Carney W, Leitzel K, Ali S, Neumann R, Lipton A. 2007. HER-2 therapy. HER-2/neu diagnostics in breast cancer. Breast Cancer Res,. vol. 9:207.

Carotenuto P, Roma C, Rachiglio AM, Botti G, D'Alessio A, Normanno N. Triple negative breast cancer: from molecular portrait to therapeutic intervention. Crit Rev Eukaryot Gene Expr. 2010;20(1):17-34.

Carpenter G, Cohen S. Epidermal growth factor. 1990. J Biol Chem; vol. 265, pp.7709–7712.

Chang H, Riese DJ, 2nd, Gilbert W, Stern DF, McMahan UJ. Ligands for ErbB-family receptors encoded by a neuregulin-like gene. Nature 1997; 387:509-12.

Cheng X, Hung MC. Breast cancer brain metastases. Cancer Metastasis Rev. 2007 Dec;26(3-4):635-43.

Clayton AJ, Danson S, Jolly S, et al. 2004. Incidence of cerebral metastases in patients treated with trastuzumab for metastatic breast cancer. Br J Cancer, vol. 91, no. 4, pp. 639–643.

Da Silva L, Clarke C, Lakhani SR. 2007. Demystifying basal-like breast carcinomas. J Clin Pathol, vol. 60, no.12, pp 1328–1332.

Da Silva L, Simpson PT, Smart CE, Cocciardi S, Waddell N, et al. 2010. HER3 and downstream pathways are involved in colonization of brain metastases from breast cancer. Breast Cancer Research, vol. 12, no. 4, pp. 1–13.

Deryugina EI, Quigley JP. Matrix metalloproteinases and tumor metastasis. Cancer Metastasis Rev. 2006 Mar;25(1):9-34.

Dontu G, Al-Hajj M, Abdallah WM, Clarke MF, Wicha MS. Stem cells in normal breast development and breast cancer. Cell Prolif 2003; 36 (Suppl 1): 59–72.

Dougher, A. M., Wasserstrom, H., Torley, L. Shridaran, L. Westdock, P. Hileman, R. E. Fromm, J. R. Anderberg, R. Lyman, S. Linhardt, R. J. Kaplan, J. Terman, B. I. 1997. "Identification of a heparin binding peptide on the extracellular domain of the KDR VEGF receptor." Growth Factors 14(4): 257-68.

Evans AJ, James JJ, Cornford EJ, et al. Brain metastases from breast cancer: 2004.identification of a high-risk group. Clin Oncol (R Coll Radiol (Great Britain); vol. 16, no. 5, pp. 345–349.

Fan P, Yue W, Wang JP, Aiyar S, Li Y, Kim TH, et al. 2009. Mechanisms of resistance to structurally diverse antiestrogens differ under premenopausal and postmenopausal conditions: evidence from in vitro breast cancer cell models. Endocrinology, vol. 150, no.5, pp. 2036–2045.

Fantl WJ, Johnson DE, Williams LT. Signalling by receptor tyrosine kinases. Annu Rev Biochem 1993;62:453–81.

Feng Y, Broder CC, Kennedy PE, Berger EA. HIV-1 entry cofactor: Functional cDNA cloning of a seven-transmembrane, G protein-coupled receptor. Science 1996; 272: 872–7.

Figarella-Branger D, Pellissier JF, Bouillot P, Bianco N, Mayan M, Grisoli F, Rougon G.Expression of neural cell-adhesion molecule isoforms and epithelial cadherin adhesion molecules in 47 human meningiomas: correlation with clinical and morphological data. Mod Pathol. 1994 Sep;7(7):752-61.

Fischer, I., J. P. Gagner, Law, M. Newcomb, E. W. Zagzag, D. 2005. "Angiogenesis in gliomas: biology and molecular pathophysiology." Brain Pathol 15(4): 297-310.

Folkman J. (1971) Tumor angiogenesis: therapeutic implications. N Engl J Med; 285:1182-1186.

Fredriksson R, Lagerstrom MC, Lundin LG, Schioth HB. The G-protein-coupled receptors in the human genome form five main families. Phylogenetic analysis, paralogon groups, and fingerprints. Mol Pharmacol 2003; 63: 1256–72.

Fukuzawa, M., Sugiura, H., Koshinaga, T., Ikeda, T., Hagiwara, N., Sawada, T. (2002). "Expression of vascular endothelial growth factor and its receptor Flk-1 in human neuroblastoma using in situ hybridization." J Pediatr Surg 37(12): 1747-50.

Fulton AM. The chemokine receptors CXCR4 and CXCR3 in cancer. Curr Oncol Rep. 2009 Mar;11(2):125-31.

Furusato B, Mohamed A, Uhlén M, Rhim JS. CXCR4 and cancer. Pathol Int. 2010 Jul;60(7):497-505

Gabos Z, Sinha R, Hanson J, et al. 2006. Prognostic significance of human epidermal growth factor receptor positivity for the development of brain metastasis after newly diagnosed breast cancer. J Clin Oncol , vol. 24, no.36, pp. 5658–5663.

Geminder H, Sagi-Assif O, Goldberg L, Meshel T, Rechavi G, Witz IP, Ben-Baruch A. A possible role for CXCR4 and its ligand, the CXC chemokine stromal cell-derived factor-1, in the development of bone marrow metastases in neuroblastoma. J Immunol. 2001 Oct 15;167(8):4747-57.

Gerhardt H, Golding M, Fruttiger M, et al. VEGF guides angiogenic sprouting utilizing endothelial tip cell filopodia. J Cell Biol 2003;161:1163–77.

Gluzman-Poltorak, Z., Cohen, T., Herzog, Y. Neufeld, G. 2000. "Neuropilin-2 is a receptor for the vascular endothelial growth factor (VEGF) forms VEGF-145 and VEGF-165 [corrected]." J Biol Chem 275(24): 18040-5.

Grandis JR, Sok JC .(2004). Signaling through the epidermal growth factor receptor during the development of malignancy. Pharmacol Ther, vol 102, pp. 37- 46.

Graumann, U., R. Reynolds, Steck, A. J., Schaeren-Wiemers, N. 2003. "Molecular changes in normal appearing white matter in multiple sclerosis are characteristic of neuroprotective mechanisms against hypoxic insult." Brain Pathol 13(4): 554-73.

Harlozinska A. Progress in molecular mechanisms of tumor metastasis and angiogenesis. Anticancer Res. 2005; 25: 3327–33.

Hattori K, Heissig B, Tashiro K, Honjo T, Tateno M, Shieh JH, Hackett NR, Quitoriano MS, Crystal RG, Rafii S, Moore MA. Plasma elevation of stromal cell-derived factor-1 induces mobilization of mature and immature hematopoietic progenitor and stem cells. Blood. 2001 Jun 1;97(11):3354-60.

Hinton CV, Avraham S, Avraham HK. Contributions of integrin-linked kinase to breast cancer metastasis and tumourigenesis. J Cell Mol Med. 2008 Sep-Oct;12(5A):1517-26.

Hinton CV, Avraham S, Avraham HK. Role of the CXCR4/CXCL12 signaling axis in breast cancer metastasis to the brain. Clin Exp Metastasis. 2010 Feb;27(2):97-105.

Hoeben A, Landuyt B, Highley MS, Wildiers H, Van Oosterom AT, De Bruijn EA. Vascular endothelial growth factor and angiogenesis. Pharmacol Rev 2004;56:549–80.

Holash J, Maisonpierre PC, Compton D, et al. Vessel cooption, regression, and growth in tumors mediated by angiopoietins and VEGF. Science 1999;284:1994–8.

Holland JD, Kochetkova M, Akekawatchai C, Dottore M, Lopez A, McColl SR.Differential functional activation of chemokine receptor CXCR4 is mediated by G proteins in breast cancer cells. Cancer Res. 2006 Apr 15;66(8):4117-24.

Howng SL, Wu CH, Cheng TS, Sy WD, Lin PC, Wang C, Hong YR. Differential expression of Wnt genes, beta-catenin and E-cadherin in human brain tumors. Cancer Lett. 2002 Sep 8;183(1):95-101.

Issa, R., Krupinski, J., Bujny, T., Kumar, S., Kaluza, J., Kumar, P., 1999. Vascular endothelial growth factor and its receptor, KDR, in human brain tissue after ischemic stroke. Lab. Invest. 79, 417–425.

Jäälinojä J, Herva R, Korpela M, Höyhtyä M, Turpeenniemi-Hujanen T. Matrix metalloproteinase 2 (MMP-2) immunoreactive protein is associated with poor grade and survival in brain neoplasms. J Neurooncol. 2000;46(1):81-90.

Jin, K.L., Mao, X.O., Nagayama, T., Goldsmith, P.C., Greenberg, D.A., 2000. Induction of vascular endothelial growth factor and hypoxiainducible factor-1 alpha by global ischemia in rat brain. Neuroscience 99, 577–585.

Jordan VC, O'Malley BW. (2007). Selective estrogen-receptor modulators and antihormonal resistance in breast cancer. J Clin Oncol, vol. 25, no.36, pp. 5815–5824.

Kang Y, Siegel PM, Shu W, Drobnjak M, Kakonen SM, Cordón-Cardo C, Guise TA, Massagué J. A multigenic program mediating breast cancer metastasis to bone. Cancer Cell. 2003 Jun;3(6):537-49.

Kaplan RN, Rafii S, Lyden D. Preparing the "soil": the premetastatic niche. Cancer Res. 2006; 66: 11089–93.

Kennecke H, Yerushalmi R, Woods R, Cheang MC, Voduc D, Speers CH, Nielsen TO, Gelmon K. Metastatic behavior of breast cancer subtypes. J Clin Oncol. 2010 Jul 10;28(20):3271-7.

Kessenbrock K, Plaks V, Werb Z. Matrix metalloproteinases: regulators of the tumor microenvironment. Cell. 2010 Apr 2;141(1):52-67.

Klein A, Olendrowitz C, Schmutzler R, Hampl J, Schlag PM, Maass N, Arnold N, Wessel R, Ramser J, Meindl A, Scherneck S, Seitz S. Identification of brain- and bone-specific breast cancer metastasis genes. Cancer Lett. 2009 Apr 18;276(2):212-20

Korkaya H, Paulson A, Iovino F, Wicha MS. 2008. HER2 regulates the mammary stem/progenitor cell population driving tumorigenesis and invasion. Oncogene, vol. 27, pp. 6120–6130.

Kremer, C., Breier, G., Risau, W., Plate, K.H., 1997. Up-regulation of flk-1/vascular endothelial growth factor receptor 2 by its ligand in a cerebral slice culture system. Cancer Res. 57, 3852–3859.

Krum, J. M., Mani, N., Rosenstein, J. M. 2008. "Roles of the endogenous VEGF receptors flt-1 and flk-1 in astroglial and vascular remodeling after brain injury." Exp Neurol 212(1): 108-17.

Krum, J.M., Mani, N., Rosenstein, J.M., 2002. Angiogenic and astroglial responses to vascular endothelial growth factor administration in adult rat brain. Neuroscience 110, 589–604.

Krum, J.M., Rosenstein, J.M., 1999. Transient coexpression of nestin, GFAP, and vascular endothelial growth factor in mature reactive astroglia following neural grafting or brain wounds. Exp. Neurol. 160, 348–360.

Kukk E, Lymboussaki A, Taira S, et al. VEGF-C receptor binding and pattern of expression with VEGFR-3 suggests a role in lymphatic vascular development. Development 1996;122:3829–37.

Kunkel P, Ulbricht U, Bohlen P, et al. Inhibition of glioma angiogenesis and growth in vivo by systemic treatment with a monoclonal antibody against vascular endothelial growth factor receptor-2. Cancer Res 2001;61:6624–8.

Kusters B, Leenders WP, Wesseling P, et al. Vascular endothelial growth factor-A(165) induces progression of melanoma brain metastases without induction of sprouting angiogenesis. Cancer Res 2002;62:341–5.

Lai R, Dang CT, Malkin MG, Abrey LE. 2004. The risk of central nervous system metastases after trastuzumab therapy in patients with breast carcinoma. Cancer; vol. 101, pp. 810–6.

Landis SH, Murray T, Bolden S, Wingo PA. Cancer statistics, 1999. CA Cancer J Clin. 1999 Jan-Feb;49(1):8-31, 1.

Lapidot T, Petit I. Current understanding of stem cell mobilization: The roles of chemokines, proteolytic enzymes, adhesion molecules, cytokines, and stromal cells. Exp Hematol 2002; 30: 973–81.

Law AJ, Shannon Weickert C, Hyde TM, Kleinman JE, Harrison PJ. 2004. Neuregulin-1 (NRG-1) mRNA and protein in the adult human brain. Neuroscience, vol. 127, pp. 125-136.

Lee SS, Ahn JH, Kim MK, Sym SJ, Gong G, Ahn SD, Kim SB, Kim WK. Brain metastases in breast cancer: prognostic factors and management. Breast Cancer Res Treat. 2008 Oct;111(3):523-30.

Lee, M.Y., Ju, W.K., Cha, J.H., Son, B.C., Chun, M.H., Kang, J.K., Park, C.K., 1999. Expression of vascular endothelial growth factor mRNA following transient forebrain ischemia in rats. Neurosci. Lett. 265, 107–110.

Lee-Hoeflich ST, Crocker L, Yao E, Pham T, Munroe X, Hoeflich KP, et al. 2008. A central role for HER3 in HER2-amplified breast cancer: implications for targeted therapy. Cancer Res, vol. 68, pp. 5878–5887.

Lewis-Tuffin LJ, Rodriguez F, Giannini C, Scheithauer B, Necela BM, Sarkaria JN, Anastasiadis PZ. Misregulated E-cadherin expression associated with an aggressive brain tumor phenotype. PLoS One. 2010 Oct 27;5(10):e13665.

Li, X., U. Eriksson, Novel VEGF family members: VEGF-B, VEGF-C and VEGF-D, Int. J. Biochem. Cell Biol. 2001, 33, 421–426.

Liang Z, Yoon Y, Votaw J, Goodman MM, Williams L, Shim H. Silencing of CXCR4 blocks breast cancer metastasis. Cancer Res. 2005 Feb 1;65(3):967-71.

Lin NU, Bellon JR, Winer EP. CNS metastases in breast cancer. J Clin Oncol 2004;22:3608-3617.

Locati M, Murphy PM. Chemokines and chemokine receptors: biology and clinical relevance in inflammation and AIDS. Annu Rev Med. 1999;50:425-40.

Loetscher P, Moser B, Baggiolini M. Chemokines and their receptors in lymphocyte traffic and HIV infection. Adv Immunol 2000; 74: 127–80.

Luster AD. Chemokines--chemotactic cytokines that mediate inflammation. N Engl J Med. 1998 Feb 12;338(7):436-45

Lymboussaki, A., Olofsson, B., Eriksson, U., Alitalo, K., 1999. "Vascular endothelial growth factor (VEGF) and VEGF-C show overlapping binding sites in embryonic endothelia and distinct sites in differentiated adult endothelia." Circ Res 85(11): 992-9.

Maharaj AS, Saint-Geniez M, Maldonado AE, D'Amore PA. Vascular endothelial growth factor localization in the adult. Am J Pathol 2006;168:639–48.

Mani, N., Khaibullina, A., Krum, J. M., Rosenstein, J. M. 2005. "Astrocyte growth effects of vascular endothelial growth factor (VEGF) application to perinatal neocortical explants: receptor mediation and signal transduction pathways." Exp Neurol 192(2): 394-406.

Mayer M. A patient perspective on brain metastases in breast cancer. Clin Cancer Res 2007;13:1623-1624.

McGrath KE, Koniski AD, Maltby KM, McGann JK, Palis J. Embryonic expression and function of the chemokine SDF-1 and its receptor, CXCR4. Dev Biol 1999; 213: 442–56.

Mendes O, Kim HT, Stoica G. Expression of MMP2, MMP9 and MMP3 in breast cancer brain metastasis in a rat model. Clin Exp Metastasis. 2005;22(3):237-46.

Mentzel, T., L. F. Brown, Dvorak, H. F. Kuhnen, C. Stiller, K. J. Katenkamp, D. Fletcher, C. D. 2001. "The association between tumour progression and vascularity in myxofibrosarcoma and myxoid/round cell liposarcoma." Virchows Arch 438(1): 13-22.

Millauer, B., Wizigmann-Voos, S., Schnurch, H., Martinez, R., Moller, N.P., Risau, W., Ullrich, A., 1993. High affinity VEGF binding and developmental expression suggest Flk-1 as a major regulator of vasculogenesis and angiogenesis. Cell 72, 835–846.

Monacci, W.T., Merrill, M.J., Oldfield, E.H., 1993. Expression of vascular permeability factor/vascular endothelial growth factor in normal rat tissues. Am. J. Physiol. 264, 995–1002.

Moser B, Loetscher P. Lymphocyte traffic control by chemokines. Nat Immunol 2001; 2: 123–8.

Müller A, Homey B, Soto H, Ge N, Catron D, Buchanan ME, McClanahan T, Murphy E, Yuan W, Wagner SN, Barrera JL, Mohar A, Verástegui E, Zlotnik A. Involvement of chemokine receptors in breast cancer metastasis. Nature. 2001 Mar 1;410(6824):50-6.

Murphy G. The ADAMs: signalling scissors in the tumour microenvironment. Nat Rev Cancer. 2008 Dec;8(12):929-41.

Murphy PM, Baggiolini M, Charo IF, Hébert CA, Horuk R, Matsushima K, Miller LH, Oppenheim JJ, Power CA. International union of pharmacology. XXII. Nomenclature for chemokine receptors. Pharmacol Rev. 2000 Mar;52(1):145-76.

Murphy PM. The molecular biology of leukocyte chemoattractant receptors. Annu Rev Immunol 1994; 12: 593–633.

Nag, S., Takahashi, J.L., Kilty, D.W., 1997. Role of vascular endothelial growth factor in blood–brain barrier breakdown and angiogenesis in brain trauma. J. Neuropathol. Exp. Neurol. 56, 912–921.

Nagasawa T, Hirota S, Tachibana K, Takakura N, Nishikawa S, Kitamura Y, Yoshida N, Kikutani H, Kishimoto T. Defects of B-cell lymphopoiesis and bone-marrow myelopoiesis in mice lacking the CXC chemokine PBSF/SDF-1. Nature. 1996 Aug 15;382(6592):635-8.

Nagy, J.A., A.M. Dvorak, H.F. Dvorak, VEGF-A(164/165) and PlGF: roles in angiogenesis and arteriogenesis, Trends Cardiovasc. Med. 2003, 13, 169– 175.

Nathoo N, Chahlavi A, Barnett GH, Toms SA. Pathobiology of brain metastases. J Clin Pathol. 2005 Mar;58(3):237-42.

Ng YS, Rohan R, Sunday ME, Demello DE, D'Amore PA. Differential expression of VEGF isoforms in mouse during development and in the adult. Dev Dyn 2001;220:112–21.

Ogawa K, Yoshii Y, Nishimaki T, Tamaki N, Miyaguni T, Tsuchida Y, Kamada Y, Toita T, Kakinohana Y, Tamaki W, Iraha S, Adachi G, Hyodo A, Murayama S. Treatment and prognosis of brain metastases from breast cancer. J Neurooncol. 2008 Jan;86(2):231-8.

Ogunshola, O.O., Stewart, W.B., Mihalcik, V., Solli, T., Madri, J.A., Ment, L.R., 2000. Neuronal VEGF expression correlates with angiogenesis in postnatal developing rat brain. Brain Res. Dev. Brain Res. 119, 139– 153.

Orimo A, Gupta PB, Sgroi DC, Arenzana-Seisdedos F, Delaunay T, Naeem R, Carey VJ, Richardson AL, Weinberg RA. Stromal fibroblasts present in invasive human breast carcinomas promote tumor growth and angiogenesis through elevated SDF-1/CXCL12 secretion. Cell. 2005 May 6;121(3):335-48.

Ottaiano A, Franco R, Aiello Talamanca A, Liguori G, Tatangelo F, Delrio P, Nasti G, Barletta E, Facchini G, Daniele B, Di Blasi A, Napolitano M, Ieranò C, Calemma R, Leonardi E, Albino V, De Angelis V, Falanga M, Boccia V, Capuozzo M, Parisi V, Botti G, Castello G, Vincenzo Iaffaioli R, Scala S. Overexpression of both CXC chemokine receptor 4 and vascular endothelial growth factor proteins predicts early distant relapse in stage II-III colorectal cancer patients. Clin Cancer Res. 2006 May 1;12(9):2795-803.

Palmieri D, Smith QR, Lockman PR, Bronder J, Gril B, Chambers AF, Weil RJ, Steeg PS. Brain metastases of breast cancer. Breast Dis. 2006-2007; 26: 139–47.

Papavassiliou, E., Gogate, N., Proescholdt, M., Heiss, J.D., Walbridge, S., Edwards, N.A., Oldfield, E.H., Merrill, M.J., 1997. Vascular endothelial growth factor (vascular permeability factor) expression in injured rat brain. J. Neurosci. Res. 49, 451–460.

Patchell RA. The management of brain metastases. Cancer Treat Rev. 2003 Dec;29(6):533-40.

Pawlowski V, Revillion F, Hebbar M, Hornez L, Peyrat JP. 2000. Prognostic value of the type I growth factor receptors in a large series of human primary breast cancers quantified with a real-time reverse transcription-polymerase chain reaction assay. Clin Cancer Res, 6, pp. 4217–4225.

Pepper MS, Ferrara N, Orci L, Montesano R. Vascular endothelial growth factor (VEGF) induces plasminogen activators and plasminogen activator inhibitor-1 in microvascular endothelial cells. Biochem Biophys Res Commun 1991;181:902–6.

Pestalozzi BC, Brignoli S. 2000. Trastuzumab in CSF. J Clin Oncol, vol. 18, no.11, pp. 2349–2351.

Pestalozzi BC, Zahrieh D, Price KN, et al. 2006. Identifying breast cancer patients at risk for Central Nervous System (CNS) metastases in trials of the International Breast Cancer Study Group (IBCSG). Ann Oncol, vol. 17, no. 6, pp. 935–944.

Peters, K.G., De Vries, C., Williams, L.T., 1993. Vascular endothelial growth factor receptor expression during embryogenesis and tissue repair suggests a role in endothelial differentiation and blood vessel growth. Proc. Natl. Acad. Sci. USA 90, 8915–8919.

Pietsch, T., Valter, M.M., Wolf, H.K., von Deimling, A., Huang, H.J., Cavenee, W.K., Wiestler, O.D., 1997. Expression and distribution of vascular endothelial growth factor protein in human brain tumors. Acta Neuropathol. 93, 109–117.

Plate, K.H., Beck, H., Danner, S., Allegrini, P.R., Wiessner, C., 1999. Cell type specific upregulation of vascular endothelial growth factor in an MCA-occlusion model of cerebral infarct. J. Neuropathol. Exp. Neurol. 58, 654–666.

Porcile C, Bajetto A, Barbero S, Pirani P, Schettini G. CXCR4 activation induces epidermal growth factor receptor transactivation in an ovarian cancer cell line. Ann N Y Acad Sci 2004; 1030: 162–9.

Prudkin L, Liu DD, Ozburn NC, Sun M, Behrens C, Tang X, Brown KC, Bekele BN, Moran C, Wistuba II. Epithelial-to-mesenchymal transition in the development and progression of adenocarcinoma and squamous cell carcinoma of the lung. Mod Pathol. 2009 May;22(5):668-78.

Razmkhah M, Talei AR, Doroudchi M, Khalili-Azad T, Ghaderi A. Stromal cell-derived factor-1 (SDF-1) alleles and susceptibility to breast carcinoma. Cancer Lett. 2005 Jul 28;225(2):261-6.

Raymond E, Faivre S, Armand JP: Epidermal growth factor receptor tyrosine kinase as a target for anticancer therapy. Drugs 2000, 60 Suppl, no.1, pp. 15-23.

Ribatti, D., Alessandri, G., Vacca, A. Iurlaro, M., Ponzoni, M., (1998). "Human neuroblastoma cells produce extracellular matrix-degrading enzymes, induce endothelial cell proliferation and are angiogenic in vivo." Int J Cancer 77(3): 449-54.

Rusnak DW, Lackey K, Affleck K, et al. 2001. The effects of the novel, reversible epidermal growth factor receptor/ErbB-2 tyrosine kinase inhibitor,GW2016, on the growth of human normal and tumor-derived cell lines in vitro and in vivo. Mol Cancer Ther. 2001, vol. 1, no. 2, (Dec 2001), pp. 85–94.

Saad AG, Yeap BY, Thunnissen FB, Pinkus GS, Pinkus JL, Loda M, Sugarbaker DJ, Johnson BE, Chirieac LR. Immunohistochemical markers associated with brain metastases in patients with nonsmall cell lung carcinoma. Cancer. 2008 Oct 15;113(8):2129-38.

Samoto K, Ikezaki K, One M, Shone T, Kohno K, Kuwano M, Fukui M: Expression of vascular endothelial growth factor and its possible relation with ueovascularization in human brain tumours. *Cancer Res* 1995, 55:1189-1193.

Sanna G, Franceschelli L, Rotmensz N, Botteri E, Adamoli L, Marenghi C, Munzone E, Cossu Rocca M, Verri E, Minchella I, Medici M, Catania C, Magni E, Goldhirsch A, Nolè F. Brain metastases in patients with advanced breast cancer. Anticancer Res. 2007; 27: 2865–9.

Scala S, Ottaiano A, Ascierto PA, Cavalli M, Simeone E, Giuliano P, Napolitano M, Franco R, Botti G, Castello G. Expression of CXCR4 predicts poor prognosis in patients with malignant melanoma. Clin Cancer Res. 2005 Mar 1;11(5):1835-41.

Schwechheimer K, Zhou L, Birchmeier W. E-Cadherin in human brain tumours: loss of immunoreactivity in malignant meningiomas. Virchows Arch. 1998 Feb;432(2):163-7.

Shabani HK, Kitange G, Tsunoda K, Anda T, Tokunaga Y, Shibata S, Kaminogo M, Hayashi T, Ayabe H, Iseki M. Immunohistochemical expression of E-cadherin in metastatic brain tumors. Brain Tumor Pathol. 2003;20(1):7-12.

Shemirani, B. and D. L. Crowe. 2000. "Head and neck squamous cell carcinoma lines produce biologically active angiogenic factors." Oral Oncol 36(1): 61-6.

Sierro F, Biben C, Martínez-Muñoz L, Mellado M, Ransohoff RM, Li M, Woehl B, Leung H, Groom J, Batten M, Harvey RP, Martínez-A C, Mackay CR, Mackay F. Disrupted cardiac development but normal hematopoiesis in mice deficient in the second CXCL12/SDF-1 receptor, CXCR7. Proc Natl Acad Sci U S A. 2007 Sep 11;104(37):14759-64.

Silverman WF, Krum JM, Mani N, Rosenstein JM. Vascular, glial and neuronal effects of vascular endothelial growth factor in mesencephalic explant cultures. Neuroscience. 1999;90(4):1529-41.

Slamon DJ, Clark GM, Wong SG, et al. 1987. Human breast cancer: correlation of relapse and survival with amplification of the HER2/neu oncogene. Science, vol. 235, pp.177–182.

Soker, S., Takashima, S., Miao, H.Q., Neufeld, G., Klagsbrun, M., 1998. Neuropilin-1 is expressed by endothelial and tumor cells as an isoformspecific receptor for vascular endothelial growth factor. Cell 92, 735– 745.

Stark AM, Anuszkiewicz B, Mentlein R, Yoneda T, Mehdorn HM, Held-Feindt J. Differential expression of matrix metalloproteinases in brain- and bone-seeking clones of metastatic MDA-MB-231 breast cancer cells. J Neurooncol. 2007 Jan;81(1):39-48.

Strugar JS, Rothbart D, Harrington W, Criscuolo GR: Vascular permeability factor in brain metastases: correlation with vasogenic brain edema and tumour angiogenesis. *J Neurosurg* 1994, 81:560-566.

Sun YX, Wang J, Shelburne CE, Lopatin DE, Chinnaiyan AM, Rubin MA, Pienta KJ, Taichman RS. Expression of CXCR4 and CXCL12 (SDF-1) in human prostate cancers (PCa) in vivo. J Cell Biochem. 2003 Jun 1;89(3):462-73.

Tachibana K, Hirota S, Iizasa H, Yoshida H, Kawabata K, Kataoka Y, Kitamura Y, Matsushima K, Yoshida N, Nishikawa S, Kishimoto T, Nagasawa T. The chemokine receptor CXCR4 is essential for vascularization of the gastrointestinal tract. Nature. 1998 Jun 11;393(6685):591-4.

Terman B, Khandke L, Dougher-Vermazan M, Maglione D, Lassam NJ, Gospodarowicz D, Persico MG, Böhlen P, Eisinger M. VEGF receptor subtypes KDR and FLT1 show different sensitivities to heparin and placenta growth factor. Growth Factors. 1994;11(3):187-95.

Tester AM, Waltham M, Oh SJ, Bae SN, Bills MM, Walker EC, Kern FG, Stetler-Stevenson WG, Lippman ME, Thompson EW. Pro-matrix metalloproteinase-2 transfection increases orthotopic primary growth and experimental metastasis of MDA-MB-231 human breast cancer cells in nude mice. Cancer Res. 2004 Jan 15;64(2):652-8.

Thelen M, Thelen S. CXCR7, CXCR4 and CXCL12: an eccentric trio? J Neuroimmunol. 2008 Jul 31;198(1-2):9-13.

Tohma Y, Yamashima T, Yamashita J. Immunohistochemical localization of cell adhesion molecule epithelial cadherin in human arachnoid villi and meningiomas. Cancer Res. 1992 Apr 1;52(7):1981-7.

Tsao, M.N., Li, Y.Q., Lu, G., Xu, Y., Wong, C.S., 1999. Upregulation of vascular endothelial growth factor is associated with radiation-induced blood–spinal cord barrier breakdown. J. Neuropathol. Exp. Neurol. 58, 1051–1060.

Ueda Y, Neel NF, Schutyser E, Raman D, Richmond A. Deletion of the COOH-terminal domain of CXC chemokine receptor 4 leads to the down-regulation of cell-to-cell contact, enhanced motility and proliferation in breast carcinoma cells. Cancer Res. 2006 Jun 1;66(11):5665-75.

Vajkoczy P, Farhadi M, Gaumann A, et al. Microtumor growth initiates angiogenic sprouting with simultaneous expression of VEGF, VEGF receptor-2, and angiopoietin-2. J Clin Invest 2002;109:777–85.

VanMeter TE, Rooprai HK, Kibble MM, Fillmore HL, Broaddus WC, Pilkington GJ. The role of matrix metalloproteinase genes in glioma invasion: co-dependent and interactive proteolysis. J Neurooncol. 2001 Jun;53(2):213-35.

Vaquero, J., Zurita, M., de Oya, S., Coca, S., 1999. Vascular endothelial growth/permeability factor in spinal cord injury. J. Neurosurg. 90, 220–223.

Vates, G. E., Hashimoto, T., Young, W. L., Lawton, M. T. 2005. "Angiogenesis in the brain during development: the effects of vascular endothelial growth factor and angiopoietin-2 in an animal model." J Neurosurg 103(1): 136-45.

Vu TH, Shipley JM, Bergers G, et al. MMP-9/gelatinase B is a key regulator of growth plate angiogenesis and apoptosis of hypertrophic chondrocytes. Cell 1998;93:411–22.

Wang J, Jarrett J, Huang CC, Satcher RL Jr, Levenson AS. Identification of estrogen-responsive genes involved in breast cancer metastases to the bone. Clin Exp Metastasis. 2007; 24: 411–22.

Xu, T., Chen, D., Chen, J. 2004. "Expression of vascular endothelial growth factor C and its correlation with lymph node metastasis in colorectal carcinoma." J Huazhong Univ Sci Technolog Med Sci 24(6): 596-8.

Xue C, Liang F, Mahmood R, Vuolo M, Wyckoff J, et al. 2006. ErbB3-dependent motility and intravasation in breast cancer metastasis. Cancer Res, vol. 66, no.3, pp.1418–1426.

Yamazaki, Y. , K. Takani, H. Atoda, T. Morita, Snake venom vascular endothelial growth factors (VEGFs) exhibit potent activity through their specific recognition of KDR (VEGF receptor 2), J. Biol. Chem. 2003 278, 51985- 51988.

Yang W, Lam P, Kitching R, Kahn HJ, Yee A, Aubin JE, Seth A. Breast cancer metastasis in a human bone NOD/SCID mouse model. Cancer Biol Ther. 2007; 6: 1289–94.

Yang W, Lam P, Kitching R, Kahn HJ, Yee A, Aubin JE, Seth A. Breast cancer metastasis in a human bone NOD/SCID mouse model. Cancer Biol Ther. 2007; 6: 1289–94.

Yano, S., H. Shinohara, Herbst, R. S. Kuniyasu, H. Bucana, C. D. Ellis, L. M. Davis, D. W. McConkey, D. J. Fidler, I. J. 2000. "Expression of vascular endothelial growth factor is necessary but not sufficient for production and growth of brain metastasis." Cancer Res 60(17): 4959-67.

Yasmeen A, Bismar TA, Al Moustafa AE ErbB receptors and epithelial-cadherin-catenin complex in human carcinomas. Future Oncol. 2006 Dec;2(6):765-81.

Yasmeen A, Bismar TA, Dekhil H, Ricciardi R, Kassab A, Gambacorti-Passerini C, Al Moustafa AE. ErbB-2 receptor cooperates with E6/E7 oncoproteins of HPV type 16 in breast tumorigenesis. Cell Cycle. 2007 Dec 1;6(23):2939-43.

Zagzag D, Amirnovin R, Greco MA, et al. Vascular apoptosis and involution in gliomas precede neovascularization: a novel concept for glioma growth and angiogenesis. Lab Invest 2000;80: 837–49.

Zeljko M, Pecina-Slaus N, Martic TN, Kusec V, Beros V, Tomas D. Molecular alterations of E-cadherin and beta-catenin in brain metastases. Front Biosci (Elite Ed). 2011 Jan 1;3:616-24.

Zhan L, Xiang B, Muthuswamy SK. 2006. Controlled activation of ErbB1/ErbB2 heterodimerspromote invasion of three-dimensional organized epithelia in an ErbB1-dependent manner: implications for progression of ErbB2-overexpressing tumors. Cancer Res, 66, no. 3, pp. 5201–5208.

Zlotnik A, Yoshie O. Chemokines: a new classification system and their role in immunity. Immunity. 2000 Feb;12(2):121-7.

Zlotnik A. Chemokines and cancer. Int J Cancer 2006b; 119: 2026–9.

Zlotnik A. Involvement of chemokine receptors in organ-specific metastasis. Contrib Microbiol 2006a; 13: 191–9.

Zou YR, Kottmann AH, Kuroda M, Taniuchi I, Littman DR. Function of the chemokine receptor CXCR4 in haematopoiesis and in cerebellar development. Nature 1998; 393: 595–9.

7

Trastuzumab-Resistance and Breast Cancer

Milos Dokmanovic and Wen Jin Wu*

Division of Monoclonal Antibodies, Office of Biotechnology Products, Office of Pharmaceutical Science, Center for Drug Evaluation and Research, U.S. Food and Drug Administration, Bethesda, Maryland, United States of America

1. Introduction

Evolution of therapeutic monoclonal antibodies significantly benefited from the recombinant DNA technologies that are used to generate chimeric, humanized, and human versions of monoclonal antibody to reduce the problem of immunogenicity and neutralization, as well as from understanding mechanisms of action mediated by monoclonal antibodies (Nelson et al., 2010; Reichert, 2009; Ranson & Sliwkowski , 2002). One of the significant advances in the application of monoclonal antibodies in oncology was the introduction and approval of trastuzumab, a humanized anti-HER2 antibody, for the treatment of HER2-positive breast cancer.

Despite initial successes and encouraging results, development of monoclonal antibody-based therapies faces several challenges (Yan et al., 2009). Among them are the selection of patients most likely to benefit from clinical trials and lack of understanding of mechanisms of resistance to monoclonal antibody-based therapies (Yan et al., 2009). Selection of patients most likely to benefit from clinical trials of monoclonal antibody-based therapies was initially based on the expression of the antigen targeted by the monoclonal antibody. The anti-HER-2 antibody trastuzumab was tested in patients whose breast tumors overexpress HER2 (Pegram et al., 1998) and the anti-epidermal growth factor receptor (EGFR) antibody cetuximab was used in patients with colorectal cancer and head and neck cancers that overexpress EGFR (Shin et al., 2001). Even with careful characterization of the antigen expression level in the patient population eligible for the clinical trials, primary resistance to monoclonal antibody-based therapies is a common problem. Up to 50% of EGFR-positive colorectal cancer patients are resistant to cetuximab (Saltz et al., 2004), and 74% of HER2-positive breast cancer patients are resistant to anti-HER2 antibody trastuzumab (Vogel et al., 2002).

It has emerged that the levels of antigen expression are not the only determinant of the patient response to monoclonal antibody therapies and that better understanding of the mechanisms of resistance to monoclonal antibodies in different patient subgroups has a potential to improve the effectiveness of the monoclonal antibody treatment. A retrospective analysis of the colorectal tumor samples from the patients that received cetuximab therapy indicated that EGFR-positive colorectal cancer patients with wild-type KRAS gene had increased overall

* Disclaimer: The information presented in this article reflects the views of the authors and does not represent the policy of the U.S. Food and Drug Administration.

survival, progression-free survival and improvement in the global health status compared to the patients whose tumors had KRAS mutations (Karapetis et al., 2008; Lievre et al., 2006). KRAS protein is a member of RAS super family of small GTP-binding proteins and a molecule downstream of the EGFR-mediated signaling cascade, and when aberrantly regulated, KRAS protein contributes to cancer development and progression (Karnoub & Weinberg, 2008). Cellular studies supported the role of KRAS mutations in the resistance to anti-EGFR antibody cetuximab (Benvenuti et al., 2007). Understanding of the role of the KRAS mutations in the resistance to the anti-EGFR antibody cetuximab has improved the selection of patients that are eligible for cetuximab treatment and as a consequence, cetuximab is currently approved for the treatment of EGFR-positive colorectal cancers that do not have KRAS mutations in codon 12 or 13. While KRAS mutations play a critical role in diminishing response to cetuximab in colorectal cancer patients, KRAS gene is infrequently mutated in breast cancer (Karnoub & Weinberg, 2008; Sanchez-Munoz et al., 2010), and it is therefore not likely to contribute to the resistance to anti-HER2 monoclonal antibody trastuzumab. The molecular basis for the resistance to anti-HER2 monoclonal antibody trastuzumab in breast cancer is still not well understood, and there are no clinically useful predictive biomarkers that can be used in conjunction with HER2 expression to predict the outcome of trastuzumab treatment in the HER2-positive breast cancer patients. Breast cancer is one of the most common cancers among women in the United States. It is the second leading cause of cancer death in women, after lung cancer. Women with HER2-overexpressing breast cancers have an increased risk of recurrence and shortened disease-free and overall survival rates (Press et al., 1993; Slamon et al., 1987; Slamon et al., 1989). Understanding the mechanism of resistance to trastuzumab and identifying the predictive biomarkers for the therapeutic resistance to trastuzumab could lead to important therapeutic advances.

Therapeutic monoclonal antibodies represent one of the most dynamic sectors in the biopharmaceutical industry (Reichert, 2009). Twelve monoclonal antibodies and antibodies-related products are licensed for the diagnosis and treatment of specific oncology indications in the U.S. (Table 1) (Note: gemtuzumab ozogamicin was withdrawn from the market in June 2010).

2. HER family of receptor tyrosine kinases

HER2 is a member of the HER family of receptor tyrosine kinases, which is composed of four type I receptors: EGFR/HER1/ErbB1, HER2/ErbB2, HER3/ErbB3, and HER4/ErbB4. All receptors share a similar structure composed of an extracellular ligand-binding region, a single transmembrane lipophilic segment and a cytoplasmic tyrosine kinase-containing domain (Zhang et al. 2007). The extracellular ligand-binding region of HER family receptors is composed of four domains (I-IV). Domains I and III are important for ligand binding. Domain II mediates receptor dimerization. Domain IV forms intramolecular interactions with the domain II and thus blocks dimerization (Garrett et al., 2003). Ligand binding to the extracellular domain of HER family members disrupts the autoinhibition conformation which results in the receptor homo- or hetero-dimerization, and transphosphorylation followed by the activation of the downstream signaling pathways which regulate cell growth and differentiation (Hudis, 2007; Hynes & Lane, 2005). The physiological ligand for HER2 has not been identified yet. HER3 function is particularly important due to its role in the development of resistance in HER2-overexpressing cancers. HER3 binds neuregulins via its extracellular region to mediate signals primarily by heterodimerization with HER2 in

Antibody name (USAN)	Antibody tradename	Therapeutic target	Antibody type	Clinical Indication	Year of approval
Ipilimumab	Yervoy	CTLA-4	IgG1/human	Advanced melanoma	2011
Ofatumumab	Arzerra	CD20	IgG1/human	Chronic lymphocytic leukemia	2009
Panitumumab	Vectibix	EGFR	IgG2/human	Colorectal cancer	2006
Cetuximab	Erbitux	EGFR	IgG1/chimeric	Colorectal cancer Head and Neck Squamous Cell Cancer	2004 2006
Bevacizumab	Avastin	VEGF-A	IgG1/humanized	Colorectal cancer	2004
I131-Tositumomab	Bexxar	CD20	IgG2/mouse	Non-Hodgkin lymphoma	2003
Y90 or I111-Ibritumomab-tiuxetan	Zevelin	CD20	IgG1/mouse	Non-Hodgkin lymphoma	2002
Alemtuzumab	Campath	CD52	IgG1/humanized	Chronic lymphocytic leukemia	2001
Gemtuzumab Ozogamicin	Mylotarg	CD33	IgG4/humanized linked to calichaemicin	Acute myeloid leukemia	2000 withdrawn in June 2010
Trastuzumab	Herceptin	HER2	IgG1/humanized	HER2-positive breast cancer	1998
Rituximab	Rituxan	CD20	IgG1/chimeric	Non-Hodgkin lymphoma	1997
Capromab pendetide	ProstaScint	PSMA	IgG1/murine	Prostate cancer imaging	1996

Table 1. FDA approved monoclonal antibodies used for diagnosis and treatment of different oncological indications.

tumors containing amplifications of HER2 (Baselga & Swain, 2009; Shi et al., 2010). In fact, HER3-HER2 is considered the most active HER signaling dimer (Tzahar et al., 1996). HER3 also plays a key role in the ability of HER2-overexpressing cells to escape the growth inhibition by the EGFR/HER2 dual-specific tyrosine kinase inhibitor (TKI) lapatinib (Sergina et al., 2007). Previously, the intracellular kinase domain of HER3 was thought to be an inactive pseudokinase, because it lacks several key conserved and catalytically important residues (Guy et al., 1994, Sierke et al., 1997). Recently however, HER3 was shown to have

kinase activity and the ability to trans-autophosphorylate its intracellular region although it is substantially less active than EGFR (Shi et al., 2010). HER2 extracellular domain adopts a fixed conformation that resembles a ligand-activated state that permits it to form a dimer in the absence of a ligand (Cho at al., 2003; Garrett et al., 2003; Hynes & Lane, 2005). This likely explains why HER2 is the preferred dimerization partner for all of the other HER receptors (Graus-Porta et al., 1997). Moreover, although none of ligands for the HER family receptors directly binds to HER2, activation of EGFR, HER3, and HER4 can facilitate transactivation of HER2 through ligand-induced heterodimerization (Carraway et al., 1994; Wada et al., 1990).
Overexpression of HER2 has been reported in different types of cancer, including breast, gastric, ovarian and salivary gland (Baselga & Swain, 2009). Gene amplification is the most common mechanism resulting in HER2 overexpression in tumors. In addition, somatic mutations in the HER2 tyrosine kinase domain are reported in lung adenocarcinomas, epithelial ovarian cancer, hepatocellular carcinoma, gastric, colorectal and breast cancers, but the activating function for these mutations has not been clarified (Bekaii-Saab et al., 2006; Lee et al., 2006; Lin at al., 2011; Shigematsu et al., 2005). Recent studies also suggest that mutational inactivation in FOXP3 tumor suppressor may contribute to HER2 promoter activation in breast cancer tissues (Zuo et al., 2007). Regardless of the causative mechanisms resulting in HER2 overexpression in certain cancer, the number of HER2 molecules expressed on the surface of these cancer cells far exceeds the number expressed on normal cells, which facilitates the formation of HER2 heterodimers and the spontaneous formation of HER2 homodimers (Yarden & Sliwkowski, 2001). The consequence of this is an excess of HER2-mediated signaling, which drives oncogenic cell survival and proliferation (Yarden & Sliwkowski, 2001).

3. Trastuzumab and mechanisms of action of trastuzumab

For the past 20 years, the development of monoclonal antibodies and tyrosine kinase inhibitors (TKIs) targeting HER2 has been intensely pursued as important cancer therapeutic strategy. There are several reasons why HER2 is an attractive target in breast cancer treatment. First, the levels of HER2 in human cancer cells are higher than that in normal tissues and the elevated levels of HER2 correlate with the pathogenesis and prognosis in breast cancer (Natali et al., 1990; Slamon et al., 1987). Second, HER2 is overexpressed in approximately 20-30% of invasive breast cancer and is associated with poor disease-free survival and poor response to chemotherapy (Gusterson et al., 1992; Paik et al., 1990; Slamon et al., 1989). Third, HER2 is overexpressed in primary tumors and in metastatic sites suggesting that anti-HER2 therapy could be effective in all disease locations (Niehans et al., 1993). Trastuzumab is a recombinant humanized monoclonal antibody directed against the extracellular domain IV of HER2 and is approved for the treatment of HER2-positive breast cancer. In 2010, the European Medicines Agency approved trastuzumab for gastric cancer patients with high expression of HER2 (Okines et al., 2010). Subsequently, in October 2010, U.S. FDA approved trastuzumab in combination with chemotherapy for HER2-positive metastatic cancer of the stomach or the gastroesophageal junction.
Trastuzumab was engineered by inserting the antigen binding loops of a murine antibody (clone 4D5) into the framework of a consensus human IgG_1 using gene conversion mutagenesis strategy (Carter et al., 1992; Pegram et al., 1999). The humanized version of 4D5 (also known as rhuMabHER2; later named trastuzumab) showed significant effects in

HER2-overexpressing breast cancer cells and in HER2-overexpressing xenograft breast cancer models either alone or in combination with other chemotherapy agents (Pegram et al., 1999). While the mechanisms by which trastuzumab induces regression of HER2-positive breast cancers are still being investigated, it is currently believed that the binding of trastuzumab to HER2 contributes to its therapeutic effect by a) inducing HER2 endocytosis followed by receptor degradation; b) inhibiting either HER2 homodimerization or heterodimerization; c) preventing the cleavage of HER2 extracellular domain by the metalloprotease ADAM10 (Hudis, 2007). Taken together, binding of trastuzumab to the extracellular domain of HER2 reduces HER2-coupled mitogenic and pro-survival signaling pathways in tumor cells, leading to the inhibition of phosphatidylinositol 3-kinase (PI3K) and mitogen-activated protein kinase (MAPK) pathways, and the induction of the cyclin-dependent kinase inhibitor, p27 (Nahta & Esteva, 2006). Furthermore, trastuzumab is an IgG_1 subtype capable of inducing antibody-dependent cell mediated cytotoxicity (ADCC). Overexpression of HER2 in human tumor cells is closely associated with the increased angiogenesis and the expression of vascular endothelial growth factor (VEGF). Trastuzumab has also been shown to inhibit tumor angiogenesis, resulting in decreased microvessel density *in vivo* and reduced endothelial cell migration *in vitro* (Nahta & Esteva, 2006).

4. HER2-overexpression and clinical indications for trastuzumab

Trastuzumab is an anti-HER2 antibody indicated for the treatment of HER2-positive breast cancer and HER2-positive metastatic gastric or gastroesophageal (GE) junction adenocarcinoma. Three testing methodologies can be used to determine the HER2 status of the tumor samples: immunocytochemistry (IHC), fluorescence in situ hybridization (FISH), and chromogenic in situ hybridization (CISH) (Wolff et al., 2007). IHC detects the level of membrane bound HER2, whereas FISH and CISH detect the level of HER2 gene amplification. The American Society of Clinical Oncology/College of American Pathologists guideline was developed to define the status of HER2-positive breast cancer and recommended the use of a combination of IHC and FISH testing (Wolff et al., 2007). According to the guideline, a positive HER2 result is the IHC staining of 3+, and a FISH result of more than six HER2 gene copies per nucleus or a FISH ratio (HER2 gene signals to chromosome 17 signals) of more than 2.2 (Wolff et al., 2007). Trastuzumab was the first monoclonal antibody therapy to be approved with a companion diagnostic assay which was used to select the patients eligible for the trastuzumab treatment (Reichert, 2009).

Trastuzumab, when used as a single agent, produced an objective response rate up to 26% in the selected HER2-positive metastatic breast cancer patients (Vogel et al., 2002). Preclinical studies of the combinations of trastuzumab and different chemotherapy agents suggested the potential for additive and/or synergistic effects in the clinical settings (Baselga et al., 1998). Clinical studies then showed that trastuzumab in combination with chemotherapy in HER2-positive metastatic breast cancers significantly improved overall response rate, median overall survival, and time to disease progression (Burstein et al., 2001; Kaufman et al., 2009; Marty et al., 2005; O'Shaughnessy et al., 2004; Pegram et al., 1998; Perez et al., 2005; Slamon et al., 2001). Clinical benefit of trastuzumab treatment in HER2-positive metastatic breast cancer provided the rationale for testing the effects of trastuzumab treatment in the early stage HER2-positive breast cancer in the adjuvant and neoadjuvant setting. The adjuvant therapy is defined as any treatment given after the primary therapy, usually surgery, to increase the chance of long term survival, whereas neoadjuvant therapy refers to the treatment given before the primary therapy. While many clinical trials are still ongoing, there are promising results for the use of trastuzumab treatment in the adjuvant and neoadjuvant settings. It was reported that one year of trastuzumab treatment after adjuvant chemotherapy significantly improved disease free survival and that trastuzumab combined concurrently with the chemotherapy improved the outcomes among HER2-positive breast cancer patients (Piccart-Gebhart et al., 2005). In addition to the use of trastuzumab in adjuvant settings, some of the clinical studies addressed the potential benefit of offering trastuzumab in the neoadjuvant settings. Results from the GeparQuattro study suggested that neoadjuvant combination of trastuzumab and different chemotherapy agents induced a high pathological complete response (pCR) rate with the minimal toxicities (Untch et al., 2010). pCR is defined as the complete absence of intact tumor cells in the resected specimen. Trastuzumab is now a standard of care in combination with chemotherapy for patients with HER2-positive breast cancer (Banerjee & Smith, 2010).

5. Resistance to the EGFR-targeted therapies

Targeting the EGFR has been intensely pursued in the past decade as a cancer treatment strategy. Small molecule tyrosine kinase inhibitors (TKIs) and anti-EGFR monoclonal antibodies are the primary approaches to inhibit EGFR-coupled signaling pathways. To date, three tyrosine kinase inhibitors, erlotinib, gefitinib, and lapatinib, have been approved for oncology indications. Cetuximab, a chimeric IgG_1 directed against the extracellular domain of EGFR, was originally generated from a murine antibody, 225 (Goldstein et al., 1995). Preclinical studies showed that cetuximab was more effective than the murine antibody 225 in inhibiting tumor growth in A431 human tumor xenografts model. Based on the preclinical studies, cetuximab was found to inhibit EGFR activation by preventing ligand binding, which inhibits EGFR dimerization and induces the EGFR internalization and downregulation (Goldstein et al., 1995; Mendelsohn, 2002). Cetuximab was approved in 2004 by FDA for the treatment of EGFR expressing metastatic colorectal cancer. In 2006, FDA approved the use of cetuximab for the treatment of locally advanced or regionally advanced head and neck squamous cell carcinomas (HNSCC). In 2006, panitumumab, a human antibody directed against the EGFR was also approved for the treatment of EGFR expressing metastatic colorectal cancer (Giusti et al., 2008; Hecht et al., 2009; Van Cutsem et al., 2007).
Molecular mechanisms contributing to the resistance to EGFR kinase inhibitors have been extensively studied. Important findings suggest that there is a strong relationship between the resistance to EGFR TKIs and the absence of an activating mutation in the intracellular kinase domain of the receptor. These EGFR kinase domain mutations, such as the point mutation, L858R, and in-frame deletion in exon 19 around codons 746–750, enhance the ligand-dependent activation of EGFR, and simultaneously increase the sensitivity to the TKIs (Han et al., 2005; Mitsudomi et al., 2005; Morgillo et al., 2007). It has also been demonstrated that the patients with the EGFR mutation-positive tumors have an improved response rate and survival after treatment with TKIs compared to the patients with tumors that express wild-type EGFR (Han et al., 2005; Mitsudomi et al., 2005). Therefore, the lack of these mutations can be considered a predictor of the treatment resistance to TKI (Morgillo et al, 2007). Mechanisms contributing to the primary resistance to EGFR TKIs also include genetic alterations, for example, EGFR variant III (EGFRvIII) and activating KRAS mutations. EGFRvIII lacks the ligand binding domain and is a constitutively activated mutant. It has also been reported that a point mutation in the exon 20 (T790M) in the kinase

domain of the EGFR gene occurs in tumors with acquired resistance to EGFR kinase inhibitors, gefitinib and erlotinib (Pao et al., 2005). Because mutations within HER2 have not been commonly found in HER2-overexpressing breast tumors (Zito et al., 2008), the mechanisms of resistance to EGFR kinase inhibitors may not be relevant to trastuzumab.
Although EGFR tyrosine kinase domain mutations may predict response to the TKIs, no mutations in the EGFR have been associated with resistance to the antibody-based therapies, cetuximab and panitumumab (Mukohara et al., 2005; Kruser & Wheeler, 2010). While EGFR gene amplification may be both predictive and prognostic and associated with the objective tumor response to cetuximab therapy, IHC based assay measuring EGFR expression may not be an accurate predictive factor for response to cetuximab therapy in colorectal cancer (Chung et al., 2005; Lievre et al., 2006), indicating that different mechanisms may contribute to cetuximab-resistance. One of the most reliable predictive biomarkers to emerge in the clinic has been that of the KRAS mutation status in colorectal cancer (Kruser & Wheeler, 2010). Lievre et al. reported that KRAS mutation status was predictive of resistance to cetuximab therapy. In this report, 30 metastatic colorectal carcinoma patients treated with cetuximab were analyzed for KRAS mutations. The authors reported that KRAS mutation was found in 43% (13 tumors) and was significantly associated with resistance to cetuximab therapy (Lievre et al., 2006). A larger study was performed to measure the KRAS mutation status in 113 patients with refractory metastatic colorectal cancer treated with cetuximab. The authors found that KRAS wild-type is a strong predictor of significant increase in progression-free survival (PFS) and overall survival (OS) in this cohort of patients (De Roock et al., 2008). Many other clinical trials have confirmed these findings, leading to a Provisional Clinical Opinion from the American Society for Clinical Oncology (ASCO) stating that all patients with metastatic colorectal carcinoma who are candidates for anti-EGFR antibody therapy should have their tumor tested for KRAS mutations in a Clinical Laboratory Improvement Amendments (CLIA)-accredited laboratory (Allegra et al., 2009). If codon 12 or 13 of KRAS is found to be mutated then patients with metastatic colorectal cancer should not receive anti-EGFR antibody therapy as a part of their treatment (Allegra et al., 2009).

6. Therapeutic resistance to trastuzumab

6.1 Clinical evidence for trastuzumab-resistance

While trastuzumab has significantly changed the outcome for the treatment of HER2-positive breast cancer, mechanisms contributing to trastuzumab-resistance are less well understood. Both primary and acquired resistance to trastuzumab pose a significant hurdle in the breast cancer therapy (Nahta & Esteva, 2006). Primary trastuzumab resistance refers to the lack of response to trastuzumab treatment in the patients with HER2-positive breast tumors who were never treated with trastuzumab before, whereas acquired resistance indicates that the patients who achieve initial response to trastuzumab acquire resistance to this antibody. In the study which evaluated the efficacy and the safety of trastuzumab as a single agent, the reported rate of primary trastuzumab-resistance was 74%, indicating that the vast majority of HER2-positive metastatic breast cancer patients demonstrate intrinsic resistance to single-agent trastuzumab (Vogel et al., 2002). Moreover, while addition of trastuzumab to chemotherapy in the cohort of HER2-positive metastatic breast cancer patients results in the higher response rates, and the extension of time to disease progression, the durations of response to trastuzumab in either the single-agent setting or in the combination with chemotherapy has been reported to be 5-9 month (Kruser & Wheeler 2010; Nahta & Esteva, 2006; Slamon et al., 2001). Therefore, the majority of patients with HER2-positive breast cancer develops acquired resistance within one year. (Kruser & Wheeler 2010; Nahta & Esteva, 2006; Slamon et al., 2001). Understanding the mechanisms of trastuzumab-resistance and developing predictive biomarkers for therapeutic resistance to trastuzumab are critical to the discovery of novel agents that could overcome trastuzumab-resistance and potentially benefit HER2-positive breast cancer patients.

6.2 Preclinical studies

6.2.1 Cellular models used for the studies of trastuzumab-resistance

There are several preclinical cellular models developed to study the mechanisms of resistance to trastuzumab. HER2-positive breast cancer cell lines were chronically exposed to trastuzumab either *in vitro* (SKBR3 cell line) or in xenograft settings (BT474 cell line) in order to develop trastuzumab-resistant clones and populations (Nahta et al., 2004a; Ritter et al., 2007). In this approach, a comparison between parental trastuzumab-sensitive and derived trastuzumab-resistant clones was carried out in order to characterize the changes in the cell signaling pathways associated with trastuzumab-resistance. Recently, the JIMT-1 cell line was established from a breast cancer patient with HER2 gene amplification and primary resistance to trastuzumab and was used to study the mechanisms of resistance to trastuzumab (Tanner et al., 2004). These trastuzumab-resistant cell lines still overexpress HER2, suggesting that resistance to trastuzumab is not due to the loss of HER2 overexpression (Diermeier et al., 2005; Dokmanovic et al., 2009; Nagy et al., 2005; Ritter et al., 2007). Interestingly, it was reported recently that chronic exposure of BT-474 cells to trastuzumab gave rise to trastuzumab-resistant clones, which lost HER2 gene amplification and HER2 overexpression (Mittendorf et al., 2009). However, it is not clear whether trastuzumab eliminated HER2-overexpressing clones leaving only HER2-negative cancer clones or that the treatment with trastuzumab inhibited HER2 expression or induced downregulation of HER2, resulting in the loss of HER2 expression and resistance to trastuzumab.

6.2.2 Molecular mechanisms of trastuzumab-resistance

Trastuzumab-resistance may be broadly divided into two mechanistic categories. The first occurs at the cell membrane where aberrant regulation of HER2 results in deregulation of HER2 signaling pathways. The second results from changes to HER2-regulated intracellular signaling molecules that result in uncoupling signaling from their upstream regulation. Examples of the latter category include PTEN loss or expression of a constitutively activated PI3K mutant, PIK3CA.

Based on *in vitro* breast cancer cell models of trastuzumab-resistance, HER2 interactions with other membrane-associated proteins contribute to resistance. For example, in the JIMT-1 trastuzumab-resistant breast cancer cell line, binding of MUC4 glycoprotein to HER2 partially masks the trastuzumab binding site in HER2, resulting in reduced trastuzumab binding and contributing to trastuzumab-resistance (Nagy et al., 2005). Trastuzumab binding to HER2 in JIMT-1 cells was restored by downregulation of MUC4 protein (Nagy et al., 2005). Formation of homodimers, and heterodimers between EGFR, HER2, and HER3 due to overexpression of HER family ligands interferes with trastuzumab-mediated growth inhibition and contributes to trastuzumab-resistance (Diermeier et al., 2005; Motoyama 2002;

Ritter et al., 2007; Valabrega et al., 2005). *In vitro* models using breast cancer cells derived for resistance to trastuzumab found that Insulin-like growth factor-I receptor (IGF-IR) heterodimerizes with and phosphorylates ErbB2 suggesting that transactivation of ErbB2 by IGF1R may contribute to resistance (Nahta et al., 2005; Lu et al., 2004). Heterotrimerization of the growth factor receptors HER2, HER3 and IGF-IR in BT-474 breast cancer cells interferes with trastuzumab-associated p27 induction and therefore contributes to trastuzumab-resistance (Huang et al., 2010). Increased activity of small GTP-binding protein Rac1 interrupts with trastuzumab-induced HER2 endocytosis and degradation, resulting in the upregulated HER2-mediated signaling in SKBR3 breast cancer cells contributing to trastuzumab-resistance (Dokmanovic et al., 2009). The Met receptor tyrosine kinase, which is aberrantly expressed in breast cancer and predicts poor patient prognosis, is frequently expressed in HER2-overexpressing breast cancer cells, as well as in HER2-positive breast cancer, and Met activation protects cells against trastuzumab by abrogating p27 induction, thus contributing to trastuzumab resistance (Shattuck et al., 2008). Moreover, HER2-overexpressing breast cancer cells rapidly up-regulate Met expression after trastuzumab treatment, promoting their own resistance (Shattuck et al., 2008). As mentioned in the previous paragraph, loss of HER2 expression in HER2-overexpression breast cancer cells could be another mechanism contributing to trastuzumab resistance (Mittendorf et al., 2009). HER2 receptor initiated downstream signaling promotes cell proliferation and cell survival by the activation of RAS-MAPK and PI3K/Akt/mTOR pathways (Hudis, 2007; Zhou et al., 2004). Addition of trastuzumab to HER2-positive trastuzumab-sensitive cells results in the activation of PTEN, which acts as a tumor suppressor to induce inhibition of Akt phosphorylation and, therefore, antagonizes the PI3K/Akt survival pathway (Nagata et al., 2004). Nagata et al. reported that reducing PTEN in breast cancer cells by antisense oligonucleotides conferred trastuzumab-resistance and that inhibition of PI3K activity enhanced trastuzumab-mediated growth inhibition in a trastuzumab-resistant xenograft model (Nagata et al., 2004). PTEN knockdown in a large scale of RNA interference screening was found to be associated with selective isolation of cell clones resistant to trastuzumab (Berns et al., 2007). Constitutive activation of PI3K, such as PIK3CA mutant, can uncouple Akt signaling from the upstream regulation resulting in trastuzumab-resistance (Berns et al., 2007).

6.3 Clinical studies

Clinical studies have focused on characterization of the HER2 status and HER2-initiated downstream signaling pathways in the samples obtained from trastuzumab-sensitive patients and trastuzumab-resistant patients. A subtype of HER2-positive tumors with distinct biological and clinical features expresses a series of carboxyl terminal fragments of HER2 known as p95HER2. It is generally accepted that the p95HER2 can arise either by proteolytic shedding of the extracellular domain of the full-length HER2 by metalloproteinases ADAM10 at a site proximal to the transmembrane domain or by translation of the mRNA encoding truncated HER2 receptor from the internal initiation codons (Arribas et al., 2011). It is believed that trastuzumab has the ability to prevent proteolytic shedding of full-length HER2 on HER2-overexpressing breast cancer cells (Hudis, 2007). p95HER2 contains a hyperactive membrane anchored fragment that lacks the extracellular domain of HER2 and drives breast cancer progression *in vivo*. Of note, expression of p95HER2 fragments in transgenic mouse models leads to the generation of the breast tumors that were more aggressive and metastatic than those driven by full-length HER2 (Pedersen et al., 2009). Expression of the p95HER2 fragment is predictive of poor prognosis and correlates with resistance to trastuzumab treatment in breast cancer patients (Arribas et al., 2011; Carney et al., 2003). This is likely due to the absence of the extracellular domain (ECD) required for trastuzumab binding (Arribas et al., 2011). The ECD of HER2 can be released into the circulation after cleavage of HER2 by the metalloproteinases ADAM10. It was reported that the prevalence of increased levels of ECD in patient serum with primary breast cancer varied between 0% and 38%, whereas in metastatic breast cancer the range was from 23% to 80% (Carney et al., 2003). Moreover, Ali et al. reported that the decrease in serum levels of HER2 ECD was positively associated with trastuzumab-sensitivity (Ali et al., 2008). In particular, in an analysis of 307 patients with metastatic breast cancer, individuals who did not achieve a significant decline (defined as ≥ 20%) in serum level of serum HER2 ECD after receiving trastuzumab had decreased benefit from trastuzumab-based therapy (Ali et al., 2008).

The analysis of *HER2* gene amplification before and after trastuzumab therapy suggested that patients who had lost *HER2* gene amplification had a significantly decreased recurrence free survival (RFS) compared with patients whose tumors remained *HER2* amplified after trastuzumab treatment (Mittendorf et al., 2009). Nagata et al. revealed that patients with PTEN-deficient breast cancers had significantly reduced responses to trastuzumab-based therapy than those with normal PTEN, suggesting PTEN deficiency may be a predictor to trastuzumab resistance (Nagata et al., 2004). Analysis of the 137 patient samples with HER2-positive metastatic breast cancer who received trastuzumab therapy revealed that activation of PI3K either by PTEN loss and/or PIK3CA mutational activation was associated with a poor response to trastuzumab and a shorter patient survival time (Esteva et al., 2010). In a neoadjuvant clinical trial, which examined the association between response to trastuzumab therapy and the status of PTEN level and PIK3CA mutations, it was found that only 15.4% of subjects with low nuclear PTEN had pathological complete response (pCR) to trastuzumab compared to 44.4% of subjects with high nuclear PTEN levels. It was reported that 20% of patients with PIK3CA activating mutations achieved pCR compared to 38.1 % of patients with wild-type PIK3 status. When the two biomarkers (PTEN level and PIK3CA status) were combined together only 18.2% of patients with low PTEN or PIK3CA achieved pCR to trastuzumab compared to 66.7 % of patients who did not have low PTEN level or PI3KAC mutations (Dave et al., 2011). Taken together, loss of PTEN and PIK3CA activating mutations are associated with trastuzumab-resistance.

Cyclin E is a critical regulator of the cell cycle G1/S transition and cyclin E levels are regulated by HER2 signaling in breast cancer cells (Mittendorf et al., 2010). Trastuzumab treatment reduces cyclin E level and activity in breast cancer cells (Mittendorf et al., 2010).

It has been recently reported that in a cohort of 34 HER2-positive breast cancer patients treated with trastuzumab-based therapy, cyclin E amplification/overexpression was associated with a worse clinical benefit and a lower progression-free survival compared with non-overexpressing cyclin E tumors, suggesting that cyclin E amplification/ overexpression may contribute to trastuzumab-resistance in HER-positive breast cancer patients (Scaltriti et al., 2011). Interestingly, in an analysis of 26 tumor samples (10 cyclin E positive and 16 cyclin E negative), cyclin E amplification only partially correlated with other clinically relevant trastuzumab-resistant markers, such as p95HER2 and PTEN loss (Scaltriti et al., 2011). This suggests that cyclin E amplification/overexpression might use a different mechanism to contribute to trastuzumab-resistance as compared to p95HER2 and PTEN loss.

7. Toxicity and trastuzumab-related cardiotoxicity

Trastuzumab is generally well tolerated with mild to moderate side effects and low incidence of chemotherapy associated adverse events (Brufsky, 2010). The side effects reported in different clinical trials include cardiomyopathy, infusion reactions, embryo-fetal toxicity, pulmonary toxicity, exacerbation of chemotherapy-induced neutropenia, diarrhea, burning sensation in the skin, rash, and nausea and vomiting, upper respiratory tract infection, increased cough. Among those side effects, the trastuzumab-related cardiotoxicity has drawn great attention for trastuzumab-based therapy.

Trastuzumab associated cardiac dysfunction was initially reported in a phase III trial, which tested the efficacy of combining chemotherapy with trastuzumab versus chemotherapy alone in metastatic breast cancer disease (Slamon et al., 2001). The addition of trastuzumab increased the incidence of chemotherapy-associated symptomatic and asymptomatic cardiac dysfunction. These manifested as severe congestive heart failure and as significant decrease in left ventricular ejection function (LVEF) (Slamon et al., 2001; Sutter et al., 2007). In the subgroup that received anthracyclines, cyclophosphamide and trastuzumab, the incidence of cardiac dysfunction was 27% compared to 8% for the subgroup that received anthracyclines and cyclophosphamide alone (Slamon et al., 2001). For the subgroup that received paclitaxel and trastuzumab the incidence of cardiac dysfunction was 13% compared to 1% for the subgroup that received paclitaxel alone (Slamon et al., 2001). Although the results of trastuzumab adjuvant trials indicate that the incidence of trastuzumab discontinuation due to cardiac disorder was low (4.3%) and that most patients with cardiac dysfunction recovered within 6 months period (Sutter et al., 2007), the finding of trastuzumab-induced cardiac dysfunction has influenced the design of subsequent trastuzumab adjuvant trials and implementation of cardiac screening prior to and during the trastuzumab adjuvant trial (Sutter et al., 2007). Meta analysis of adjuvant trastuzumab clinical trials have assessed the incidence of cardiac dysfunction and found a favorable benefit to risk ratio for trastuzumab treatment in the early breast cancer (Viani et al., 2007).

Cancer chemotherapy, in particular anthracycline therapy, was known to be associated with cardiac dysfunction, and trastuzumab treatment increased the incidence of chemotherapy-induced cardiac dysfunction in the early trials with metastatic breast cancer patients (Slamon et al., 20001). Subsequent analysis indicated that trastuzumab-associated cardiac toxicity was clinically different than cardiac dysfunction associated with anthracyclines treatment (Ewer et al., 2005). Currently, trastuzumab-associated cardiac dysfunction is recognized as type II chemotherapy related cardiac dysfunction (Ewer & Lipmann, 2005). Clinical studies indicate that the increase in patient plasma troponin I levels, which has been proposed as an early marker of high dose chemotherapy (HDCT)-induced cardiac dysfunction, is associated with a risk of trastuzumab-induced cardiac dysfunction and the lack of left ventricular ejection fraction (LVEF) recovery (Cardinale et al., 2010). The evidence from the clinical trials indicate that trastuzumab-induced cardiomyopathy is not dose dependent, and that it is increased when trastuzumab is administered concurrently with anthracyclines, and that it is at least partially reversible (Ewer et al., 2005).

HER2 signaling in heart is essential for cardiac development and function, as well as for the prevention of dilated cardiomyopathy (Negro et al., 2004). While the mechanisms contributing to trastuzumab-induced cardiac toxicity are still incompletely understood, it appears that blocking HER2 with anti-HER2 antibodies increases the production of reactive oxygen species and reduces human cardiomyocyte cell viability (Gordon et al., 2009). In other studies, treatment of rat cardiomyocytes with anti-HER2 antibodies increased mitochondria-dependent apoptosis by modulating the levels of Bcl-XL and Bcl-xS (Grazette et al., 2004). Consistent with the above studies, HER2 knockout mice have ventricular trabeculation deterioration, dilated cardiomyopathy, and increased sensitivity to anthracyclines toxicity (Lee et al., 1995; Negro et al., 2004). Molecular mechanisms by which trastuzumab induces cardiac dysfunction still remain elusive.

8. Strategies to overcome trastuzumab-resistance

Most examples of acquired therapeutic resistance to receptor tyrosine kinase inhibitors (TKIs) include development of mutations within the targeted receptors. For example, mutations in BCR/ABL in chronic myeloid leukemia and c-kit in gastrointestinal stromal tumors confer resistance to a specific BCR/ABL, c-kit kinase inhibitor Imatinib (Gleevec) (Litzow, 2006). Improvement of the binding of small molecules to their targets has been successfully used as a strategy to overcome resistance to imatinib (Guilhot et al.,2007; le Coutre et al.,2008).

While KRAS mutations have been found to be associated with primary resistance to cetuximab for the treatment of colorectal cancer, no predictive markers are currently used in the clinic to differentiate HER2-positive breast cancers that would respond favorably to trastuzumab from trastuzumab-resistant disease. Interestingly, KRAS, which signals downstream of both EGFR and HER2 receptors, is usually not mutated in HER2-positive breast cancer (Karnoub & Wenberg, 2008). Therefore, KRAS is not likely to contribute to therapeutic resistance to trastuzumab. Furthermore, mutations in HER2 have not been associated with resistance to trastuzumab. Based on these data, the strategies used to overcome therapeutic resistance to TKIs may not apply to trastuzumab-resistance.

8.1 Small molecule inhibitors used for the treatment of trastuzumab-resistant disease

Many new small molecule inhibitors are under clinical development to treat trastuzumab-resistant breast cancers. Early clinical studies suggest that TKIs that specifically target EGFR and HER2 have anti-tumor effects. Lapatinib, a reversible inhibitor targeting the ATP binding site of the tyrosine kinase domain of EGFR and HER2, has a mechanism of action distinct from trastuzumab. Based on the evidence obtained from preclinical and clinical studies, lapatinib activity is not dependent on the PTEN, p95HER2, and PI3K mutation status (Bartsch et al., 2007; Nahta & Esteva, 2006). Preclinical studies indicate that lapatinib is effective in inducing apoptosis in trastuzumab-resistant HER2-overexpressing breast cancer cells (Konecny et al, 2006; Nahta et al., 2007). Results from a phase I study of lapatinib in a cohort of EGFR and/or HER2 overexpressing breast cancer patients indicate that lapatinib was well tolerated and produced partial responses in patients with trastuzumab-resistant breast cancer (Burris et al., 2005). Taken together, these studies provided the rationale for clinical studies to evaluate the effect of lapatinib plus trastuzumab on duration of response. A randomized study of lapatinib alone versus the combination of lapatinib and trastuzumab in patients with trastuzumab-resistant HER2-positive metastatic breast cancer indicate that the combination of trastuzumab and lapatinib is superior to lapatinib alone for progression free survival (Blackwell et al., 2010).

Other TKIs in clinical development include neratinib which is a potent and irreversible TKI inhibitor of both EGFR and HER2. Neratinib showed promising results in clinical studies with HER2-positive breast cancer patients that were either heavily pretreated or not pretreated with trastuzumab (Burstein et al., 2010).

HER2 activates the PI3K/Akt/mammalian target of rapamycin pathway (mTOR), which represents a central signaling pathway that promotes proliferation, invasion, and survival of breast cancer cells (Zhou et al., 2004). Activation of the PI3K pathway either by loss of PTEN or by an activating mutation in PI3K, PIK3CA, is associated with lower response to anti-HER2 targeting agents, including trastuzumab (Berns et al., 2007; Nagata et al., 2004). Preclinical testing of combination of trastuzumab and PI3K, Akt or mTOR targeting agents showed that they have the potential to inhibit the growth of trastuzumab-resistant breast cancer cells and xenografts (Lu et al., 2007; Serra et al., 2008). These preclinical data are supported by recently published data of phase I trial where the oral mTOR inhibitor, everolimus, in combination with trastuzumab and vionorelbine had anti-tumor activity in HER2-positive metastatic breast cancer patients that progressed on trastuzumab (Jerusalem et al., 2011). Two additional mTOR inhibitors, rapamycin and temsirolimus, are also in clinical trials targeting trastuzumab-resistant breast cancers.

The chaperon Hsp90 has been implicated in the stabilization of a number of cellular proteins that play central roles in signaling transduction processes (Pratt & Toft, 2003). It has been reported that the intracellular domain of HER2 binds to Hsp90 and binding of Hsp90 to HER2 not only serves to maintain its physiological conformation, but also to restrain HER2 from forming active signaling dimer (Citri et al, 2004). Tanespimycin is a geldanamycin derivative that inhibits Hsp90 function in tumor cells, as well as in murine models (Zsebik et al., 2005). Cellular studies established that tanespimycin treatment either alone or in combination with trastuzumab inhibited cell growth and induced cell death in trastuzumab-sensitive and in trastuzumab-resistant cell lines (Zsebik et al., 2005). The inhibition of cell growth by tanespimycin was associated with decrease in membrane bound HER2 levels, most likely due to ubiquitination and lysosomal pathway dependent HER2 protein degradation (Raja et al., 2008). A phase I clinical testing of a combination of trastuzumab and tanespimycin showed safe and active in trastuzumab-resistant breast cancer and induced antitumor activity in HER2-positive metastatic breast cancers (Modi et al., 2007).

The following table provides information with regards to clinical trials testing multiple agents for the treatment of trastuzumab-resistant breast cancers. More detailed information can be found in the U.S. National Cancer Institute's website at http://www.cancer.gov/clinicaltrials.

8.2 Monoclonal antibodies indicated for the treatment of trastuzumab-resistant disease

Pertuzumab is an IgG_1 monoclonal antibody that binds to domain II of extracellular segment of HER2. Domain II mediates homo- and hetero-dimerization of HER2 with other members of the HER family. Therefore, binding of HER2 with pertuzumab prevents HER2-mediated dimerization and inhibits HER2-coupled signaling (Nahta et al., 2004b). Unlike pertuzumab, trastuzumab binds to domain IV of extracellular segment of HER2 receptor (Franklin et al., 2004). Cellular studies indicate that the combination of these two anti-HER2 antibodies exhibited synergistic effects in inhibiting breast cancer cell survival (Nahta et al., 2004b).

Clinical trial combination therapy for trastuzumab-resistant HER2 positive breast cancer	Molecular targets	Phase of clinical study
XL147/trastuzumab/paclitaxel	PI3K/HER2/microtubules	I,II
BKM120/trastuzumab	PI3K/HER2	I,II
AUY922/trastuzumab	Hsp90/HER2	I,II
GRN163L/trastuzumab	Telomerase/ErbB2	I
Everolimus/trastuzumab/vinorelbine	mTOR/HER2/tubulin	III
Rapamycin/trastuzumab	mTOR/HER2	II
Temsirolimus/neratinib	mTOR/EGFR, HER2	I,II
Panobinostat/trastuzumab	Histone deacetylase (HDAC)/HER2	I,II
BIBW2992/vinorelbine	EGFR, HER2/tubulin	III
BMS-754807/trastuzumab	Insulin-like growth factor-I receptor, insulin receptor/HER2	I,II

Table 2. Ongoing clinical trials testing multiple agents for trastuzumab-resistant breast cancer.

Addition of pertuzumab after progression to ongoing trastuzumab in xenografts synergistically increased tumor inhibition compared with trastuzumab alone (Friess et al., 2005). Taken together, these data suggest that trastuzumab and pertuzumab have complementary mechanisms of action and that the addition of pertuzumab to trastuzumab may improve clinical efficacy as a result of potentially broader blockade of the HER tumor cell proliferation and survival signaling (Friess et al., 2005). A Phase II trial of combination of pertuzumab and trastuzumab in HER2-positive patients that progressed on trastuzumab therapy indicated that the combination was active and well tolerated and adverse events were mild to moderate (Baselga et al., 2010). Data from this Phase II clinical trial indicated that objective response rate was 24.2%, the clinical benefit rate was 50%, and progression-free survival was 5.5 months in the cohort of patients (Baselga et al., 2010). Additionally, IMC-1121B (anti-VEGFR-2 monoclonal antibody) and IMC-18F1 (anti-VEGFR-1 monoclonal antibody) have been tested in clinical trials in combination with capecitabine, a chemotherapeutic agent that inhibits DNA synthesis and slows growth of tumor tissue, for the treatment of trastuzumab-resistant disease (National Cancer Institute, 2011; Schwartz et al., 2010; Spratin et al., 2010;).

8.3 Optimization of antibody structures

Advanced recombinant DNA technologies allow researchers to engineer therapeutic antibodies on a more rational basis. This can yield more homogeneous and stable molecules with additional properties such as increased cytotoxicity, dual-targeting, monovalent monoclonal antibodies, and enhanced penetration into solid tumors (Beck et al., 2010; Jin et al., 2008).

The variable region (Fv) of a monoclonal antibody is responsible for the binding of antibody to the antigens. Affinity maturation technology has been used to improve the binding affinity and specificity of Fv to the target. Targeting c-Met with antibodies had been difficult because most antibodies had intrinsic agonistic activity (Prat et al., 1998). A one-armed (OA) variant of the anti-c-Met antibody 5D5 was found to act as a pure antagonist and had the ability to inhibit the growth of cells dependent on SF/HGF-c-Met autocrine and paracrine signaling (Jin et al., 2008; Nguyen et al., 2003). Data have shown that monovalent 5D5 antibody potently inhibited glioma growth in an orthotopic *in vivo* model (Martens et al., 2006).

The constant region (Fc) of an antibody is essential for the interaction between antibody and Fc receptors presenting on immune cells (Bruhns et al., 2009). Fc functions can be modulated by altering glycosylation status and binding affinity to Fc receptors, resulting in changes in antibody-dependent cellular cytotoxicity (ADCC), serum half-life, anti-inflammatory properties, and complement activation. Musolino et al. reported that the response to trastuzumab in metastatic breast cancer correlates with expression of the high affinity allele of the activating FcγRIIIa (CD16a)-158V/V (Musolino et al., 2008). It was recently reported that MGAH22, an anti-HER2 monoclonal antibody, was engineered in the Fc domain to increase binding to both alleles of the CD16a (Nordstrom et al., 2010). It was also reported that MGAH22 had enhanced activity against HER2-expressing tumors in hCD16a-158F transgenic mice (Nordstrom et al., 2010). A preclinical study showed that MGAH22 conferred enhanced activity against HER2-positive breast tumor cells, including cells resistant to trastuzumab (Nordstrom et al., 2010). Furthermore, MGAH22 exhibited greater ADCC against HER2-expressing cancer cells with lower EC_{50} (Nordstrom et al., 2010). According to the information obtained from the website of the National Cancer Institute, MGAH22 is currently in phase I clinical trials for the treatment of the patients with the HER2-positive cancers, including breast cancer, that have not responded to the standard treatment (National Cancer Institute, 2011, http://www.cancer.gov/clinicaltrials).

Multiple signaling pathways contribute to cancer development and progression. Bispecific antibodies, which are directed against two antigens that drive cancer progression, might yield better therapeutic efficacy than inhibition of a single target (Chames & Baty, 2009). Bispecific antibodies can be obtained by combining the variable domains of two already characterized monoclonal antibodies (two V_L domains on the light chain and two V_H domains on the heavy chain) using the dual variable domain IgG (DVD-IgG) technology.

This technology enables the different specificities of two monoclonal antibodies to be engineered into a single functional, dual-specific, tetravalent IgG like molecule (Beck et al., 2010). A different approach consists of engineering an additional paratope, the antigen-binding site of an antibody, in the variable domain of an existing antibody, which results in simultaneous binding to two different antigens (Beck et al., 2010; Bostrom et al., 2009). The bispecific antibody (MM-111) was developed to target both ErbB2 and ErbB3. MM-111 was indicated to displace heregulin from ErbB3 and thereby prevents receptor phosphorylation, resulting in the inhibition of tumor growth. MM-111 in combination with trastuzumab is currently in a clinical trial to treat trastuzumab-resistant breast cancer (Arnett et al., 2011; National Cancer Institute, 2011, http://www.cancer.gov/clinicaltrials).

Polyclonal or oligoclonal antibodies refer to the recombinant polycolonal or oligoclonal antibodies directed against the same or different targets. For example, the Rhesus D blood group antigen-specific polyclonal antibody rozrolimupab (Sym001; Symphogen A/S), which is a mixture of 25 unique recombinant monoclonal antibodies, is currently in Phase II clinical trials for the treatment of chronic and acute idiopathic thrombocytopenic purpura (Beck et al, 2010; Swann, et al 2008;). Hopefully, in the near future we will see more optimized monoclonal antibodies entering the clinical trials to treat trastuzumab-resistant disease.

8.4 Antibody-drug conjugates (ADC)

An important approach to delivering a lethal quantity of cytotoxic agent to the cancer cells is to select an antibody that specifically binds to a cancer-specific antigen that can mediate a rapid rate of endocytosis of antibody conjugate and accumulate them at a high concentration in cancer cells, thus resulting in cancer cell-specific killing while minimizing damage to normal cells (Chen at al., 2005; Senter, 2009). Antibody-drug conjugates are monoclonal antibody-based products that are covalently attached to the cytotoxic agent by chemical linkers (Alley et al., 2010). It is now a common strategy to develop monoclonal antibody-cytotoxic drug conjugates to improve the efficacy of both the monoclonal antibody and the cytotoxic agent for cancer indications (Chen at al, 2005; Senter, 2009). Antibody-drug conjugates consist of three different elements: the monoclonal antibody, linker, and cytotoxic agent. Three different classes of cytotoxic agents, including calicheamicin-based, maytansinoid-based, and auristatin-based cytotoxic agents, are commonly used as drugs to be conjugated to antibodies. Calicheamicin is a natural product and has been the subject of extensive research for drug delivery, due to its ability to bind to DNA in the minor groove, resulting in DNA cleavage. Maytansinoid derivatives and auristatin represent other classes of highly potent drugs that have been widely utilized for antibody-drug conjugate development. Both cytotoxic agents, maytansinoid derivatives and auristatin, act by binding to tubulin to mediate inhibition of tubulin polymerization (Chari, 2008; Doronina et al, 2006; Doronina et al. 2003). Traditionally, the antibody in an antibody-drug conjugate functions as a vehicle to carry drugs to the tumor site and drugs with high systemic toxicity are selected as payload in the antibody-drug conjugate. Gemtuzumab ozogamicin (Mylotarg), an anti-CD33 antibody conjugated to calicheamicin, was granted marketing approval for the treatment of relapsed acute myeloid leukemia in 2000. It was withdrawn from the U.S. market in June 2010 when a clinical trial showed that the drug failed to demonstrate clinical benefit to the patients enrolled in clinical trials.

Trastuzumab-DM1 (T-DM1) is an antibody-drug conjugate that was generated by linking the maytansinoid derivative maytansin to trastuzumab via a thioether linker (Lewis Phillips et al., 2008). Testing of T-DM1 in a panel of HER2-positive trastuzumab-sensitive and trastuzumab-resistant cell lines indicated that T-DM1 was cytotoxic in both trastuzumab-sensitive and trastuzumab-resistant breast cancer cell lines (Lewis Phillips et al. 2008). T-DM1 also inhibited tumor growth and caused tumor regression in trastuzumab resistant animal xenograft models (Lewis Phillips et al. 2008). T-DM1 was reported to retain the mechanisms of action of trastuzumab and was also active against lapatinib-resistant cell lines and tumors (Junttila et al., 2010). A Phase I clinical trial testing of T-DM1 reported that T-DM1 was associated with clinical activity in HER2-positive patients who had progressed on trastuzumab-based therapy (Krop et al., 2010). A Phase II study recently reported that T-DM1 had robust single-agent activity in metastatic breast cancer patients who had progressed on the previous HER2-directed therapy (Burris III et al., 2011). These clinical studies provide the evidence that the HER2 pathway remains a valid therapeutic target following disease progression on trastuzumab and suggest that antibody-drug conjugates are a novel and effective approach that can be used to treat trastuzumab-resistant disease.

8.5 Development of novel therapeutic approaches: Mechanisms of resistance-based design of antibody drug conjugates

Significant effort has been made to understand the mechanisms of resistance to trastuzumab. Many different small molecules, for example PI3 kinase inhibitors and c-Src inhibitors have been shown to be able to revert trastuzumab-resistant phenotypes in preclinical settings (Junttila et al., 2009; Zhuang et al., 2010). Table 3 summarizes some of the novel proposed molecular targets involved in trastuzumab-resistance and small molecules that are able to override trastuzumab-resistant phenotypes based on the preclinical studies.

Molecular target implicated in trastuzumab resistance	Inhibitor for the target (preclinical studies)	Reference for the preclinical studies
Rac1	NSC23766	Dokmanovic et al., 2009
EGFR	Lapatinib Neratinib	Nahta et al.,2007 Burstein et al.,2010
PI3K	GDC-0941 LY294002 Wortmannin SF1126	Junttila et al., 2009 Clark et al., 2002 Nagata et al., 2004 Ozbay et al., 2010
Akt	Triciribine (API-2)	Lu et al.,2007
mTOR	RAD001(everolimus)	Lu et al.,2007
PI3K/mTOR	NVP-BEZ235	Serra et al., 2008
PDK-1/Akt	OSU-03012	Tseng et al., 2006
HSP90	SNX-2112 17-AAG	Chandarlapaty et al., 2010 Modi et al., 2007
TGF-β1	LY2109761	Wang et al., 2008
Src	Dasatinib	Zhuanget al., 2010
Proteasome	LLnL	Lu et al., 2004
Hyaluronan synthesis	4-MU (methylumbelliferon)	Palyi-Krekk et al., 2007
Fatty acid synthase	C-75	Vazquez-Martin et al., 2007

Table 3. Emerging molecular targets implicated in the trastuzumab-resistance and their respective inhibitors.

TGF-β is a secreted ligand that binds to type I and type II TGF-β receptors and induces the secretion of HER family ligands, such as TGF-α, amphiregulin, and heregulin. Secreted HER family ligands may enhance the association of p85 subunit of PI3K with HER3 and activate PI3K/Akt (Wang et al., 2008). Treatment with TGF-β or expression of TGF-β type I receptor in HER2-overexpressing cells reduced their sensitivity to the HER2 antibody trastuzumab. Inhibition of TGF-β type I receptor by LY2109761, a TGF-β receptor type I and type II dual inhibitor, restored sensitivity to trastuzumab (Wang et al., 2008). Rac1 is a Ras-like small GTPase which is believed to be associated with breast cancer progression and metastasis (Sahai & Marshall, 2002). Inhibition of Rac1 activity by Rac1 specific inhibitor, NSC23766, resulted in the restoration of the trastuzumab-mediated HER2 endocytic degradation and inhibition of the cell growth in trastuzumab-resistant cells (Dokmanovic et al., 2009). It has been reported that the inhibition of c-Src activity by dasatinib partially restored trastuzumab sensitivity in trastuzumab-resistant breast cancer cells (Zhuang et al., 2010). 4-MU inhibition of hyaluronan synthase enhanced trastuzumab-mediated growth inhibition in trastuzumab-resistant JIMT-1 xenografts (Palyi-Krekk et al., 2007). Inhibition of fatty acid syntheses (FASN) re-sensitized the trastuzumab-resistant SKBR3 cells to trastuzumab-mediated cell death (Vazquez-Martin et al., 2007).

Several other approaches were utilized to interfere with the molecular pathways associated with trastuzumab-resistance in the preclinical studies. It has been recently reported that the overexpression of FoxM1, an oncogenic transcription factor, confers resistance to the trastuzumab (Carr et al., 2010). Attenuation of FoxM1 expression either by small interfering RNA or by an alternate reading frame (ARF)-derived peptide inhibitor increased the sensitivity to trastuzumab (Carr et al., 2010). Damiano et al. report that a novel toll-like receptor 9 agonist, which is also referred as the immune modulatory oligonucleotide (IMO), exerts antiangiogenic effects by cooperating with anti-EGFR or anti-VEGF antobodies, (Damiano et al., 2009). It was also shown that IMO and trastuzumab exert a cooperative antiangiogenic effect on trastuzumab-resistant breast cancer xenografts and that combining IMO and trastuzumab may be a potential strategy for the treatment of trastuzumab-resistant breast cancers (Damiano et al., 2009). The Y-box binding protein-1 (YB-1) is an oncogenic transcription/translation factor mediating expression of growth promoting genes such as EGFR and HER2. YB-1 is activated by phosphorylation at Serine 102 residue, and a decoy cell permeable peptide (CPP) functions as interference peptide to prevent endogenous YB-1 phosphorylation and activation. This results in the down-regulation of both HER-2 and EGFR transcript level and protein expression (Law et al., 2010). Interestingly, treatment with CPP has been reported to enhance sensitivity and overcome resistance to trastuzumab in cells expressing amplified HER-2, suggesting that CPP may be a novel approach for the treatment of trastuzumab-resistant breast cancers (Law et al., 2010).

Even though there were multiple mechanisms of trastuzumab-resistance proposed from the preclinical studies, the question remains how the knowledge gained from these cellular and animal models can be translated into the next generation of monoclonal antibodies to overcome therapeutic resistance to trastuzumab. Based on literature and data from our laboratory (Dokmanovic et al., 2009), we propose a new approach by designing an antibody-drug conjugate (ADC) based on mechanisms of trastuzumab resistance. In this ADC, trastuzumab is conjugated by a small molecule that has ability to inhibit the cellular target(s) that has been demonstrated to contribute to trastuzumab-resistance. This proposed strategy may increase the magnitude and duration of the response to trastuzumab treatment.

9. Conclusions

Treatment with trastuzumab significantly improves outcomes for women with HER2-positive breast cancer. However, therapeutic resistance to trastuzumab poses a significant challenge in the treatment of human breast cancer. Pre-clinical studies conducted in the past few years have improved our understanding of molecular mechanisms contributing to the trastuzumab-resistance, and potential predictive biomarkers, such as the serum levels of extracellular cellular domain (ECD) of HER2, the status of p95HER2 and IGF-IR, and loss of PTEN, have been reported. However, no predictive markers are currently used in the clinic to differentiate HER2-positive breast cancers that would respond favorably to trastuzumab from trastuzumab-resistant disease. Validation of novel predictive biomarkers must be performed with clinical samples in the context of prospective clinical trial in which prognostic or predictive questions can be answered (Hirsch & Wu, 2007; Murphy et al., 2005). Resistance to monoclonal antibody therapeutics represents a common obstacle to the clinical efficacy for monoclonal antibody-based therapy. Understanding the molecular mechanisms of trastuzumab-resistance will lead to the discovery of new therapeutic targets, as well as more effective approaches. Innovative strategies to optimize antibody structures to develop next generation of monoclonal antibodies, such as antibody-drug conjugates, bispecific antibodies, and antibodies with either enhanced or silenced effector function, will also play a critical role in overcoming therapeutic resistance to monoclonal antibodies.

10. Acknowledgment

We thank Drs. Dianne S. Hirsch, David M. Frucht, and Patrick G. Swann for the critical review of this manuscript. Disclaimer: The information presented in this article reflects the views of the authors and does not represent the policy of the U.S. Food and Drug Administration.

11. References

Ali, SM., Carney, WP., Esteva, FJ., Fornier, M., Harris, L., Kostler, WJ., Lotz, J-P., Luftner, D., Pichon, MF., Lipton, A. & Serum HER-2/neu Study Group. Serum HER-2/neu and relative resistance to trastuzumab-based therapy in patients with metastatic breast cancer. (2008). *Cancer,* Vol.113, No.6, (September 2008), pp. (1294-1301).

Allegra, CJ., Jessup, JM., Somerfield, MR., Hamilton, SR., Hammond, EH., Hayes, DF., McAllister, PK., Morton RF. & Schilsky, RL. (2009). American Society of Clinical Oncology provisional clinical opinion: testing for KRAS gene mutations in patients with metastatic colorectal carcinoma to predict response to anti-epidermal growth factor receptor monoclonal antibody therapy. *Journal of Clinical Oncology,* Vol.27, No.12, (April 2009), pp. (2091–2096).

Alley, SC., Okeley, NM. & Senter, PD. (2010). Antibody-drug conjugates: targeted drug delivery for cancer. *Current Opinion in Chemical Biology,* Vol.14, No.4, (August 2010), pp. (529-537).

Arnett, SO., Teillaud, JL., Wurch, T., Reichert, JM., Dunlop, C. & Huber, M. (2011)..IBC's 21st Annual Antibody Engineering and 8th Annual Antibody Therapeutics International Conferences and 2010 Annual Meeting of The Antibody Society December 5-9, 2010, San Diego, CA. *mAbs,*Vol. 3,No.2, (March 2011), pp. (133-152).

Arribas, J., Baselga, J., Pedersen, K. & Parra-Palau, JL. (2011). P95HER2 and Breast Cancer. *Cancer Research,* Vol.71, No.5, (March 2011), pp. (1515-1519).

Banerjee, S. & Smith, IE. (2010). Management of small HER2-positive breast cancers. *The Lancet Oncology,* Vol.11, No.12, (December 2010), pp. (1193-1199).

Bartsch, R., Wenzel, C., Zielinski, CC. & Steger, GG. (2007).HER-2-positive breast cancer: hope beyond trastuzumab. *BioDrugs,* Vol.21, No.2, pp.(69-77).

Baselga, J., Norton, L., Albanell, J., Kim YM. & Mendelsohn, J. (1998). Recombinant humanized anti-HER2 antibody (Herceptin) enhances the antitumor activity of paclitaxel and doxorubicine against HER2/neu overexpressing human breast cancer xenografts. *Cancer Research,* Vol.58, No.13, (July 1998), pp. (2825-2831).

Baselga, J. & Swain, SM. (2009). Novel anticancer targets: revisiting ERBB2 and discovering ERBB3. *Nature Reviews Cancer,* Vol. 9, No.7, (July2009), pp. (463-475).

Baselga, J., Gelmon, KA., Verma, S., Wardley, A., Conte, P., Miles, D., Bianchi, G., Cortes, J., McNally, VA., Ross, GA., Fumoleau, P. & Gianni, L. (2010). Phase II trial of pertuzumab and trastuzumab in patients with human epidermal growth factor receptor 2-positive metastatic breast cancer that progressed during prior trastuzumab therapy. *Journal of Clinical Oncology,* Vol.28, No.7, (March 2010), pp. (1138-1144).

Bekaii-Saab, T., Williams, N., Plass, C., Calero, MV. & Eng, C. (2006). A novel mutation in the tyrosine kinase domain of ERBB2 in hepatocellular carcinoma. *BMC Cancer,* Vol.6, (December 2006), pp.278.

Beck, A., Wurch, T., Bailly, C. & Corvaia, N. (2010). Strategies and challenges for the next generation of therapeutic antibodies. *Nature Reviews Immunology,*Vol.10, No.5, (May 2010), pp.(345-352).

Benvenuti, S., Sartore-Bianchi, A., Di Nicolantonio, F., Zanon, C., Moroni, M., Veronese, S., Siena, S. & Bardelli, A. (2007) .Oncogenic activation of the RAS/RAF signaling pathway impairs the response of metastatic colorectal cancers to anti-epidermal growth factor receptor antibody therapies. *Cancer Research,* Vol.67, No.6, (March 2007), pp. (2643-2648).

Berns, K., Horlings, HM., Hennessy, BT., Madiredjo, M., Hijmans, EM., Beelen, K., Linn, SC., Gonzalez-Angulo, AM., Stemke-Hale, K., Hauptmann, M., Beijersbergen, RL., Mills, GB., van de Vijver, MJ. & Bernards ,R. (2007). A functional genetic approach identifies the PI3K pathway as a major determinant of trastuzumab resistance in breast cancer. *Cancer Cell,* Vol.12, No.4, (October 2007), pp. (395-402).

Blackwell, KL., Burstein, HJ., Storniolo, AM., Rugo, H., Sledge, G., Koehler, M., Ellis, C., Casey, M., Vukelja, S., Bischoff, J., Baselga, J. & O'Shaughnessy, J. (2010). Randomized study of Lapatinib alone or in combination with trastuzumab in women with ErbB2-positive, trastuzumab-refractory metastatic breast cancer. *Journal of Clinical Oncology,* Vol.28, No.7, (March 2010), pp. (1124-1130).

Bostrom, J., Yu, SF., Kan, D., Appleton, BA., Lee, CV., Billeci, K., Man, W., Peale, F., Ross, S., Wiesmann, C. & Fuh, G.(2009). Variants of the antibody herceptin that interact with HER2 and VEGF at the antigen binding site. *Science,* Vol.323, No.5921, (March 2009), pp.(1610–1614).

Brufsky, A. (2010). Trastuzumab-based therapy for patients with HER2-positive breast Cancer: from early scientific development to foundation of care. *American Journal of Clinical Oncology,* Vol.33, No.2, (April 2010), pp. (186-195).

Bruhns, P., Iannascoli, B., England, P., Mancardi, DA., Fernandez, N., Jorieux, S. & Daëron, M. (2009).Specificity and affinity of human Fcgamma receptors and their polymorphic variants for human IgG subclasses. *Blood,* Vol.113, No.16, (April 2009), pp.(3716–3725).

Burris HA 3 rd., Rugo HS., Vukelja SJ., Vogel CL., Borson RA., Limentani S., Tan-Chiu E., Krop IE., Michaelson RA.,Girish S., Amler L., Zheng M., Chu YW., Klencke B.,& O'Shaughnessy, JA.(2011). Phase II study of the antibody-drug conjugate trastuzumab-DM1 for the treatment of human epidermal growth factor receptor 2(HER2)-positive breast cancer after prior HER2-directed therapy. *Journal of Clinical Oncology,* Vol.29, No.4, (February 2011), pp. (398-405).

Burris, HA 3rd., Hurwitz, HI., Dees, EC., Dowlati, A., Blackwell, KL., O'Neil, B., Marcom, PK., Ellis, MJ., Overmoyer, B., Jones, SJ., Harris, JL., Smith, DA., Koch, KM., Stead,

A., Mangum, S. & Spector, NL.(2005). Phase I safety, pharmacokinetics, and clinical activity study of lapatinib (GW572016), a reversible dual inhibitor of epidermal growth factor receptor tyrosine kinases, in heavily pretreated patients with metastatic carcinomas. *Journal of Clinical Oncology,* Vol.23, No.23, (August 2005), pp. (5305-5313).

Burstein, HJ., Kuter, I., Campos, SM., Gelman, RS., Tribou, L., Parker, LM., Manola, J., Younger, J., Matulonis, U., Bunnell, CA., Partridge, AH., Richardson, PG., Clarke, K., Shulman, LN. & Winer, EP. (2001). Clinical activity of trastuzumab and vinorelbine in women with HER2-overexpressing metastatic breast cancer. *Journal of Clinical Oncology,* Vol.19, No.10, (May 2001), pp. (2722-2730).

Burstein, HJ., Sun, Y., Dirix, LY., Jiang, Z., Paridaens, R., Tan, AR., Awada, A., Ranade, A., Jiao, S., Schwartz, G., Abbas, R., Powell, C., Turnbull, K., Vermette, J., Zacharchuk, C. & Badwe, R. (2010). Neratinib, an irreversible ErbB receptor tyrosine kinase inhibitor, in patients with advanced ErbB2-positive breast cancer. *Journal of Clinical Oncology,* Vol.28, No.8, (March 2010), pp. (1301-1307).

Cardinale, D., Colombo, A., Torrisi, R., Sandri, MT., Civelli, M., Salvatici, M., Lamantia, G., Colombo, N., Cortinovis, S., Dessanai, MA., Nole, F., Veglia, F. & Cipolla, CM. (2010). Trastuzumab-induced cardiotoxicity: clinical and prognostic implications of troponin I evaluation. *Journal of Clinical Oncology,* Vol.28, No.25, (September 2010), pp. (3910-3916).

Carney, WP. Neumann, R., Lipton, A., Leitzel K., Ali, S. & Price, CP. (2003).Potential clinical utility of serum HER2/neu oncoprotein concentrations in patients with breast cancer. *Clinical Chemistry*, Vol.49, No.10, (October 2003), pp. (1579-1598).

Carr, JR., Park, HJ. Wang, Z., Kiefer, MM. & Raychaudhuri, P. (2010). FoxM1 mediates resistance to herceptin and paclitaxel. *Cancer Research,* Vol.70, No.12, (June 2010), pp. (5054-5063).

Carraway, KL 3rd. & Cantley, LC. (1994). A neu acquaintance for erbB3 and erbB4: a role for receptor heterodimerization in growth signaling. *Cell,* Vol.78, No.1, (July 1994), pp.(5–8).

Carter, P., Presta, L., Gorman, CM., Ridgway, JB., Henner, D., Wong, WL., Rowland, AM., Kotts, C., Carver, ME.& Shepard, HM.(1992). Humanization of an anti-p185HER2 antibody for human cancer therapy. *Proceedings of the National Academy of Sciences of the United States of America,* Vol.89, No.10, (May 1992), pp.(4285-4289).

Chames, P. & Baty, D. (2009). Bispecific antibodies for cancer therapy: the light at the end of the tunnel? *mAbs*, Vol.1, No.6, (November-December 2009), pp.539–547.

Chandarlapaty, S., Scaltriti, M., Angelini, P., Ye, Q., Guzman, M., Hudis, CA., Norton, L., Solit, DB., Arribas, J., Baselga, J.& Rosen, N.(2010). Inhibitors of HSP90 block p95-HER2 signaling in Trastuzumab-resistant tumors and suppress their growth. *Oncogene,* Vol.29, No.3, (January 2010), pp.(325-334).

Chari, RV.(2008). Targeted cancer therapy: conferring specificity to cytotoxic drugs. *Accounts of Chemical Research,* Vol.41,No.1, (January 2008), pp.(98-107).

Chen, J., Jaracz, S., Zhao, X., Chen, S.& Ojima, I. (2005). Antibody-cytotoxic agent conjugates for cancer therapy. *Expert Opinion on Drug Delivery,* Vol.2, No.5, (September 2005),pp. (873-890).

Cho, HS., Mason, K., Ramyar, KX., Stanley, AM., Gabelli, SB., Denney, DW Jr. & Leahy, DJ. (2003). Structure of the extracellular region of HER2 alone and in complex with the Herceptin Fab. *Nature,* Vol.421, No.6924, (February 2003), pp. (756-760).

Chung, KY., Shia, J., Kemeny, NE., Shah, M., Schwartz, GK., Tse, A., Hamilton, A., Pan, D., Schrag, D., Schwartz, L., Klimstra, DS., Fridman, D., Kelsen, DP. & Saltz, LB. (2005). Cetuximab shows activity in colorectal cancer patients with tumors that do not express the epidermal growth factor receptor by immunohistochemistry. *Journal of Clinical Oncology,* Vol.23, No.9, (March 2005), pp. (1803–1810).

Citri, A., Gan, J., Mosesson, Y., Vereb, G., Sz¨oll˝osi, J.& Yarden, Y. (2004). Hsp90 restrains ErbB2/HER2 signalling by limiting heterodimer formation. *EMBO Reports,* Vol.5, No.12, (December 2004), pp.(1165-1170).

Clark, AS., West, K., Streicher, S. & Dennis, PA. (2002). Constitutive and inducible Akt activity promotes resistance to chemotherapy, trastuzumab, or tamoxifen in breast cancer cells. *Molecular Cancer Therapeutics,* Vol.1, No.9, (July 2002), pp. (707-717).

Damiano, V., Garofalo, S., Rosa, R., Bianco, R., Caputo, R., Geraldi, T., Merola, G., Racioppi, L., Garbi, C., Kandimalla, ER., Agrawal S.& Tortora, G. (2009). A novel toll-like receptor 9 agonist cooperates with trastuzumab in trastuzumab-resistant breast tumors through multiple mechanisms of action. *Clinical Cancer Research,* Vol.15, No.22, (November 2009), pp. (6921-6930).

Dave, B., Migliaccio, I., Gutierrez, MC., Wu, MF., Chamness, GC., Wong, H., Narasanna, A., Chakrabarty, A., Hilsenbeck, SG., Huang, J., Rimawi, M., Schiff, R., Arteaga, C., Osborne, CK. & Chang, JC. Loss of phosphatase and tensin homolog or phosphoinositol-3 kinase activation and response to trastuzumab or lapatinib in human epidermal growth factor receptor 2-overexpressing locally advanced breast cancer. (2011). *Journal of Clinical Oncology,* Vol.29, No.2, (January 2011), pp.(166-173).

De Roock, W., Piessevaux, H., De Schutter, J., Janssens, M., De Hertogh, G., Personeni, N., Biesmans, B., Van Laethem, JL., Peeters, M., Humblet, Y., Van Cutsem, E. & Tejpar, S.(2008). KRAS wild-type state predicts survival and is associated to early radiological response in metastatic colorectal cancer treated with cetuximab. *Annals of Oncology,* Vol.19, No.3, (March 2008), pp. (508–515).

Diermeier, S., Horvath, G., Knuechel-Clarke, R., Hofstaedter, F., Szollosi, J. & Brockhoff, G. (2005). Epidermal growth factor receptor coexpression modulates susceptibility to Herceptin in HER2/neu overexpressing breast cancer cells via specific erbB-receptor interaction and activation. *Experimental Cell Research,* Vol.304, No.2, (April 2005), pp.(604–619).

Dokmanovic, M., Hirsch, DS., Shen, Y. & Wu, WJ. (2009). Rac1 contributes to trastuzumab resistance of breast cancer cells: Rac1 as a potential therapeutic target for the treatment of trastuzumab-resistant breast cancer. *Molecular Cancer Therapeutics,* Vol.8, No.6, (June 2009), pp. (1557-1569).

Doronina, SO., Mendelsohn, BA., Bovee, TD., Cerveny, CG., Alley, SC., Meyer, DL., Oflazoglu, E., Toki, BE., Sanderson, RJ., Zabinski, RF., Wahl, AF. & Senter, PD. (2006).Enhanced activity of monomethylauristatin F through monoclonal antibody delivery: effects of linker technology on efficacy and toxicity. *Bioconjugate Chemistry,* Vol.17,No.1, (January-February 2006), pp.(114-124).

Doronina, SO., Toki, BE., Torgov, MY., Mendelsohn, BA., Cerveny, CG., Chace, DF., DeBlanc, RL., Gearing, RP., Bovee, TD., Siegall, CB., Francisco, JA., Wahl, AF., Meyer, DL. & Senter, PD. (2003). Development of potent monoclonal antibody auristatin conjugates for cancer therapy. *Nature Biotechnology,* Vol.21, No.7, (July 2003), pp.(778-784).

Esteva, FJ., Guo, H., Zhang, S., Santa-Maria, C., Stone, S., Lanchbury, JS., Sahin, AA., Hortobagyi, GN.& Yu, D. (2010). PTEN, PIK3CA, p-AKT, and p-p70S6K status: association with trastuzumab response and survival in patients with HER2-positive metastatic breast cancer. *The American Journal of Pathology,* Vol. 177, No. 4, (October 2010), pp. (1647-1656).

Ewer, MS., Vooletich, MT., Durand, JB., Woods, ML., Davis, JR., Valero, V. & Lenihan, DJ. (2005).Reversibility of trastuzumab-related cardiotoxicity: new insights based on clinical course and response to medical treatment. *Journal of Clinical Oncology,* Vol.23, No.31, (November 2005), pp. (7820-7826).

Ewer, MS. & Lippman, SM. (2005). Type II chemotherapy-related cardiac dysfunction: time to recognize a new entity. *Journal of Clinical Oncology,* Vol.23, No.13, (May 2005), pp. (2900-2902).

Franklin, MC., Carey, KD., Vajdos FF., Leahy, DJ., de Vos, AM. & Sliwkowski, MX. (2004). Insights into ErbB signaling from the structure of the ErbB2-pertuzumab complex. *Cancer Cell,* Vol.5, No.4, (April 2004), pp. (317-328).

Friess, T., their, M., Scheuer, W. et al. (2005). Combination treatment with pertuzumab and trastuzumab against Calu-3 human NSCLC xenograft tumors is superior to monotherapy. *Presented at the 17th Annual Meeting of the American Association for Cancer Research–National Cancer Institute–European Organisation for Research and Treatment of Cancer*, Philadelphia, PA, November 14-18, 2005

Garrett, TP., McKern, NM., Lou, M., Elleman, TC., Adams, TE., Lovrecz, GO., Kofler, M., Jorissen, RN., Nice, EC., Burgess, AW. & Ward, CW. (2003). The crystal structure of truncated ErbB2 ectodomain reveals an active conformation, poised to interact with other ErbB receptors. *Molecular Cell,* Vol.11, No.2, (February 2003), pp. (495-505).

Giusti, RM., Shastri, K., Pilaro, AM., Fuchs, C., Cordoba-Rodriguez, R., Koti, K., Rothmann, M., Men, AY., Zhao, H., Hughes, M., Keegan, P., Weiss, KD. & Pazdur, R. (2008). U.S. Food and Drug Administration approval: panitumumab for epidermal growth factor receptor-expressing metastatic colorectal carcinoma with progression following fluoropyrimidine-, oxaliplatin-, and irinotecan-containing chemotherapy regimens. *Clinical Cancer Research,* Vol.14, No.5, (March 2008), pp.(1296–1302).

Goldstein, NI., Prewett, M., Zuklys, K., Rockwell, P.& Mendelsohn, J. (1995). Biological efficacy of a chimeric antibody to the epidermal growth factor receptor in a human tumor xenograft model. *Clinical Cancer Research,* Vol.1, No.11, (November 1995), pp. (1311–1318).

Gordon, LI., Burke, MA., Singh, A.T.., Prachand, S., Lieberman, ED., Sun, L., Naik, TJ., Prasad, SV. & Ardehali, H. (2009). Blockage of the erbB2 receptor induces cardiomyocyte death through mitochondrial and reactive oxygen species-dependent pathways. *The Journal of Biological Chemistry,* Vol.284, No.4, (January 2009), pp. (2080-2087).

Graus-Porta, D., Beerli, RR., Daly, JM. & Hynes, NE. (1997). ErbB-2, the preferred heterodimerization partner of all ErbB receptors, is a mediator of lateral signaling. *EMBO Journal*, Vol.16, No.7, (April 1997), pp.(1647-1655).

Grazette, LP., Boecker, W., Matsui, T., Semigran, M., Force, TL., Hajjar, RJ. & Rosenzweig, A.(2004). Inhibition of ErbB2 causes mitochondrial dysfunction in cardiomyocytes.: implications for Herceptin-induced cardiomyopathy. *Journal of American College of Cardiology*, Vol.44, No.11, (December 2004), pp. (2231-2238).

Guilhot, F., Apperley, J., Kim, DW., Bullorsky, EO., Baccarani, M., Roboz, GJ., Amadori, S., de Souza, CA., Lipton, JH., Hochhaus, A., Heim, D., Larson, RA., Branford, S., Muller, MC., Agarwal, P., Gollerkeri, A. & Talpaz, M. (2007). Dasatinib induces significant hematologic and cytogenetic responses in patients with imatinib-resistant or -intolerant chronic myeloid leukemia in accelerated phase. *Blood*, Vol.109, No.10, (May 2007), pp.(4143-4150).

Gusterson, BA., Gelber, RD., Goldhirsch, A., Price, KN., Save-Soderborgh, J., Anbazhagan, R., Styles, J., Rudenstam, CM., Golouh, R., Reed, R., Martinez-Tello, F., Tiltman, A., Torhorst, J., Grigolato, P., Bettelheim, R., Neville, AM., Burki, K., Castiglione, M., Collins, J., Lindtner, J. & Senn, HJ for the International (Ludwig)Breast Cancer Study Group. (1992). Prognostic importance of c-erbB-2 expression in breast cancer. International (Ludwig) Breast Cancer Study Group. *Journal of Clinical Oncology*, Vol.10, No.7, (July 1992), pp.(1049-1056).

Guy, PM., Platko, JV., Cantley, LC., Cerione, RA. & Carraway, KL 3rd. (1994). Insect cell-expressed p180erbB3 possesses an impaired tyrosine kinase activity. *Proceedings of the National Academy of Sciences of the United States of America*, Vol.91, No.17, (August 1994), pp.(8132–8136).

Han, SW., Kim, TY., Hwang, PG., Jeong, S., Kim, J., Choi, IS., Oh, DY., Kim, JH., Kim, DW., Chung, DH., Im, SA., Kim,YT., Lee, JS., Heo, DS., Bang, YJ. & Kim, NK. (2005). Predictive and prognostic impact of epidermal growth factor receptor mutation in non-small-cell lung cancer patients treated with gefitinib. *Journal of Clinical Oncology*, Vol.23, No.11, (April 2005), pp.(2493–2501).

Hecht, JR., Mitchell, E., Chidiac, T., Scroggin, C., Hagenstad, C., Spigel, D., Marshall, J., Cohn, A., McCollum, D., Stella, P., Deeter, R., Shahin, S. & Amado, RG. (2009). A randomized phase IIIB trial of chemotherapy, bevacizumab, and panitumumab compared with chemotherapy and bevacizumab alone for metastatic colorectal cancer. *Journal of Clinical Oncology*, Vol.27, No.5, (February 2009), pp. (672–680).

Hirsch, DS. & Wu, WJ.(2007). Cdc42: an effector and regulator of ErbB1 as a strategic target in breast cancer therapy. *Expert Review of Anticancer Therapy*, Vol.7,No.2, (February 2007), pp.(147-157).

Huang, X., Gao, L., Wang, S., McManaman, JL., Thor, AD., Yang, X., Esteva, FJ. & Liu, B. (2010). Heterotrimerization of the growth factor receptors erbB2, erbB3 and insulin-like growth factor-i receptor in breast cancer cells resistant to herceptin. *Cancer Research*, Vol.70, No.3, (February 2010), pp.(1204-1214).

Hudis, CA. (2007). Trastuzumab-mechanism of action and use in clinical practice. *The New England Journal of Medicine*, Vol.357, No.1, (July 2007), pp. (39-51).

Hynes, NE. & Lane, HA. (2005). ERBB receptors and cancer: the complexity of targeted inhibitors. *Nature Reviews Cancer*, Vol.5, No.5, (May 2005), pp.(341-354).

Jerusalem, G., Fasolo, A., Dieras, V., Cardoso, F., Bergh, J., Vittori, L., Zhang, Y., Massacesi, C., Sahmoud, T. & Gianni, L. (2011). Phase I trial of oral mTOR inhibitor everolimus in combination with trastuzumab and vinoirelbine in pre-treated patients with HER2-overexpressing metastatic breast cancer. *Breast Cancer Research and Treatment,* Vol.125, No.2, (January 2011), pp. (447-455).

Jin, H., Yang, R., Zheng, Z., Romero, M., Ross, J., Bou-Reslan, H., Carano, RA., Kasman, I., Mai, E., Young, J., Zha, J., Zhang, Z., Ross, S., Schwall, R., Colbern, G. & Merchant, M. (2008). MetMAb, the one-armed 5D5 anti-c-Met antibody, inhibits orthotopic pancreatic tumor growth and improves survival. *Cancer Res.earch,* Vol.68, No.11 (Jun 2008), pp. (4360-4368).

Junttila, TT., Li, G., Parsons, K., Phillips, GL. & Sliwkowski, MX. (2010). Trastuzumab-DM1 (T-DM1) retains all the mechanisms of action of trastuzumab and efficiently inhibits growth of lapatinib insensitive breast cancer. *Breast Cancer Research and Treatment,* (August 2010).

Junttila, TT., Akita, RW., Parsons, K., Fields, C., Lewis Phillips, GD., Friedman, LS., Sampath, D. & Sliwkowski, MX. (2009). Ligand-independent HER2/HER3/PI3K complex is disrupted by trastuzumab and is effectively inhibited by the PI3K inhibitor GDC-0941. *Cancer Cell,* Vol.15, No.5, (May 2009), pp. (429-440)

Karapetis, CS., Khambata-Ford, S., Jonker, DJ., O'Callaghan, CJ., Tu, D., Tebbutt, NC., Simes, RJ., Chalchal, H., Shapiro, JD., Robitaille, S., Price, TJ., Shepherd, L., Au, HJ., Langer, C., Moore, MJ. & Zalcberg, JR. (2008). K-ras mutations and benefit from cetuximab in advanced colorectal cancer. *The New England Journal of Medicine,* Vol.359, No.17, (October 2008), pp. (1757-1765).

Karnoub, AE. & Weinberg, RA. (2008). Ras oncogenes: split personalities. *Nature Reviews Molecular Cell Biology,* Vol. 9, No.7, (July 2008), pp. (517-531).

Kaufman B., Mackey, JR., Clemens, MR., Bapsy, PP., Vaid, A., Wardley, A., Tjulandin, S., Jahn, M., Lehle, M., Feyereislova, A., Revil, C.,& Jones, A. (2009). Trastuzumab plus anastrozole versus anastrozole alone for the treatment of postmenopausal women with human epidermal growth factor receptor 2-positive, hormone receptor-positive metastatic breast cancer: results from the randomized phase III TAnDEM study. (2009). *Journal of Clinical Oncology,* Vol.27, No.33, (November 2009), pp. (5529-5537).

Konecny, GE., Pegram, MD., Venkatesan, N., Finn, R., Yang, G., Rahmeh, M., Untch, M., Rusnak, DW., Spehar, G., Mullin, RJ., Keith, BR., Gilmer, TM., Berger, M., Podratz, KC. & Slamon DJ. (2006). Activity of the dual kinase inhibitor lapatinib (GW572016) against HER-2-overexpressing and trastuzumab-treated BC cells. *Cancer Research,* Vol.66, No.3, (February 2006), pp. (1630-1639).

Krop, IE., Beeram, M., Modi, S., Jones, SF., Holden, SN., Yu, W., Girish, S., Tibbitts, J., Yi, J H., Sliwkowski, MX., Jacobson, F., Lutzker, SG. & Burris, HA. (2010). Phase I study of trastuzumab-DM1, an HER2 antibody-drug conjugate, given every 3 weeks to patients with HER2-positive metastatic breast cancer. *Journal of Clinical Oncology,* Vol.28, No.16, (June 2010), pp. (2698-2704).

Kruser, TJ. & Wheeler,DL. (2010). Mechanisms of resistance to HER family targeting antibodies. *Experimental Cell Research,* Vol.316, No.7, (April 2010), pp.(1083-1100).

Law, JH., Li, Y., To, K., Wang, M., Astanehe, A., Lambie, K., Dhillon, J., Jones, SJ., Gleave, ME., Eaves, CJ. & Dunn, SE. (2010). Molecular decoy to the Y-box binding protein-1 suppresses the growth of breast and prostate cancer cells whilst sparing normal cell viability. *PLOS One,* Vol.5, No.9, (September 2010), pp. e12661.

le Coutre, P., Ottmann, OG., Giles, F., Kim, DW., Cortes, J., Gattermann, N., Apperley, JF., Larson, RA., Abruzzese, E., O'Brien, SG., Kuliczkowski, K., Hochhaus, A., Mahon, FX., Saglio, G., Gobbi, M., Kwong, YL., Baccarani, M., Hughes, T., Martinelli, G., Radich, JP., Zheng, M., Shou, Y. & Kantarjian, H. (2008). Nilotinib (formerly AMN107), a highly selective BCR-ABL tyrosine kinase inhibitor, is active in patients with imatinib-resistant or -intolerant accelerated-phase chronic myelogenous leukemia. *Blood,* Vol.111, No.4, (February 2008), pp.(1834-1839).

Lee, KF., Simon, H., Chen, H., Bates, B., Hung, MC. & Hauser, C. (1995). Requirement for neuregulin receptor erbB2 in neural and cardiac development. *Nature,* Vol.378, No.6555, (November 1995), pp. (394-398).

Lee, JW., Soung, YH., Seo, SH., Kim, SY., Park, CH., Wang, YP., Park, K., Nam, SW., Park, WS., Kim, SH., Lee, JY., Yoo, NJ.& Lee, SH. (2006). Somatic mutations of ERBB2 kinase domain in gastric, colorectal, and breast carcinomas. *Clinical Cancer Research,* Vol.12, No.1, (January 2006), pp. (57–61).

Lewis Phillips, GD., Li, G., Dugger, DL., Crocker, LM., Parsons, KL., Mai, E., Blattler, WA., Lambert, JM., Chari, RV., Lutz, RJ., Wong, WL., Jacobson, FS., Koeppen, H., Schwall ,RH., Kenkare-Mitra, SR., Spencer, SD. & Sliwkowski, MX. (2008). Targeting HER2-positive breast cancer with trastuzumab-DM1, an antibody-cytotoxic drug conjugate. *Cancer Research,* Vol.68, No.22, (November 2008), pp. (9280-9290).

Lievre, A., Bachet, JB., Le Corre, D., Boige, V., Landi, B., Emile, JF., Cote, JF., Tomasic, G., Penna, C., Ducreux, M., Rougier, P., Penault-Llorca, F. & Laurent-Puig, P. (2006). KRAS mutation status is predictive of response to cetuximab therapy in colorectal cancer. *Cancer Research,* Vol.66, No.8, (April 2006), pp. (3992-3995).

Lin, WL., Kuo, WH., Chen FL., Lee, MY., Ruan, A., Tyan, YS., Hsu, JD., Chiang, H. & Han, CP. (2011). Identification of the Coexisting HER2 Gene Amplification and Novel Mutations in the HER2 Protein-Overexpressed Mucinous Epithelial Ovarian Cancer. *Annals of Surgical Oncology,* (February 2011).

Litzow, MR. (2006). Imatinib resistance: obstacles and opportunities. *Archives of Pathology and Laboratory Medicine,* Vol.130, No.5, (May 2006), pp.(669-689).

Lu, CH., Wyszomierski, SL., Tseng, LM., Sun, MH., Lan, KH., Neal, CL., Mills, GB., Hortobagyi, GN., Esteva, FJ. & Yu, D. (2007). Preclinical testing of clinically applicable strategies for overcoming trastuzumab resistance caused by PTEN deficiency. *Clinical Cancer Research,* Vol.13, No.19, (October 2007), pp. (5883-5888).

Lu, Y., Zi, X. & Pollak, M. (2004). Molecular mechanisms underlying IGF-I-induced attenuation of the growth-inhibitory activity of trastuzumab (Herceptin) on SKBR3 breast cancer cells. *International Journal of Cancer,* Vol.108, No.3, (January 2004), pp. (334-341).

Martens, T., Schmidt, NO., Eckerich, C., Fillbrandt, R., Merchant, M., Schwall, R., Westphal, M., Lamszus, K. (2006). A novel one-armed anti-c-Met antibody inhibits glioblastoma growth in vivo. *Clinical Cancer Research,* Vol.12, No.20 Pt1, (October 2006) pp. (6144-6152).

Marty, M., Cognetti, F., Maraninchi, D., Snyder, R., Mauriac, L., Tubiana-Hulin, M., Chan, S., Grimes, D., Anton, A., Lluch, A., Kennedy, J., O'Byrne, K., Conte, P., Green, M.,

Ward, C., Mayne, K., & Extra, JM. (2005). Randomized phase II trial of the efficacy and safety of trastuzumab combined with docetaxel in patients with human epidermal growth factor receptor 2-positive metastatic breast cancer administered as first-line treatment: the M77001 study group. *Journal of Clinical Oncology,* Vol.23, No.19, (July 2005), pp. (4265-4274).

Mendelsohn, J. (2002). Targeting the epidermal growth factor receptor for cancer therapy. *Journal of Clinical Oncology,* Vol.20, No.18 Suppl, (September 2002), pp. (1S–13S).

Mittendorf, EA., Wu, Y., Scaltriti, M., Meric-Bernstam, F., Hunt, KK., Dawood, S., Esteva, FJ., Buzdar, AU., Chen, H., Eksambi, S., Hortobagyi, GN., Baselga, J. & Gonzalez-Angulo, AM.(2009). Loss of HER2 amplification following trastuzumab-based neoadjuvant systemic therapy and survival outcomes. *Clinical Cancer Research,* Vol.15, No.23, (December 2009), pp. (7381-7388).

Mittendorf, EA., Liu, Y., Tucker, SL., Mckenzie, T., Qiao, N., Akli, S., Biernacka, A., Liu, Y., Meijer, L., Keyomarsi, K. & Hunt, KK. (2010). A novel interaction between HER2/neu and cyclin E in breast cancer. *Oncogene,*Vol. 29, No.27, (July 2010), pp. (3896-3907).

Mitsudomi, T., Kosaka, T., Endoh, H., Horio, Y., Hida, T., Mori, S., Hatooka, S., Shinoda, M., Takahashi, T. & Yatabe, Y. (2005). Mutations of the epidermal growth factor receptor gene predict prolonged survival after gefitinib treatment in patients with non-small-cell lung cancer with postoperative recurrence. *Journal of Clinical Oncology,* Vol.23, No.11, (April 2005), pp. (2513–2520).

Modi, S., Stopeck, AT., Gordon, MS., Mendelson, D., Solit, DB., Bagatell, R., Ma, W., Wheler, J., Rosen, N., Norton, L., Cropp, GF., Johnson, RG., Hannah, AL. & Hudis, CA. (2007). Combination of trastuzumab and tanespimycin (17-AAG, KOS-953) is safe and active in trastuzumab-refractory HER-2 overexpressing breast cancer: a phase I dose-escalation study. *Journal of Clinical Oncology,* Vol. 25, No.34, (December 2007), pp. (5410-5417).

Morgillo, F., Bareschino, MA., Bianco, R., Tortora, G. & Ciardiello, F. (2007). Primary and acquired resistance to anti-EGFR targeted drugs in cancer therapy. *Differentiation,* Vol.75, No.9, (November 2007), pp. (788–799).

Motoyama, AB., Hynes, NE. & Lane, HA. (2002).The efficacy of ErbB receptor-targeted anticancer therapeutics is influenced by the availability of epidermal growth factor-related peptides. *Cancer Research,* Vol.62, No.11, (June 2002), pp. (3151–3158).

Mukohara, T., Engelman, JA., Hanna, NH., Yeap, BY., Kobayashi, S., Lindeman, N., Halmos, B., Pearlberg, J., Tsuchihashi, Z., Cantley, LC., Tenen, DG., Johnson, BE. & Jänne, PA. (2005). Differential effects of gefitinib and cetuximab on non - small-cell lung cancers bearing epidermal growth factor receptor mutations. *Journal of the National Cancer Institute,* Vol.97, No.16, (August 2005), pp. (1185-1194).

Murphy, N., Millar, E. & Lee, CS. (2005).Gene expression profiling in breast cancer: towards individualizing patient management. Pathology, Vol.37, No.4, (August 2005), pp.(271-277).

Musolino, A., Naldi, N., Bortesi, B., Pezzuolo, D., Capelletti, M., Missale, G., Laccabue, D., Zerbini, A., Camisa, R., Bisagni, G., Neri, TM. & Ardizzoni, A. (2008). Immunoglobulin G fragment C receptor polymorphisms and clinical efficacy of trastuzumab-based therapy in patients with HER-2/neu-positive metastatic breast cancer. *Journal of Clinical Oncology,* Vol.26, No.11, (April 2008), pp. (1789-1796)

Nagata, Y., Lan, KH., Zhou, X., Tan, M., Esteva, FJ., Sahin, AA., Klos, KS., Li, P., Monia, BP., Nguyen, NT., Hortobagyi, GN., Hung, MC. & Yu, D. (2004). PTEN activation contributes to tumor inhibition by trastuzumab, and loss of PTEN predicts trastuzumab resistance in patients. *Cancer Cell,* Vol.6, No.2, (August 2004), pp. (117-127).

Nagy, P., Friedlander, E., Tanner, M., Kapanen, AI., Carraway, KL., Isola, J. & Jovin, TM.(2005). Decreased accessibility and lack of activation of ErbB2 in JIMT-1, a herceptin-resistant, MUC4-expressing breast cancer cell line. *Cancer Research,* Vol.65, No.2, (January 2005), pp. (473-482).

Nahta, R., Takahashi, T., Ueno, NT., Hung, MC. & Esteva, FJ. (2004a). $P27^{kip1}$ down-regulation is associated with trastuzumab resistance in breast cancer cells. *Cancer Research,* Vol.64, No.11, (June 2004), pp. (3981-3986).

Nahta, R., Hung, MC. & Esteva, FJ. (2004b). The HER-2 targeting antibodies trastuzumab and pertuzumab synergistically inhibit the survival of breast cancer cells. *Cancer Research,* Vol.64, No.7, (April 2004), pp. (2343-2346).

Nahta, R., Yuan, LX., Zhang, B., Kobayashi, R. & Esteva, FJ. (2005). Insulin-like growth factor I receptor/human epidermal growth factor receptor 2 heterodimerization contributes to trastuzumab resistance of breast cancer cells. *Cancer Research,* Vol. 65, No. 23, (December 2005), pp.(11118-11128).

Nahta, R. & Esteva, FJ. (2006). Herceptin: mechanisms of action and resistance. *Cancer Letters,* Vol.232, No.2, (February 2006), pp. (123-138).

Nahta, R., Yuan, LX., Du, Y. & Esteva, FJ. (2007). Lapatinib induces apoptosis in trastuzumab-resistant breast cancer cells: effects on insulin-like growth factor I signaling. *Molecular Cancer Therapeutics,* Vol.6, No.2, (February 2007), pp. (667-674).

Natali, PG., Nicotra, MR., Bigotti, A., Venturo, I., Slamon, DJ., Fendly, BM. & Ullrich, A. (1990). Expression of the p185 encoded by HER2 oncogene in normal and transformed human tissues. *International Journal of Cancer,* Vol.45, No.3, (March 1990), pp. (457-461).

Negro, A., Brar, BK. & Lee, KF. (2004). Essential roles of Her2/erbB2 in cardiac development and function. *Recent Progress in Hormone Research,* Vol.59, pp. (1-12).

Nelson, AL., Dhimolea, E. & Reichert, JM. (2010). Development trends for human monoclonal antibody therapeutics. *Nature Reviews Drug Discovery,* Vol.9, No.10, (October 2010), pp. (767-774).

Nguyen, TH., Loux, N., Dagher, I., Vons, C., Carey, K., Briand, P., Hadchouel, M., Franco, D., Jouanneau, J., Schwall, R. & Weber, A. (2003). Improved gene transfer selectivity to hepatocarcinoma cells by retrovirus vector displaying single-chain variable fragment antibody against c-Met. *Cancer Gene Therapy,* Vol. 10, No.11, (November 2003), pp.(840-849).

Niehans, GA., Singleton, TP., Dykosk,i D., & Kiang, DT. (1993). Stability of HER-2/neu expression over time and at multiple metastatic sites. *Journal of the National Cancer Institute,* Vol.85, No.15, (August 1993), pp. (1230-1235).

Nordstrom, JL., Huang, L., Yang, Y., Tuaillon, N., Stavenhagen, JB., Stewart, S., Moore, PA., Johnson, S., Koenig, S., Bonvini; E.(2010). Preclinical antitumor activity of an Fc domain-optimized HER2 monoclonal antibody (mAb). Abstract (e13135) of 2010 American Society of Clinical Oncology Annual Meeting, Chicago, IL June 2010.

O'Shaughnessy, JA., Vukelja, S., Marsland, T., Kimmel, G., Ratnam, S. & Pippen, JE. (2004). Phase II study of trastuzumab plus gemcitabine in chemotherapy-pretreated patients with metastatic breast cancer. *Clinical Breast Cancer,* Vol.5, No.2, (June 2004), pp. (142-147).

Ohashi K., Marion PL., Nakai H., Meuse L., Cullen JM., Bordier BB., Schwall R., Greenberg HB., Glenn JS. & Kay MA. (2000) .Sustained survival of human hepatocytes in mice: A model for in vivo infection with human hepatitis B and hepatitis delta viruses. *Nature Medicine,* Vol. 6, No.3, (Mar 2000), pp.(327-331).

Okines, AF. & Cunningham, D. (2010).Trastuzumab in gastric cancer. *European Journal of Cancer,* Vol.46, No.11, (July 2010), pp. (1949–1959).

Ozbay, T., Durden, DL., Liu, T., O'Regan, RM. & Nahta, R. (2010). In vitro evaluation of pan-PI3-kinase inhibitor SF1126 in trastuzumab-sensitive and trastuzumab-resistant HER2-over-expressing breast cancer cells. *Cancer Chemotherapy and Pharmacology,* Vol.65, No.4, (March 2010), pp. (697-706).

Paik, S., Hazan, R., Fisher, ER., Sass, RE., Fisher, B., Redmond, C., Schlessinger, J., Lippman, ME., & King, CR. (1990). Pathologic findings from the National Surgical Adjuvant Breast and Bowel Project: prognostic significance of erbB-2 protein overexpression in primary breast cancer. *Journal of Clinical Oncology,* Vol.8, No.1, (January 1990), pp. (103-112).

Palyi-Krekk, Z., Barok, M., Isola, J., Tammi, M., Szollosi, J. & Nagy, P. (2007). Hyaluronan-induced masking of ErbB2 and CD44-enhanced trastuzumab internalization in trastuzumab resistant breast cancer. *European Journal of Cancer,* Vol.43, No.16, (November 2007), pp. (2423-2433).

Pao, W., Miller, VA., Politi, KA., Riely, GJ., Somwar, R., Zakowski, MF., Kris, MG. & Varmus, H. (2005). Acquired resistance of lung adenocarcinomas to gefitinib or erlotinib is associated with a second mutation in the EGFR kinase domain. *PLoS Med,* Vol.2, No.3, (March 2005), pp. e73.

Prat, M., Crepaldi, T., Pennacchietti, S., Bussolino, F.& Comoglio, PM. (1998). Agonistic monoclonal antibodies against the Met receptor dissect the biological responses to HGF. *Journal of Cell Science,* Vol. 111, No. Pt2, (January 1998), pp. (237-247).

Pedersen, K., Angelini, PD., Laos, S., Bach-Faig, A., Cunningham, MP., Ferrer-Ramon, C., Luque-Garcia, A., Garcia-Castillo, J., Parra-Palau, JL., Scaltriti, M., Ramon y Cajal, S., Baselga, J. & Arribas, J. (2009). A naturally occurring HER2 carboxy-terminal fragment promotes mammary tumor growth and metastasis. *Molecular and Cellular Biology,* Vol.29, No.12, (June 2009), pp. (3319-3331).

Pegram, MD., Lipton, A., Hayes, DF., Weber, BL., Baselga, JM., Tripathy, D., Baly, D., Baughman, SA., Twaddell, T., Glaspy, JA.& Slamon, DJ.(1998). Phase II study of receptor-enhanced chemosensitivity using recombinant humanized anti-p185 HER2/neu monoclonal antibody plus cisplatin in patients with HER2/neu-overexpressing metastatic breast cancer refractory to chemotherapy treatment. *Journal of Clinical Oncology,* Vol.16, No.8, (August 1998), pp. (2659-2671).

Pegram, M., Hsu, S., Lewis, G., Pietras, R., Beryt, M., Sliwkowski, M., Coombs, D., Baly, D., Kabbinavar, F. & Slamon, D. (1999). Inhibitory effects of combinations of HER-2/neu antibody and chemotherapeutic agents used for treatment of human breast cancer. *Oncogene,* Vol.18, No.13, (April 1999), pp. (2241-2251).

Perez, EA., Suman, VJ., Rowland, KM., Ingle, JN., Salim, M., Loprinzi, CL., Flynn, PJ., Mailliard,JA., Kardinal, CG., Krook, JE., Thrower, AR., Visscher, DW. & Jenkins, RB. (2005). Two concurrent phase II trials of paclitaxel/carboplatin/trastuzumab (weekly or every-3-week schedule) as first-line therapy in women with HER2-overexpressing metastatic breast cancer: NCCTG study 983252.*Clinical Breast Cancer,* Vol.6, No.5, (December 2005), pp. (425-432).

Piccart-Gebhart, MJ., Procter, M., Leyland-Jones, B., Goldhirsch, A., Untch, M., Smith, I., Gianni, L., Baselga, J., Bell, R., Jackisch, C., Cameron, D., Dowsett, M., Barrios, CH., Steger, G., Huang, CS., Andersson, M., Inbar, M., Lichinitser, M., Lang, I., Nitz, U., Iwata, H., Thomssen, C., Lohrisch, C., Suter, TM., Ruschoff, J., Suto, T.,Greatorex, V., Ward, C., Straehle, C., McFadden, E., Dolci, MS., & Gelber, RD. for the Herceptin Adjuvant (HERA) Trial Study Team. (2005). Trastuzumab after adjuvant chemotherapy in HER2 –positive breast cancer. *The New England Journal of Medicine,* Vol.353, No.16, (October 2005), pp. (1659-1672).

Pratt, WB.& Toft, DO. (2003). Regulation of signaling protein function and trafficking by the hsp90/hsp70-based chaperone machinery. *Experimental Biology and Medicine (Maywood),* Vol.228 ,No.2, (February 2003) pp.(111–133).

Press, MF., Pike, MC., Chazin, VR., Hung, G., Udove, JA., Markowicz, M., Danyluk, J., Godolphin, W., Sliwkowski, M., Akita, R., Paterson, MC. & Slamon, DJ. (1993). Her-2/neu expression in node-negative breast cancer: direct tissue quantitation by computerized image analysis and association of overexpression with increased risk of recurrent disease. *Cancer Research,* Vol.53, No.20, (October 1993), pp. (4960-4970) .

Raja, SM., Clubb, RJ., Bhattacharyya, M., Dimri, M.,Cheng, H., Pan, W.,Ortega-Cava, C., Lakku-Reddi, A., Naramura, M., Band, V. & Band, H. A combination of Trastuzumab and 17-AAG induces enhanced ubiquitination and lysosomal pathway-dependent ErbB2 degradation and cytotoxicity in ErbB2-overexpressing breast cancer cells. *Cancer Biology& Therapy,* Vol.7, No.10, (October 2008), pp. (1630-1640)

Ranson, M. & Sliwkowski, MX. (2002). Perspectives on anti-HER antibodies. *Oncology,* Vol. 63,Suppl 1, (November 2002), pp. (17-24).

Reichert, JM. (2009). Global antibody development trends. *mABs,* Vol.1, No.1, (January/February 2009), pp. (86-87).

Ritter, CA., Perez-Torres, M., Rinehart, C., Guix, M., Dugger, T., Engelman, JA. & Arteaga, CL. (2007). Human breast cancer cells selected for resistance to trastuzumab *in vivo* overexpress epidermal growth factor receptor and ErbB ligands and remain dependent on the ErbB receptor network. *Clinical Cancer Research,* Vol.13, No.16, (August 2007), pp. (4909-4919).

Sahai E.& Marshall, CJ. (2002). RHO-GTPases and cancer. *Nature Reviews Cancer.,* Vol. 2, No.2, (February 2002), pp. (133-142).

Saltz, LB., Meropol, NJ., Loehrer, PJ Sr., Needle, MN., Kopit, J. & Mayer, RJ. (2004). Phase II trial of cetuximab in patients with refractory colorectal cancer that expresses the epidermal growth factor receptor. *Journal of Clinical Oncology,* Vol.22, No.7, (April 2004), pp. (1201-1208).

Sanchez-Munoz, A., Gallego, E., de Luque, V., Perez-Rivas, LG., Vicioso, L., Ribelles, N., Lozano, J. & Alba, E. (2010). Lack of evidence for KRAS oncogenic mutations in triple-negative breast cancer. *BMC Cancer,* Vol.10, (April 2010), pp. 136.

Scaltriti, M., Eichhorn, PJ., Cortes, J., Prudkin, L., Aura, C., Jimenez, J., Chandarlapaty, S., Serra, V., Prat, A., Ibrahim, YH., Guzman, M., Gili, M., Rodriguez, O., Rodriguez, S., Perez, J., Green, SR., Mai, S., Rosen, N., Hudis, C. & Baselga, J. (2011).Cyclin E amplification/overexpression is a mechanism of trastuzumab resistance in HER2^{+} breast cancer patients. *Proceedings of the National Academy of Sciences of the Unites States of America,* Vol.108, No.9, (March 2011), pp. (3761-3766).

Schwartz, JD., Rowinsky, EK., Youssoufian, H., Pytowki, B. & Wu, Y. (2010). Vascular endothelial growth factor receptor-1 in human cancer: concise review and rationale for development of IMC-18F1 (Human antibody targeting vascular endothelial growth factor receptor-1). *Cancer,* Vol.116, No.4Suppl, (February 2010), pp. (1027-1032).

Senter, PD. (2009). Potent antibody drug conjugates for cancer therapy. *Current opinion in chemical biology,* Vol.13, No.3, (June 2009), pp. (235-244).

Sergina, NV., Rausch, M., Wang, D., Blair, J., Hann, B., Shokat, KM. & Moasser, MM. (2007). Escape from HER-family tyrosine kinase inhibitor therapy by the kinase-inactive HER3. *Nature,* Vol.445, No.7126, (January 2007), pp. (437–441).

Serra, V., Markman, B., Scaltriti, M., Eichhorn, PJ., Valero, V., Guzman, M., Botero, ML., Llonch, E., Atzori, F., Di Cosimo, S., Maira, M., Garcia-Echeverria, C., Parra, JL., Arribas, J. & Baselga, J. (2008). NVP-BEZ235, a dual PI3K/mTOR inhibitor, prevents PI3K signaling and inhibits the growth of cancer cells with activating PI3K mutations. *Cancer Research,* Vol.68, No. 19, (October 2008), pp. (8022-8030).

Shattuck, DL., Miller, JK., Carraway, KL 3rd.& Sweeney, C. (2008). Met receptor contributes to trastuzumab resistance of Her2-overexpressing breast cancer cells. *Cancer Research,* Vol. 68, No. 5 (March 2008), pp.(1471-1477).

Shi, F., Telesco, SE., Liu, Y., Radhakrishnan, R. & Lemmon, MA. (2010). ErbB3/HER3 intracellular domain is competent to bind ATP and catalyze autophosphorylation. *Proceedings of the National Academy of Sciences of the United States of America,* Vol.107, No.17, (April 2010), pp. (7692-7697).

Shigematsu, H., Takahashi, T., Nomura, M., Majmudar, K., Suzuki, M., Lee, H., Wistuba, II., Fong, KM., Toyooka, S., Shimizu, N., Fujisawa, T., Minna, JD. & Gazdar, AF. (2005). Somatic mutations of the HER2 kinase domain in lung adenocarcinoma. *Cancer Research,* Vol.65, No.5, (March 2005), pp. (1642-1646).

Shin, DM., Donato, NJ., Perez-Soler, R., Shin, HJ., Wu, JY., Zhang, P., Lawhorn, K., Khuri, FR., Glisson, BS., Myers, J., Clayman, G., Pfister, D., Falcey, J., Waksal, H., Mendelsohn, J. & Hong, WK. (2001). Epidermal growth factor receptor-targeted therapy with C225 and cisplatin in patients with head and neck cancer. *Clinical Cancer Research,* Vol.7, No.5, (May 2001), pp. (1204-1213).

Sierke, SL., Cheng, K., Kim, HH. & Koland, JG. (1997). Biochemical characterization of the protein tyrosine kinase homology domain of the ErbB3 (HER3) receptor protein. *Biochemistry Journal,* Vol.322, No.Pt 3, (March 1997), pp. (757–763).

Slamon, DJ., Clark, GM., Wong, SG., Levin, WJ., Ullrich, A. &McGuire, WL. (1987). Human breast cancer: correlation of relapse and survival with amplification of the HER-2/neu oncogene. *Science,* Vol.235, No.4785, (January 1987), pp. (177-182).

Slamon, DJ., Godolphin, W., Jones, LA., Holt, JA., Wong, SG., Keith, DE., Levin, WJ., Stuart, SG., Udove, J., Ullrich, A. & Press, MF. (1989). Studies of the HER-2/neu proto-oncogene in human breast and ovarian cancer. *Science,* Vol.244, No.4905, (May 1989), pp. (707-712).

Slamon, DJ., Leyland-Jones, B., Shak, S., Fuchs, H., Paton, V., Bajamonde, A., Fleming, T., Eiermann, W., Wolter, J., Pegram, M., Baselga, J. & Norton, L. (2001). Use of chemotherapy plus a monoclonal antibody against HER2 for metastatic breast cancer that overexpresses HER2. *The New England Journal of Medicine,* Vol.344, No.11, (March 2001), pp. (783-792).

Spratlin, JL., Cohen, RB., Eadens, M., Gore, L., Camidge, DR., Diab, S., Leong, S., O'Bryant, C., Chow, LQ., Serkova, NJ., Meropol, NJ., Lewis, NL., Chiorean, EG., Fox, F., Youssoufian, H., Rowinsky, EK.& Eckhardt, SG. (2010). Phase I pharmacological and biological study of ramucirumab (IMC-1121B), a fully human immunoglobulin G1 monoclonal antibody targeting the vascular endothelial growth factor receptor-2. *Journal of Clinical Oncology,* Vol.28, No.5, (February 2010), pp. (780-787).

Sutter, TM., Procter, M., van Veldhuisen, DJ., Muscholl, M., Bergh, J., Carlomagno, C., Perren, T., Passalacqua, R., Bighin, C., Klijn, J.G.M., Ageev, FT., Hitre, E., Groetz, J., Iwata, H., Knap, M., Gnant, M., Muehlbauer, S.,Spence, A., Gelber, RD. & Piccart-Gebhart ,MJ. (2007). Trastuzumab-associated cardiac adverse effects in the herceptin adjuvant trial. *Journal of Clinical Oncology,* Vol.25, No.26, (September 2007), pp. (3859-3865).

Swann, PG., Tolnay, M., Muthukkumar, S., Shapiro, MA., Rellahan, BL. & Clouse, KA. (2008). Considerations for the development of therapeutic monoclonal antibodies. *Current Opinion in Immunology,* Vol.20, No.4, (August 2008), pp. (493–499).

Tanner, M., Kapanen, AI., Junttila, T., Raheem, O., Grenman, S., Elo, J., Elenius, K. & Isola, J. (2004). Characterization of a novel cell line established from a patient with Herceptin-resistant breast cancer. *Molecular Cancer Therapeutics,* Vol.3, No.12, (December 2004), pp. (1585-1592).

Tseng, PH., Wang, YC., Weng, SC., Weng, JR., Chen, CS., Brueggemeier, RW., Shapiro, CL., Chen, CY., Dunn, SE., Pollak, M. & Chen, CS. (2006). Overcoming trastuzumab resistance in HER2-overexpressing breast cancer cells by using a novel celecoxib-derived phosphoinositide-dependent kinase-1 inhibitor. *Molecular Pharmacology,* Vol.70, No.5, (November 2006), pp. (1534-1541).

Tzahar, E., Waterman, H., Chen, X., Levkowitz, G., Karunagaran, D., Lavi, S., Ratzkin, BJ. & Yarden, Y. (1996). A hierarchical network of interreceptor interactions determines signal transduction by Neu differentiation factor/neuregulin and epidermal growth factor. *Molecular and Cellular Biology,* Vol.16, No.10, (October 1996), pp. (5276–5287).

Untch, M., Rezai, M., Loibl, S., Fasching, PA., Huober, J., Tesch, H., Bauerfeind, I., Hilfrich, J., Eidtmann, H., Gerber, B., Hanusch, C., Kuhn, T., du Bois, A., Blohmer, JU., Thomssen, C., Dan Costa, S., Jackisch, C., Kaufmann, M., Mehta, K., & von Minckwitz, G. (2010). Neoadjuvant treatment with trastuzumab in HER2-positive breast cancer: results from the GeparQuattro study. *Journal of Clinical Oncology,* Vol.28, No.12, (April 2010), pp. (2024-2031).

Valabrega, G., Montemurro, F., Sarotto, I., Petrelli, A., Rubini, P., Tacchetti, C., Aglietta, M., Comoglio, PM. & Giordano, S. (2005). TGF alpha expression impairs Trastuzumab-induced HER2 downregulation. *Oncogene,* Vol.24, No.18, (April 2005), pp. (3002-3010).

Van Cutsem, E., Peeters, M., Siena, S., Humblet, Y., Hendlisz, A., Neyns, B., Canon, JL., Van Laethem, JL., Maurel, J., Richardson, G., Wolf, M. & Amado, RG. (2007). Open-label phase III , trial of panitumumab plus best supportive care compared with best supportive care alone in patients with chemotherapy-refractory metastatic colorectal cancer. *Journal of Clinical Oncology*, Vol.25, No.13, (May 2007), pp. (1658–1664).

Vazquez-Martin, A., Colomer, R., Brunet, J. & Menendez, JA. (2007). Pharmacological blockage of fatty acid synthase (FASN) reverses acquired autoresistance to trastuzumab (Herceptin) by transcriptionally inhibiting "HER2 super-expression" occurring in high-dose trastuzumab-conditioned SKBR3/Tzb100 breast cancer cells. *International Journal of Oncology*, Vol.31, No.4, (October 2007), pp. (769-776).

Viani, GA., Afonso, SL., Stefano, EJ., De Fendi, LI. & Soares, FV. (2007). Adjuvant trastuzumab in the treatment of her-2-positive early breast cancer: a meta-analysis of published randomized trials. *BMC Cancer*, Vol.7, (August 2007), pp.153.

Vogel, CL., Cobleigh, MA., Tripathy, D., Gutheil, JC., Harris, LN., Fehrenbacher, L., Slamon, DJ., Murphy, M., Novotny, WF., Burchmore, M., Shak, S., Stewart, SJ. & Press, M. (2002). Efficacy and safety of trastuzumab as a single agent in first-line treatment of HER2-overexpressing metastatic breast cancer. *Journal of Clinical Oncology*, Vol.20, No.3, (February 2002), pp. (719-726).

Wada, T., Qian, XL. & Greene, MI. (1990). Intermolecular association of the p185neu protein and EGF receptor modulates EGF receptor function. *Cell*, Vol.61, No.7, (June 1990), pp. (1339–1347).

Wang, SE., Xiang, B., Guix, M., Olivares, MG., Parker, J., Chung, CH., Pandiella, A. & Arteaga, CL. (2008). Transforming growth factor beta engages TACE and ErbB3 to activate phosphatidylinositol-3 kinase/Akt in ErbB2-overexpressing breast cancer and desensitizes cells to trastuzumab. *Molecular and Cellular Biology*, Vol.28, No.18, (September 2008), pp. (5605-5620).

Wolff, AC., Hammond, ME., Schwartz, JN., Hagerty, KL., Allred, DC., Cote, RJ., Dowsett, M., Fitzgibbons, PL., Hanna, WM., Langer, A., McShane, LM., Paik, S., Pegram, MD., Perez, EA., Press, MF., Rhodes, A., Sturgeon, C., Taube, SE., Tubbs, R., Vance, GH., van de Vijver, M., Wheeler, TM. & Hayes, DF. (2007). American Society of Clinical Oncology/College of American Pathologist guideline recommendations for human epidermal growth factor receptor 2 testing in breast cancer. *Journal of Clinical Oncology*, Vol.25, No.1, (January 2007), pp. (118-145).

Yan, L., Ehrlich, PJ. , Gibson, R., Pickett, C. & Beckman, RA. (2009).How can we improve antibody-based cancer therapy? *mAbs*, Vol.*1, No. 1,* (January/February 2009), pp. (67-70).

Yarden, Y. & Sliwkowski, M.X. (2001).Untangling the ErbB signalling network. *Nature Reviews Molecular Cell Biology*, Vol.2, No.2, (February 2001), pp. (127–137).

Zhang, H., Berezov, A., Wang, Q., Zhang, G., Drebin, J., Mural,i R.& Greene, MI. (2007). ErbB receptors: from oncogenes to targeted cancer therapies. *The Journal of Clinical Investigation*, Vol.117, No.8, (August 2007), pp. (2051-2058).

Zhou, X., Tan, M., Stone Hawthorne, V., Klos, KS., Lan, KH., Yang, Y., Yang, W., Smith, TL., Shi, D. & Yu, D.(2004). Activation of the Akt/mammalian target of rapamycin/4E-BP1 pathway by ErbB2 overexpression predicts tumor progression in breast cancers. *Clinical Cancer Research*, Vol.10, No.20, (October 2004), pp. (6779-6788).

Zhuang, G., Brantley-Sieders, DM., Vaught, D., Yu, J., Xie, L., Wells, S., Jackson, D., Muraoka-Cook, R., Arteaga, C. & Chen, J. (2010). Elevation of receptor tyrosine kinase ephA2 mediates resistance to trastuzumab therapy. *Cancer Research,* Vol.70, No.1, (January 2010), pp. (299-308).

Zito, CI., Riches, D., Kolmakova, J., Simons, J., Egholm, M. & Stern, DF.(2008). Direct resequencing of the complete ERBB2 coding sequence reveals an absence of activating mutations in ERBB2 amplified breast cancer. *Genes, Chromosomes and Cancer*, Vol.47, No.7, (July 2008), pp. (633- 638).

Zuo, T., Wang, L., Morrison, C., Chang, X., Zhang, H., Li, W., Liu, Y., Wang, Y., Liu, X., Chan, MW., Liu, JQ., Love, R., Liu, CG., Godfrey, V., Shen, R., Huang, T.H.., Yang, T., Park, BK., Wang, CY., Zheng, P. & Liu, Y. (2007). FOXP3 is an X-linked breast cancer suppressor gene and an important repressor of the HER-2/ErbB2 oncogene. *Cell,* Vol.129, No.7, (June 2007), pp. (1275-1286).

Zsebik, B., Citri, A., Isola, J., Yarden, Y., Szollosi, J. & Vereb, G. (2006). Hsp90 inhibitor 17-AAG reduces ErbB2 levels and inhibits proliferation of the trastuzumab resistant breast tumor cell line JIMT-1. *Immunology Letters,* Vol.104, No.1-2, (April 2006), pp. (146-155).

8

EGFR-Ligand Signaling in Breast Cancer Metastasis: Recurring Developmental Themes

Nicole K. Nickerson[1], Jennifer L. Gilmore[1], Kah Tan Allen[1], David J. Riese II[2], Kenneth P. Nephew[1,3] and John Foley[1,3,4]
[1]*Medical Sciences Program, Indiana University School of Medicine, Bloomington, IN*
[2]*Harrison School of Pharmacy, Auburn University, Auburn, AL*
[3]*Indiana University Cancer Center Indiana University School of Medicine, Indianapolis, IN*
[4]*Department of Dermatology, Indiana University School of Medicine, Indianapolis, IN*
United States of America

1. Introduction

1.1 ErbB receptors, ligands and signaling

Breast cancer affects nearly 1 out of 9 women worldwide. The quality of treatment for breast cancer has improved to the point that close to 80% of patients in countries with advanced healthcare delivery systems survive the disease (1). Yet over 20% of breast cancer patients succumb to the disease, and the majority of these have metastatic breast cancer cells that occupy and compromise the function of distal organs (1). There has been an intensive effort to improve treatments for metastatic breast cancer. Novel treatment strategies have arisen from the study of the molecular and cellular biology of breast cancer cell lines. These studies have produced a group of agents called targeted therapeutics because they are often directed at a single molecule rather than a general process such as DNA replication or cytoskeletal function. The ErbB family represents a target that is present in breast cancer. Therapeutics to ErbB2 have been used to treat aggressive breast cancer for over a decade with considerable success (2). However, therapeutics that primarily target the EGFR have not been used extensively in breast cancer, and there are some improved agents for the receptor that are just entering the clinic. Recent conclusions from studies of metastatic breast cancer suggest new possibilities for the use of EGFR therapeutics. This review will describe the members of the EGFR signaling family, discuss the cellular context in which they function in development, and correlate this with the biological role of these molecules in breast cancer metastasis.

1.2 ErbB family members

The ErbB family consists of 4 receptors: ErbB1 or more commonly called EGFR, ErbB2/ Her2, ErbB3 and ErbB4 (3). Signaling is generated when EGFR and ErbB4 bind to their ligands. In contrast, the ErbB2 extracellular binding domain fails to bind any of the 15 agonists, and in ErbB3 the kinase domain is not functional. Upon ligand stimulation, EGFR and ErbB4 receptors can transduce their signals as homodimers or heterodimers; however, the signal generation from ErbB2 or ErbB3 require heterodimerization with another ErbB family member (3).

The ErbB receptors are stimulated by 15 ligands but the situation is complicated because several of these agonists can bind more than one receptor. The EGFR exclusive agonists are epidermal growth factor (EGF), transforming growth factor alpha (TGF-α), amphiregulin (AREG) and Epigen (Epi) (3, 4). ErbB4 is specifically bound and activated by Neuregulins (NRG) 3, 4, 5 (3, 4). Heparin-binding EGF-like growth factor (HB-EGF), epiregulin (EREG), and β-cellulin (BTC) bind and activate both the EGFR and ErbB4 (3, 4). NRG 1 and 2 binds both ErbB3 and ErbB4 and NRG 1 can bind the EGFR with low affinity (3, 4).

All of the ErbB agonists are synthesized as plasma membrane bound integral membrane proteins (5). In some cases, the transmembrane ligands stimulate ErbB signaling on adjacent cells through a juxtracrine mechanism which may mediate the stromal-epithelial interactions (6) (7). Most ErbB signaling requires proteolytic cleavage termed ectodomain shedding for the ligand to be released and available to bind receptors that may be on the same cell (autocrine signaling), or on neighboring cells (paracrine signaling) (5). The proteases that mediate the process are from the "a disintegrin and metalloproteinase " or (ADAM) family (8, 9). There are 40 members of the ADAM protein family that function in cell adhesion and ectodomain shedding. These ADAMs are integral membrane proteins in which the extracellular region contains a protease as well as a disintegrin domain that modulates integrin binding (9). ADAMs can be activated by a wide range of stimuli that signal through G-protein-coupled receptors and these signals are often transduced by Src (10). The shedding of AREG, EREG, HB-EGF, Epigen, TGFα and NRG 1&2 is typically catalyzed by the single family member ADAM 17, whereas BTC and EGF are cleaved by ADAM 10 (8). In addition, ADAM 17 cleaves many other cytokines, growth factors, receptors, adhesion molecules and extracellular matrix proteins, suggesting its activity may be a key determinate of cellular behavior (9). Nevertheless, emerging data suggest that EGFR ligands can be shed by other proteases such as the ADAM thrombospondin (ADAMTS) family that is structurally related to the ADAM family, but is secreted and the disintgrin domain is replaced by a thrombospondin domain that binds to matrix (11, 12). Also, it is likely that other metalloproteinases secreted from cells in a paracrine relationship are capable of releasing ligands (13).

Over the past two decades the expression of ErbB receptors, ligands, and their activating proteases in normal breast and breast cancers have been intensively studied. Various mRNA detection methods and immunohistochemistry studies have concluded that the entire ErbB family is expressed in various breast cancers. In fact, it appears the vast majority of the family is expressed in the mammary epithelia (14-16). Since newer therapeutics that target the EGFR are being considered for use in cases of advanced breast cancer, in the rest of this review we will focus on how this receptor is activated and describe its role in development and cancer progression.

1.3 EGFR homodimer signaling

EGF was the first ligand identified and due its abundance in the mouse salivary gland and relative ease of purification from this source (17). EGF has historically been used for receptor binding, signaling, trafficking, and cell fate studies resulting in a model of receptor signaling that is in many ways considered to be the prototype for receptor tyrosine kinases (18-20). The binding of EGF to the EGFR exposes the dimerization arm in the extracellular domain that permits interaction with another EGFR receptor or hetrodimerization with other ErbBs. Ligand binding also induces a conformational change in the receptor that activates the intracellular kinase domain, which in turn can phosphorylate tyrosine residues on the adjacent C-terminal tail of the dimerized ErbB receptor. The 10 phosphorylated tyrosine residues serve as docking sites for adapter proteins or other signal transduction components, resulting in activation of Ras, MAPK, src, STAT 3/5 and PLCγ/PKC and the PI3 kinase-AKT-pro survival pathway. Activation of these signaling pathways by ErbB dimers has profound impact on proliferation, resistance to apoptosis, differentiation, as well as motility/migration associated behaviors. Not all tyrosine phosphorylation of EGFR C-terminal tail results in stimulation of downstream signaling pathways. For example, phosphorylation of the 974 residue triggers enodcytosis of the receptor, and phospho 1045 binds to Cbl, mediating ubquitination of the receptor and subsequent proteosomal degradation (4, 21). Trafficking studies suggest that ~50% of EGF stimulated EGFR is degraded, whereas the remainder is recycled back to the plasma membrane (22). Thus, activation of the EGFR by EGF directly stimulates a broad group of cellular signaling pathways, many of which converge on elements of the ERK/MAPK pathway (3), but this signaling is dampened by receptor turnover. The rapid turnover of the EGF stimulated EGFR is believed to limit stimulation of cellular proliferation, permitting a balance with various differentiation-inducing stimuli present in a normal tissue (3, 22, 23). In cancers, autocrine EGFR homodimer signaling is substantially attenuated, shifting the cell fate balance towards proliferation and survival rather than differentiation, apoptosis and senescence.

1.4 Attenuating EGFR signaling with heterodimerization

Probably the most well understood attenuation of EGFR signaling occurs when the receptor heterodimerizes with the ErbB 2 receptor (24, 25). It is believed that EGFR heterodimerization with ErbB2 frequently occurs in a number of breast cancers (26, 27). Despite being unable to bind ligand, the ErbB2 dimerization arm is constitutively exposed, which allows this receptor to more efficiently dimerize with other liganded ErbB family members (4). The resulting ErbB2 containing heterodimers attenuate EGFR signal transduction in several ways (28-32). First, the affinity of this ErbB2 complex for ligands is enhanced. Second, the ErbB2 phosphotyrosine domains bind most adapter proteins with higher affinity than those of the ErbB homodimers, resulting in more efficient signal transduction. Third, ErbB2/EGFR heterodimers are slowly endocytosed, and are more frequently recycled to the plasma membrane than the EGF stimulated homodimers. By virtue of its strong interactions with adapter proteins and altered trafficking downstream of endocytosis, an EGFR/ErbB2 heterodimer can amplify and extend the duration of EGFR ligand signaling, leading to proliferation and survival at the expense of other cell fates (28-31).

In contrast to the fairly well established understanding of ErbB2 containing heterodimers, there have been few studies on the EGFR heterodimerized with ErbB4 or ErbB3. Co-immuno precipitation experiments have confirmed the presence of the ErbB4/EGFR in a lung epithelial cells and type II pneumocytes; however, the specific function of this complex was not determined (33, 34). Co-expression of ErbB4 and EGFR plasmids in model NIH 3T3 fibroblasts or CHO lines, provided evidence of dimerization of these receptors, and suggested that this complex could induce cellular transformation in the presence of EGF or NRG1. Further analysis of the CHO system found that the ErbB4/EGFR heterodimer specifically induced B-Raf kinase activity, which was speculated to induce transformation by increasing the activity of the ERK/MAPK pathway (35). Recently, ErbB3/EGFR heterodimers have been identified in pancreatic cancer cell lines (36, 37). It appeared that the ErbB3/EGFR complex may be a more effective stimulus of proliferation in pancreatic cancer cell lines than EGFR homodimers (36). Additionally, these studies suggest the ligand AREG is able to stimulate activity of the ErbB3/EGFR heterodimer (36, 37). Unfortunately, the comprehensive binding, signal transduction and trafficking studies completed for ErbB2 containing receptor complexes have not been completed for EGFR/ErbB4 or ErbB3 heterodimers. This information, coupled with the identification of the specific cell types and tumors that express heterodimers and the function of these complexes will be important considerations for expanded use of ErbB targeted therapeutics.

1.5 Other EGFR ligands

As studies of receptor binding, conformation, phosphorylation, and trafficking are completed for each ligand, it is becoming clear that each agonist induces signaling that can be viewed as a variation of the basic EGF-EGFR homodimer scenario. This attenuated signaling produced by each ligand has the potential to induce subtle differences in downstream signaling, which would be expected to result in altered gene expression and cellular behavior. In the preceding section, the emerging differences in signaling are detailed for each of the ligands that bind the EGFR.

1.5.1 TGFα

Next to EGF, the most intensively studied ligand has been TGFα. Similar to EGF, TGFα exclusively binds to and activates the EGFR. Binding studies suggest that TGFα binds to the receptor with similar affinity as EGF (32). However, conclusions from structural studies involving ligand-receptor complex data indicates there are subtle differences in the conformation of the extracellular ligand-binding domain (sub domain II) induced by TGFα as compared to EGF (4). It is unclear whether this conformational change induced by TGFα could generate alterations in EGFR kinase activity or accessibility of C-terminal tyrosines. Although not comprehensively studied at this point, some of our early studies with breast cancer cell lines suggest that TGFα does not induce the extensive receptor phosphorylation observed with mouse salivary gland derived EGF (Fig 1). Additionally, it has been long recognized that TGFα induces different trafficking of the receptor than EGF (38). Close to 100% of receptors internalized after TGFα treatment are recycled to the plasma membrane (22). At physiological pH of 7.4 in the extracellular environment, TGFα and EGF have similar binding affinities for the EGFR (22, 38). However, at pH close to 5 such as in the endosome, TGFα has decreased affinity for the EGFR (22, 38). It appears that dissociation of the ligand from the EGFR in the endosome permits the receptor to be recycled back to the plasma membrane where it can be reengaged by ligand. It is thought that the three additional histidines found in the receptor binding domain of TGFα provide a greater sensitivity to pH for agonist-receptor interactions (38). In fact, mutations that add histidines to this region of EGF decreased ligand-receptor binding at low pH (39, 40). Together, the altered ligand induced receptor conformation, phosphorylation and trafficking appear to result in TGFα being a more potent stimulator of proliferation of EGFR expressing cell lines than EGF.

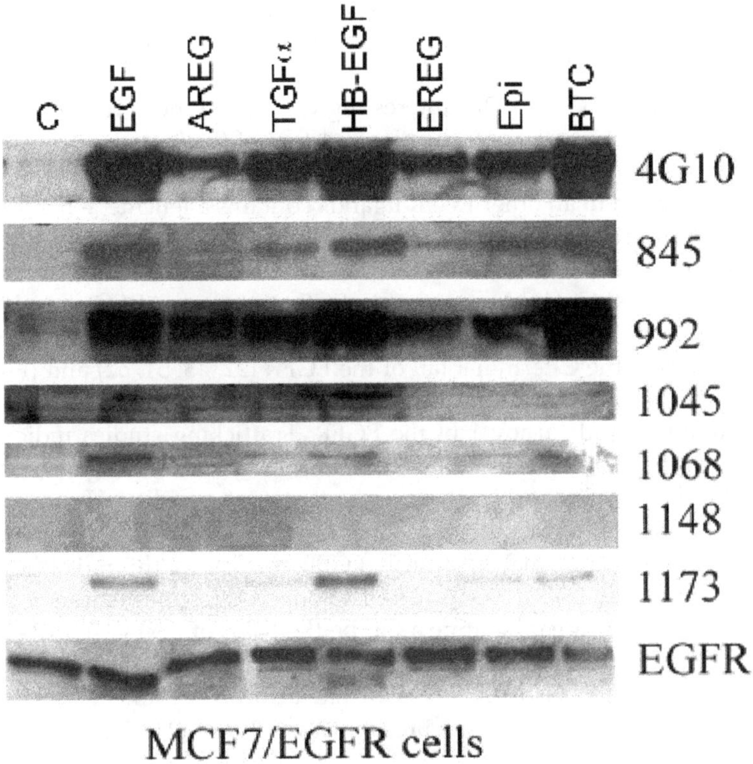

Fig. 1. EGFR phosphorylation after ligand stimulation.
The human breast cancer cell line MCF7 was engineered to overexpress high levels of the EGFR after retroviral transduction. Cells were grown to 80% confluence and placed on ice for 30 minutes. Ligands (R&D, Minneapolis) were applied for 10 minutes to the media and then the media was removed, cells washed and proteins extracted. The EGFR was concentrated with Concanavalin A beads and extracted with Laemmli sample and applied to gels and western blotted with specific antibodies to phosphorylated tyrosines listed on the left. The various ligands used are listed on the top of the figure (C) represents vehicle treated cells.

1.5.2 AREG

The differential impact on breast cancer cell behavior that AREG exhibits compared to EGF has drawn considerable attention to the concept that various EGFR ligands have discrete functions (41-43). Among the ErbB receptors, AREG appears to exclusively bind and activate the EGFR. In addition, the ligand contains a heparin-binding domain N-terminal to the receptor binding region (44, 45). It appears that interaction with heparin-sulfated proteoglycans on the plasma membrane enhances the ability of exogenous AREG to activate the EGFR (46). What has been a matter of controversy has been the relative strength of AREG binding to the EGFR as compared to other ligands. The initial identification of human AREG by Shoyab and colleagues, reported the fully processed ligand isolated from breast cancer cells had reduced affinity for the human EGFR, as compared to salivary gland derived mouse EGF (44). In contrast, subsequent studies with human recombinant ligands found that AREG has similar affinity for the EGFR as EGF and TGFα (47, 48). Inducing further complexity, additional analyses of ligand receptor interactions have suggested that recombinant AREG does not induce efficient dimerization of the EGFR, as compared to recombinant EGF and TGFα (49). Interestingly, proteolytic processing of AREG in mammalian cells may eliminate the C-terminal portion of the ligand binding domain that is required for high affinity for the receptor (50). In addition, the terminal portion of the receptor binding domain in all other EGFR ligands contains a leucine, whereas a methionine is found in AREG, and this is speculated to reduce affinity for the receptor (50).

More recent studies have focused on the distinct downstream signaling and cellular behavior induced by AREG. Unlike exogenous EGF treatment, AREG stimulation of model cell lines and breast cancer cell lines is unable to induce efficient phosphorylation of many of the tyrosine residues in the C-terminal tail of the EGFR (22, 43, 51, 52) and (Fig. 1). Notably, the Cbl binding 1045 tyrosine residue is not efficiently phosphorylated by AREG and this ligand fails to induce rapid turnover of the EGFR. Trafficking studies indicate that AREG liganded EGFR is rapidly internalized, but then is recycled back to the plasma membrane. In addition, AREG binding to the EGFR is very resistant to acidic pH suggesting that the ligand does not disengage in the endosome as does TGFα (22). It appears that AREG may be unique among the ligands in that it induces EGFR trafficking through Rab 4 and Rab 11 containing endosomes (22, 43). AREG induces prolonged phosphorylation of ERK relative to EGF (41, 52). This altered signaling appears to be the basis of AREG stimulating the loss of cell-cell adhesion and increase motility/migration associated behaviors in breast and other epithelial cells (41, 53). AREG overexpression has also been found to selectively activate interleuken-1 induced NFκβ signaling in breast epithelial cells (41-43).

1.5.3 Epigen

This was the last ErbB family member identified in 2000, and it has not been as intensively studied as other ligands. The ligand activates the EGFR and does not activate ErbB3 or ErbB4 when these receptors are expressed in isolation (54, 55). However, epigen can activate ErbB4 and ErbB3 when these receptors are co-expressed with ErbB2 (54, 55). Epigen appears to have ~100 fold less affinity for the EGFR relative to recombinant human EGF. Not surprisingly, we found that epigen induced modest phosphorylation of breast cancer cells (Fig. 1). The binding of epigen to the EGFR appears to be sensitive to pH similar to TGFα. Modeling suggests that additional histidines in the receptor binding domain are responsible for the dissociation of the ligand from the EGFR at low pH (54, 55). In comparison with EGF, epigen induced significantly weaker ubiquitylation and degradation of EGFR, and once internalized, it appears that the receptor is efficiently recycled to the plasma membrane. As expected for lower affinity ligands, epigen is a more potent mitogen than EGF and displays prolonged MAPK signaling (54, 55).

1.5.4 HB-EGF

Exogenous HB-EGF is a high affinity ligand for the EGFR but it also binds and activates ErbB4 (32). Exogenous HB-EGF does not as robustly stimulate phosphorylation of ErbB4 as it does the EGFR (56). In addition, pro-HB-EGF serves as the diptheria toxin receptor in human cells (6). Similar to EGF, exogenous HB-EGF induces extensive EGFR tyrosine phosphorylation in most cell types studied (22, 56), and we found this to be the case for breast cancer cells (Fig. 1). Upon binding to and activation by HB-EGF, the EGFR is rapidly endocytosed and the majority of ligand engaged receptors are trafficked to lysosomes and degraded (22). The binding of HB-EGF to the EGFR was resistant to low pH. HB-EGF shows similar effects on cell proliferation and migration to those exhibited by EGF (57).

As its name implies, HB-EGF has a heparin-binding region N-terminal to the EGF domain. This domain has been shown to interact with heparin sulfated plasma membrane proteins such as the tetraspanin, CD9 and the extracellular matrix binding/cell differentiation marker protein CD44 (6, 57). In particular the heparin-mediated interaction between HB-EGF and CD9 appear to be crucial to juxtacrine signaling by the proligand (58). Finally, the associations between the heparin binding domain and cell membrane associated heparin sulfated proteoglycans appear to be crucial to localizing HB-EGF to regions of cell-cell contact. Furthermore, the interaction with these heparin-sulfated proteoglycans prevented proteolytic cleavage of the pro-ligand, whereas exogenous heparin increased shedding of HB-EGF (7, 58). In contrast to the impact of shed ligand, juxtacrine signaling by the pro HB-EGF appears to be antiproliferative (58).

1.5.5 β-cellulin

Exogenous β-cellulin is a high affinity ligand for the EGFR and ErbB4 (32). In general, exogenous β-cellulin phosphorylates the EGFR to a similar extent as EGF in model cell types, and this is what we observed with breast cancer cells (Fig. 1) (22, 59). This exogenous ligand also stimulates total ErbB4 phosphorylation to an extent similar to NRG1, but there may be differences in phosphorylation of specific tyrosine residues (60). Upon binding to and activation by β-cellulin, the EGFR is rapidly endocytosed and trafficked to lysosomes where the majority of it is degraded (22). The binding of β-cellulin to the EGFR was resistant to low pH. Exogenous β-cellulin was slightly less efficient than EGF at inducing proliferation in some specific cell types (60). There have been some reports that β-cellulin binds to heparin and may participate in juxtacrine signaling (61).

1.5.6 EREG

Unlike the other dual receptor ligands HB-EGF and BTC, EREG is a low affinity ligand for the EGFR (32). EREG typically induces much less phosphorylation of the EGFR than EGF in model cell lines (62-65). In breast cancer cells, we found that the epiregulin induced phosphorylation of the various tyrosines on the EGFR to an extent similar to AREG and the low affinity ligand epigen (Fig. 1). EREG is not as effective as NRG or BTC in stimulating ErbB4 phosphorylation (62-65). The ligand appears to preferentially activate heterodimers and efficiently induces EGFR heterodimers with all three other receptors (65). Upon binding to and activation by EREG, the EGFR is rapidly endocytosed, but then is recycled back to the plasma membrane, and its binding to the receptor was resistant to low pH (22). Exogenous EREG was more efficient than EGF at inducing proliferation in some cell types (63, 65). Also EREG does not induce as great of activation of the MAPK pathway as EGF, but the duration of MAPK phosphorylation was increased relative to the prototype ligand (63, 65).

Thus, the expression of specific EGFR ligands could influence the progression of breast cancer in several ways. First, three of the ligands (HB-EGF, BTC and EREG) could induce ErbB4 signaling on breast cancer cells themselves or their microenvironment, whereas the other 4 ligands EGF, TGFα, AREG and epigen would only induce EGFR signaling. Second, if juxtacrine EGFR signaling between breast cancer cells may require interaction with heparin sulfate proteoglycans, only HB-EGF and AREG would be likely mediators of this signaling.

Juxacrine EGFR signaling might be antiproliferative and also only occur in breast cancer that lacked active sheddases that released HB-EGF and AREG. Third, EGFR signaling induced by soluble ligands appears to be dependent on the relative ratio of receptor degradation versus recycling to the plasma membrane. For example, those ligands whose binding leads to rapid receptor degradation (EGF, HB-EGF and BTC) would activate high levels of downstream signal transduction, but this would likely be of short duration. In contrast, the ligands that induce recycling of the internalized receptor to the plasma membrane would produce longer duration EGFR signaling. In the context of autocrine signaling in breast cancer cells, the longer duration EGFR signaling is likely to more efficiently induce mitogenesis. What remains to be determined is whether the duration of EGFR signaling differentially impacts other cellular behaviors relevant to breast cancer progression such as resistance to apoptosis, and the stimulation of invasive/motile behaviors. Finally, in the context of paracrine signaling it is not clear how EGFR turnover influences the supportive functions of stromal and immune cells of the tumor microenvironment.

2. EGFR/ErbB signaling in development

2.1 ErbB signaling and mammary gland development

The majority of research on mammary gland development is performed in the mouse model due to its biologically and histologically similarity with humans, and the power of transgenic knockout murine models (66). Embryonic mammary gland development in the mouse begins around embryonic day 10.5 (E 10.5), where bilateral milk lines are formed from front to hind paws. Between E11.5 and E12.5, five placodes on each milk line develop with eventual epithelial bud formation at each placode. These epithelial buds remain quiescent until E15.5, where minor branching permits the migration of mammary epithelia into the fat pad, and mesenchymal differentiation forms the overlying nipple epidermis. This rudimentary mammary gland will remain quiescent until after birth (67). The majority of mammary gland growth and development occurs in postnatal life during puberty and pregnancy, and ErbB signaling impacts this phase.

The primary hormone that drives post-natal mammary gland development is the nuclear steroid hormone, estrogen. Estrogen stimulates proliferation of luminal cells within the mammary ducts, causing ductal elongation and branching (68). Progesterone also increases cellular proliferation of the mammary ducts, and acts synergistically with estrogen during periods of high hormone levels such as pregnancy (68). Prolactin, a non-steroid hormone released from the pituitary gland, is active in mammary gland development, late in pregnancy, stimulating alveolar development and triggering milk production during lactation (69).

The mouse mammary gland begins pubertal outgrowth between 3-4 weeks of age, and is complete at 8-12 weeks of age. The gland requires both longitudinal ductal growth, as well as ductal branching to fully infiltrate the mammary fat pad. Pubertal growth is directed by the cells within structures called terminal end buds (TEBs), which are a bulbous expansion of the epithelia. The TEBS are found at the distal end of each growing duct, and consist of 3 to 4 cell layers, including cap cells that make up the 'basal' layer and multiple layers of interior luminal-like body cells that line the duct. Signaling within the cells of the TEBs and the surrounding stroma will determine the extent of continued ductal branching (70) (71). From this point, the mammary gland will show minimal growth with each estrous cycle. Upon pregnancy, estrogen and progesterone drive another large spurt of growth resulting in extensive ductal branching. Progesterone also works with prolactin to signal differentiation of the secretory or alveolar cells throughout the duct system, which produces the large volumes of milk post parturition (72, 73). Termination of lactation will eventually lead to involution, where large-scale apoptosis will eliminate the secretory alveoli and remodel the remaining ducts of the mammary gland, returning the structure to a state similar to that of the virgin gland.

2.1.1 Role of EGFR in mammary gland growth

In virgin mice, EGFR, ErbB2, and ErbB3 are present in the developing ductal structure while there is minimal ErbB4. During pregnancy, this pattern changes to greatly increase expression of ErbB4 in the mammary epithelium, while ErbB4 levels will again regress during lactation and involution (74). Even though three of the receptors are present during growth, there is minimal ErbB phosphorylation observed until ductal morphogenesis begins. During pubertal growth, phosphorylated EGFR and ErbB2 are detected, which suggested that these receptors may mediate the impact of estradiol (E2) on the gland (75).

The EGFR-/- mice die within 8-days after birth and show a wide range of dysfunctional epithelia, but their mammary glands were similar to their wild-type littermates. Transplantation of pre-pubertal glands from EGFR-/- mice into cleared fat pads of wild-type littermates failed to infiltrate the structure, but glands from wild-type mice produced normal ductal systems (76). In contrast, when a purified mammary epithelium from the EGFR-/- mouse was implanted into cleared fat pads with mammary stroma from wild-type mice it produced a normal ductal tree, whereas the opposite combination of wild-type epithelium and EGFR-/- stroma failed to penetrate the fat pad. Thus, postnatal mammary ductal growth is dependent on the presence of the EGFR in mammary stromal fibroblasts. It appears that signaling by the receptor triggers the production of stromal growth factors important to TEBs in ductal elongation (76).

The EGFR ligands EGF, TGFα, and AREG, are found in different locations within the TEB during ductal growth. Using immunohistochemical techniques, TGFα is found exclusively in the basal cap cell layer while the luminal cells express only EGF (70). AREG has been found in both the basal cap cells and the luminal cell layers of TEBs (77). Luekette and colleagues produced knockout mice for each of these ligands separately or as double and triple knockouts. While all three mice null for the individual ligands and their various crosses were fertile, not all had distinct mammary phenotypes. Double-knockout mice for EGF and TGFα, but which contained AREG, displayed normal ductal growth and TEB formation. Mice that were single-knockout for AREG or a triple-knockout for all ligands displayed almost a complete lack of ductal growth into the fat pad at 8-12 weeks (78). In the AREG-/- mice, mammary epithelial failed to fill the fat pad even after multiple pregnancies, strongly suggesting that AREG-EGFR signaling mediated the impact of estrogen on mammary ductal growth. This suggests that EGF and TGFα are dispensable for mammary gland growth, while AREG plays a vital role in glandular development. Recombination grafts indicated that estrogen stimulated pubertal mammary gland growth will not occur without AREG signaling to the stroma (79). The AREG gene is regulated by estrogen receptor alpha (ERα), which apparently accounts for its requirement in postnatal mammary gland development (80, 81). Whether there are any ligand specific effects of the AREG ligand in mammary development have not been explored.

Studies performed with mice deficient for ADAM-17 have shown cardiac insufficiencies, a constellation of epithelial defects and die soon after birth similar to the phenotype of EGFR -/- mice. The ADAM17-/- mice have small, immature mammary glands with minimal branching or ductal growth (82). To verify the requirement of ADAM-17, the defective growth of ADAM-17-null mammary epithelia can be rescued in the presence of exogenous AREG, EGF, or TGFα (82). In conclusion, estrogen induced growth of the mammary pad requires mammary epithelial cell ADAM-17 to shed AREG which then, is necessary to stimulate EGFR signaling in the stromal fibroblasts.

2.1.2 Breast epithelial stem cell and ErbB signaling

Potential mammary gland stem and progenitor cells have been identified using a series of methodologies used to identify the hierarchy of cells that produces that mature hematopoetic system. A single human mammary gland stem cell has been shown to regenerate all the cellular components of the human mammary gland, as well as produce milk proteins in immunocompromised mice (83-86). This work, coupled with mouse work has given rise to an epithelial hierarchy illustrated in figure 2. In this hierarchy, the mammary stem cells give rise to " the common or bipotent" progenitor; the bipotent progenitor gives rise to a luminal progenitor, as well as a cell type that gives rise to mature myoepthelial cells; and the luminal progenitor produces derivatives that ultimately differentiate into mature duct and alveolar cells (83-86).

The reproducible isolation of stem and progenitor cells from mammary epithelia has permitted profiling the various cell types for the expression of the receptors involved in post-natal mammary gland growth and breast cancer progression (85). The subpopulation containing putative mammary multipotent stem cells appear to lack expression of estrogen and progesterone receptors, whereas the EGFR is expressed in ~12% of this fraction. Nearly 50% of the luminal progenitor inclusive population expressed high levels of EGFR. The relatively small subset of the differentiated luminal cell segment (ductal and alveolar cells) express the EGFR (83-86). Of possible significance is that both the mammary stem cell and luminal progenitor population are routinely propagated in a media supplement containing EGF. Whether this implies that propagation of these stem and progenitor cells are dependent on EGFR signaling or simply that there is a requirement for generalized receptor tyrosine kinase activity remains to be determined.

Taken together, the post-natal development of the mammary gland is regulated in large part by the EGFR. EGFR signaling in stromal fibroblasts is required for the estrogen-stimulated invasion mammary epithelium into the stromal fat pad that establishes the adult virgin mammary gland. It appears that the stromal EGFR signaling is mediated primarily by the estrogen-controlled ligand, AREG. Interestingly, the EGFR and its ligands are expressed in the mammary epithelia, but the recombination experiments suggest that autocrine receptor activity in this compartment is dispensable for the establishment of the adult mammary gland. At this time, it is not clear if autocrine EGFR signaling in a mammary epithelial stem or progenitor cells might be required for maintenance of the organ throughout adult life.

2.2 EGFR signaling and cardiac development

Careful reexamination of the EGFR-/- mice along with observations from the Waved-2 mice (these express a mutant form of the receptor with only 10% kinase activity) found defective

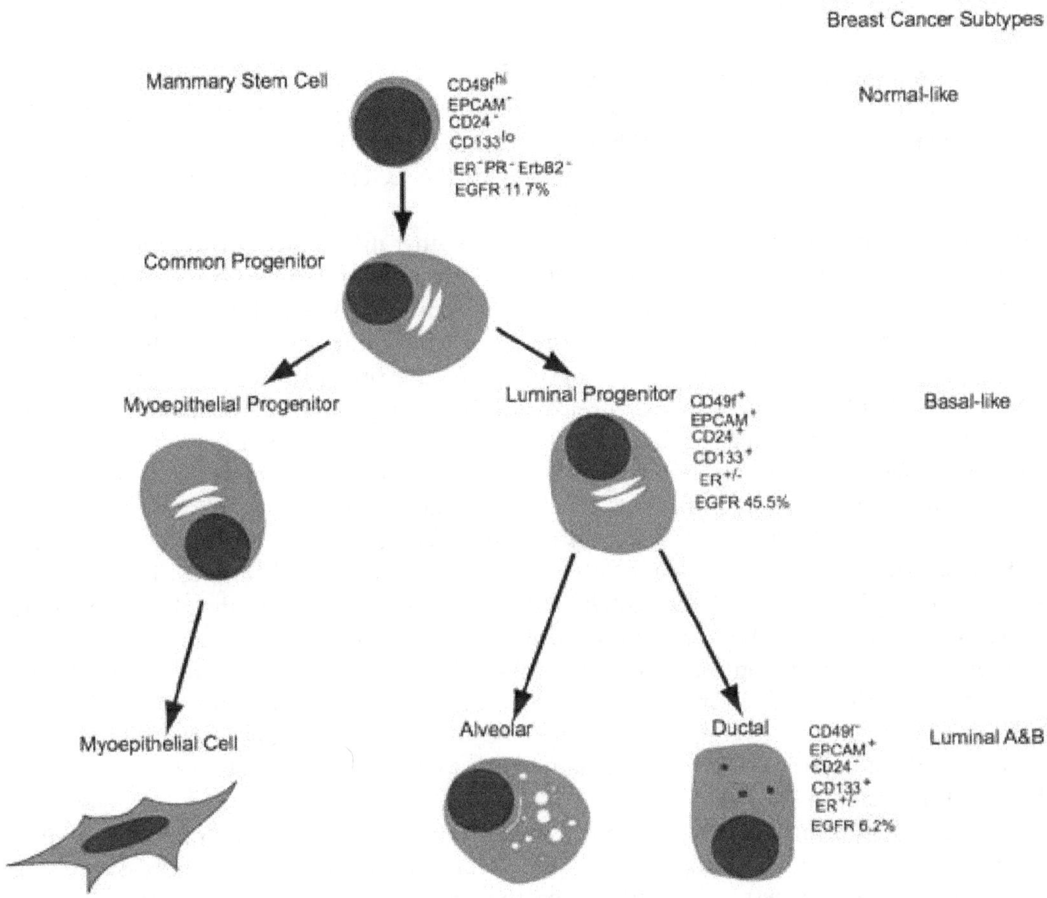

Fig. 2. Hierarchy of mammary epithelial cells.
The various cells of the mammary epithelium and their relationships are represented. To the right, is the expression pattern of the various cell surface markers. Below this is the ErbB and ERα expression along with breast cancer cell types the various cells are related to.

cardiac valve morphogenesis and maturation (94, 96). HB-EGF KO mice also exhibit defective maturation of cardiac valves, suggesting that this may be the relevant ligand that induces EGFR signaling in this process. Also, the HB-EGF-/- cardiac defect was phenocopied in the ADAM-17, suggesting that this protease released the ligand during cardiac development (97).

In the context of cellular behaviors, it appears that the EGFR signaling system plays a role in differentiation. In the EGFR, HB-EGF and ADAM-17 KO mice which have hyperplastic valves it appears that the impact of this signaling is distinct from a proliferation and migration defect observed with the other ErbB knockouts. It is thought that HB-EGF-EGFR signaling decreases BMP expression, the factor which drives cardiac valve maturation, and hence is a differentiation factor (97).

2.3 EGFR signaling and nervous system

In the mouse, EGFR is highly expressed during brain development (E-7 to E-17) and is present on multipotent precursors of both neurons and glia, as well as developing astrocytes and some neurons (98, 99). The initial reports of the EGFR knockout did not identify a nervous system defect. However, reexamination of the KOs with extended post natal survival due to breeding of the knockout allele onto other mouse strains was able to identify brain defects (98). Among the defects identified were smaller or thinner forebrain regions, including the cerebral cortex, olfactory bulb and neocortex (98). Both HB-EGF and TGFα are expressed in portion of the fore brain during late embryonic and early postnatal life (98, 100). Modest histological defects were observed in the prefrontal cortex of mice with a conditional KO of HB-EGF in the forebrain, and these mice displayed behavior and defects in dopamine metabolism that have been observed in schizophrenia (98).

The defects observed in the forebrain of the EGFR-KO mice appear to result from disruption of the cellular interactions required to support neurons. There was substantial neuronal apoptosis in the early postnatal forebrain regions affected (98). However, this occurred in EGFR-expressing and non-receptor bearing neurons. In addition, there was a delay in the appearance of glial fibrulary acidic protein (GFAP) positive astrocytes in the glial limitans and white matter tracks of the fore brain. Although EGFR ligands can stimulate both the proliferation of astrocytes and recruitment of these cells from multipotent precursor cells, the major defect of the knockout mice appears to have a defect in the migration these glial cells from germinal centers. It is speculated that the delay in formation of contacts between neurons and astrocytes results in a deficiency of trophic support, resulting in neuronal cell death in the forebrain (98, 99).

EGFR expression is high in developing astrocytes, but the receptor is not present in mature astrocytes of the healthy adult brain. Upon injury or disease, EGFR expression is up regulated in reactive astrocytes (101). Reactive astrocytes lengthen processes produce plasma membrane pseudopodia and increase expression GFAP in response to all forms of CNS injury or disease (102). Stimulation of the EGFR on reactive astrocytes results in the upregulation of motility chemokines and extracellular matrix remodeling genes that are likely to contribute to glial scarring (101). Intriguingly, the use of EGFR tyrosine kinase inhibitors reduced nerve loss and lead to greater nerve fiber regeneration in optic nerve crush a model of a glial scarring (101). Thus, EGFR signaling in astrocytes facilitates neuronal survival during development, but receptor activity in reactive astrocytes actually contributes to neuron loss in pathologies.

2.4 EGFR signaling and bone

Bone phenotypes had not been reported in the original characterization ErbB receptor KO mice. However, work on the problem of malignancy-associated hypercalcemia had long established that TGFα increased the formation of bone resorbing osteoclasts in bone marrow cultures and whole animals (103, 104). The EGFR is expressed on both chondrocytes and cells of the osteoblast lineage in animals and humans (105). However, the function of the receptor was not established until a human EGFR gene-knockin mouse was created (106). This human EGFR transgene had a limited expression in mouse tissues that normally express the receptor, probably due to the presence of the Neo gene in the first intron of the construct. The human EGFR was expressed in the heart and nervous system and provided a rescue of the murine EGFR KO, but the receptor was not expressed in epithelia and bone. The human EGFR knockin mice were growth retarded and the skeletal phenotype appeared to be largely due to premature hypertrophy of the growth plate cartilages. Although routine histology did not reveal defects in the bones, growth of the knockin osteoblasts *in vitro* resulted in the increased formation of calcified nodules, which represent the end point of differentiation for these cells. Thus, in both cartilage and bone, EGFR signaling inhibits differentiation and helps maintain chondrocytes and osteoblasts in a proliferative state. At this point, it is unknown if any other ErbB receptors play a functional role in bone development or physiology.

Further insight into the role of EGFR in bone resulted from a study of global changes in osteoblast gene expression induced by the main serum calcium regulator, PTH. Activation of the PTH receptor on osteoblasts rapidly upregulates AREG mRNA expression 10 to 20-fold, as well as increasing the TGFα and HB-EGF ligands (107, 108). In addition, PTH signaling induces shedding of ADAM-17 controlled ligands in the kidney (109). Further experiments indicated that addition of exogenous AREG to osteoblasts stimulated their proliferation. However ligand-EGFR signaling also inhibited osteoblast differentiation and dramatically decreased mineralization of osteoblast cell lines. Consistent with the role for AREG in stimulating the proliferation of osteoblasts, 4-week-old AREG-knockout mice exhibited less trabecular bone in the tibia than wild type littermates (107). These experiments suggested that EGFR signaling may mediate the impact of PTH on the recruitment and expansion of cells committed to the osteoblast lineage, but excessive signaling by this system could prevent these cells from undergoing terminal differentiation and forming mineralized bone. The inhibition of osteoblast differentiation and subsequent mineralized bone matrix deposition by-EGFR signaling may contribute to the uncoupling of bone formation from the accelerated bone resorbtion

3. EGFR and breast cancer

3.1 ErbB and EGFR expression in primary tumors

The development of platforms capable of simultaneously evaluating gene expression from a large portion of the genome have lead to identification of gene expression profiles that correlate with various established and some novel classes of breast cancer. These profiles have produced further insights into the impact of ErbB family members in breast cancer progression. Based on these studies, breast cancers are now divided into the following subclasses: ErbB2 amplified, luminal A, luminal B, normal breast-like, and basal (110-112). The ErbB2 amplified, basal and luminal B subtypes had substantially worse prognosis than the normal breast-like and luminal A.

3.1.1 ErbB2 amplified tumors

Among the molecular subclasses of breast cancer, the ErbB2 amplified, has the most well established functional role for an ErbB member in disease development and progression. The ErbB2 amplified tumors typically express ErbB3 and cell line experiments suggest the

ErbB2/ErbB3 heterodimers stimulate proliferation of these cells through the PI3 kinase-AKT pathway (113). Despite the identification of the ErbB2 co-receptor, the precise ligand activating the ErbB3 has not been established. In addition, the correlation between high ErbB2 expression and poor prognosis suggests that ErbB2 contributes to metastasis and how the receptor contributes to these processes, is still under investigation (110-112).

3.1.2 ER+ tumors: luminal A&B

Luminal A tumors express ERα along with GATA binding protein 3, X-box binding protein 1, trefoil factor 3, and other estrogen-regulated genes and high levels of the luminal keratins K8 and 18 (110-112). Luminal B tumors tend to express the above markers at slightly reduced levels, but have an upregulated cassette of genes, including proliferation related genes such as Myb and components involved in DNA replication. There is no specific ErbB family member included in luminal A or B signature. Further evaluations of ERα+ tumors have indicated that the majority of these tumors lack ErbB2 and EGFR expression, but close examination of data from microarray and PCR studies suggest there are occasional luminal type tumors that express these receptors (16, 110-112). A large fraction of ERα+ tumors also contain ErbB4 (110-112), and there is some indication this receptor may be involved in a reciprocal regulatory loop with ERα signaling (114). Surprisingly, AREG was not in the original gene set that defined ERα+ luminal tumors. A follow up interrogation of data that was used to relate disease outcome to cancer subclasses identified a correlation between higher levels of AREG expression, ERα, and the luminal A subclass (115). Also, this analysis indicated that ADAM-17 levels were low in the luminal A class relative to other tumor subtypes. These observations suggest that although most ERα+ luminal A breast cancers express AREG, they lack the EGFR; therefore, autocrine signaling by this ligand receptor system should not be present in most of these tumors. Because the tumor cells express low levels of ADAM-17 it is unclear whether AREG could even participate in paracrine signaling between luminal A breast cancer cells and the tumor stroma. There is a possibility that other proteases produced by the tumor cell or microenvironment lead to shedding of AREG by luminal A breast cancers but whether this signaling impacts progression is unclear.

3.1.3 Normal-like breast cancers

The gene expression signature of these tumors clustered with the normal breast samples. These tumors had a signature that was not associated with epithelial cell types. They instead express high levels of collagen receptors, lipoprotein lipase and glycerol-3-phosphate dehydrogenase normally found in stromal cells or adipocytes. High levels of AREG and moderate levels of ADAM-17 were observed in occasional samples from this group of tumors, but the EGFR was absent. At this time there is no evidence that ErbB signaling plays any role in the biology of these tumors (110-112).

3.1.4 Basal tumors

These tumors lack the expression of the estrogen, progesterone and ErbB2 receptor-for this reason they are often called triple receptor negative tumors-and these cancers express some markers consistent with the myoepithelial cells that are in contact with the basement membrane. These tumors express high levels of the epithelial markers kertatin 5 and 14 (basal keratins), P cadherin as well as troponin (110-112). Basal breast cancers are correlated with poor survival, high rates of distant metastasis and are generally high grade, large tumors. Once the category became established, antibody labeling studies indicated that 50 to 70% of the basal cancers expressed high levels of EGFR immunoreactivity (116). Low levels of EGFR expression is correlated with reduced numbers of distant metastasis (117). These tumors also frequently express elevated levels of TGFα and ADAM-17 (115).

Within basal breast cancers there could be a fraction that exhibits autocrine TGFα-EGFR signaling. The correlation of ADAM-17, TGFα and EGFR with poor prognosis implicates some role for this signaling system in metastasis. At this time, functional testing of TGFα in basal breast cancer models has not been completed. One major question that remains is: does TGFα participate in autocrine tumor cell signaling or paracrine tumor-stroma interactions. Future studies will identify which prometastatic cellular behaviors are activated by TGFα-EGFR signaling, providing insight into whether receptor-targeted therapeutics might provide benefit in a metastasis prevention paradigm.

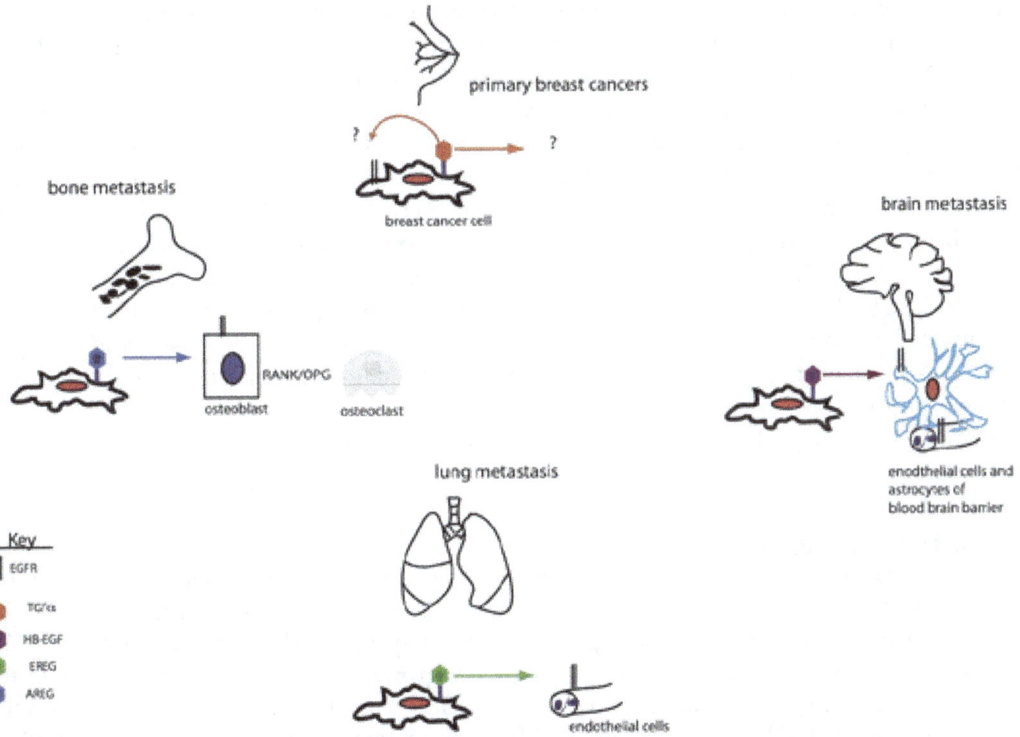

Fig. 3. Summary of EGFR-ligand signaling in models of basal breast cancer metastases. The specific ligand involved in primary tumors and metastatic site are indicated by the colored hexagons. The cell type that responds to the signal is also indicated. Paracrine signaling interactions appear to be important to metastases, whereas the relative role of autocrine versus paracrine signaling has not been explored in primary basal breast cancer.

3.2 ErbB signaling in breast cancer metastasis

Metastasis requires a set of cellular behaviors that are distinct from primary tumor formation. To spread from the site of the primary tumor to distant organs cancer cells must:

1) move out of the primary tumor and invade through local connective tissue; 2) enter capillaries (intravasation); 3) survive in the blood stream; 4) exit the blood stream (extravasation) and invade into a new organ; 5) survive in the new organ possibly as a micro metastasis; 6) adapt to the new organ and grow as a macrometastasis (virulence) (118, 119). These steps can be viewed as two generalized processes: 1) invasion, which is movement of cancer cells through normal tissue and entry into the blood stream, and 2) colonization, which is escape from the blood stream and growth in a distant organ. Substantial progress is being made in identifying metastasis genes that mediate these generalized steps of the process. Metastasis genes are thought dispensable for primary tumor initiation and growth, but are crucial to the novel processes involved in the spread of cancer (119). In general, genes that facilitate invasion for carcinomas such as breast cancer are associated with EMT. Some of the genes involved in invasion are expressed in primary tumors. Colonization is considered to be the most inefficient part of the metastatic process and the growth of a cancer cells in a novel organ is likely to require novel changes in gene expression. Thus, the expression of colonization/virulence-associated metastasis genes are thought to be limited tumors within the specific target organ, rather than being present in most primary tumors (118, 119). Due to less availability, comprehensive gene expression studies of metastases have lagged behind the studies of primary tumors. As a result, alternative strategies for identifying gene signatures that are functionally involved with metastasis have been developed. For breast cancer metastases, Massague and colleagues selected *in vitro* various subclones of the aggressive breast cancer cell line MDA-MB-231. They found that many of the subclones had differing capacities to colonize various organs after intracardiac injection into mice (12, 119-123). Gene expression profiles were generated from the subclones that colonized specific organs, and these were compared to signatures from subclones that colonized the other organs. These signatures were then compared to larger data bases generated from human primary tumors that had ultimately metastasized to the organ of interest producing a refined signature. Subsequent functional analysis of these gene signatures has resulted in the identification of specific EGFR ligands as breast cancer metastasis genes.

3.2.1 EREG and lung metastases

The identification of a lung metastatic signature was derived from subclones of the MDA-MB-231 (LM) breast cancer cells that produced lesions in the lung after intracardiac injection. Among the genes that emerged from this analysis was the ErbB ligand, EREG (121, 123). Knockdown of EREG alone failed to slow the growth of LM as primary tumors in the mammary fat pad or in lung. However, knockdown of EREG in conjunction with cyclooxigenase 2 (COX2), MMP1 and MMP2 (these genes had also been identified as upregulated in the LM signature) had a dramatic impact on both primary tumor growth and subsequent metastasis to lungs. The decreased primary tumor growth in the cells with reduced levels of EREG, COX2, MMP1 and MMP2 appeared to result from reduced angiogenesis. The LM cells recruited abundant dilated tortuous and leaky blood vessels, and the repression of these 4-genes resulted in reduced capillary branching, length and dye effusion. However, VEGF levels were not reduced in the quadruple knockdown tumors relative to controls. Also, no differences were observed in pericyte recruitment to the capillaries between the LM cells and the quadruple knockdowns, suggesting that capillary defects were the result of altered endothelial cell behavior. Also, these multiple knockdowns exhibited reduced ability to colonize lungs after intravenous injection as compared to the parental LM cells. Close evaluation of the lungs of animals injected with the quadruple knockdown cells found abundant cells trapped in the vasculature, suggesting a failure in extravasation. The deficiencies in quadruple knockdown extravasation were also observed with an *in vitro* assay. Consistent with the knockdown studies, single therapeutic agents that targeted EGFR (such as cetuximab, an EGFR blocking antibody), COX2 (celecoxib) or MMPs (GM6001) also had modest impact on behavior of the LM cells grown as primary tumor and their spontaneous metastases to the lung. However, combinations of two agents slowed the growth of primary tumors and reduced subsequent lung colonization. The efficacy of cetuximab suggests that EREG is stimulating this the EGFR and not ErbB4. The fact that LM cells lacked upregulation of VEGF production, (an EGFR regulatory target in most cancer cells) was interpreted as evidence that EREG functioned in paracrine signaling with endothelial cells rather than being engaged in autocrine signaling.

Although microvasculature defects do not appear to be a major component of the various EGFR-/- or other ErbB-knockout mice, studies of normal and tumor capillaries *in vitro* suggest signaling by family members has an influence on angiogenesis. Intriguingly, ErbB receptor expression is altered in tumor capillary endothelial cells as compared to those in normal vessels. ErbB 2, 3, 4 but minimal EGFR is found in most normal endothelial cells in culture (124). In contrast, tumor endothelial cells acquire the EGFR and down regulate ErbB3 expression both *in vitro* and *in vivo*. Endothelial cells in culture also express EGFR and ErbB4 ligands HB-EGF and NRG-1 (124-126). It is thought that HB-EGF signaling through both the EGFR and Erbb4 helps recruit pericytes to capillaries to stabilize the structures (125). The addition of exogenous EGF to tumor endothelial cells *in vitro* increases their proliferation (124). Shedding of HB-EGF and activation of the EGFR leads to down regulation of tight junction proteins and migration of normal endothelial cells (127). Also, NRG-1-ErbB4 signaling stimulates endothelial cell proliferation, migration and angiogenesis in animals; however, NRG-1 inhibits proliferation of tumor derived endothelial cells (124, 126). In light of the impact of EGFR signaling on tumor endothelial cells, breast cancer cell upregulation of EREG would contribute to the recruitment of a leaky vasculature that is common to aggressive tumors. In addition, EREG-EGFR/ErbB4 signaling might contribute to intrasavation and extrasavation by down regulation adhesion molecules between endothelial cells within capillaries. The question that remains is whether the low affinity ligand EREG might be more efficient at stimulating proliferation, migration and downregulation of junctional complexes than the high affinity ligand, HB-EGF normally present in endothelial cells.

3.2.2 HB-EGF and brain metastasis

A brain metastasis signature was derived using methods similar to those described for lung metastasis (120, 128). Among the genes that emerged as upregulated in brain metastatic cells was the ErbB ligand, HB-EGF (120). Treating mice cardiac-injected with brain seeking sublines MDA-MB-231 and CN34-BrM2C with cetuximab resulted in reduced numbers of brain metastases. Knockdown of both EREG and HB-EGF, or cetuximab treatment, reduced migration of MDA-MB-231 and CN34-BrM2C through consecutive monolayers of endothelial cells and astrocytes in a model of blood brain barrier extravasation. Brain endothelial cells and astrocytes both express the EGFR (100, 127). Activation of the EGFR has been shown to down regulate components of tight junctions in brain endothelial cells (127). This coupled with EGFR signaling induced upregulation of motility, chemokines and extracellular matrix remodeling genes in astrocytes would likely aid in extrasavation of breast cancer cells through the blood brain barrier into the parenchyma. Beyond this EGFR signaling produces reactive astrocytes that are components of the microenvironment of brain metastases. This raises the question of whether breast cancer generated EGFR ligands could play a role in breast cancer cell virulence in the brain by generating increased numbers of reactive astrocytes (129). HB-EGF is the EGFR ligand most abundantly expressed in the brain and endothelial cells, suggesting it may be the most well suited agonist to mediate in paracrine interactions among cancer cells, capillaries and the brain parenchyma.

3.2.3 AREG and bone metastasis

Tumor cell colonization of bone may be a less complex process than that of lung and brain because the capillaries in bone called sinusoids, have large openings in them to facilitate entrance of bone marrow derivatives into the circulation (119). It is thought that cancer cells may be able to exit through these openings dispensing with the intricacies of extravasation from continuous capillaries.

The growth of breast cancer macrometastases is described as a vicious cycle (130, 131). In this cycle, breast cancer cells exploit the natural renewal process based on the paracrine interactions between the bone forming osteoblast and the bone resorbing osteoclast. In normal bone, osteoblasts regulate osteoclast numbers and activity by releasing chemokines that recruit osteoclast precursors and then differentiate and activate them with a cell surface ligand for the receptor for activation of NFκβ (RANKL). Osteoblasts also produce a soluble decoy receptor osteoprotegrin (OPG) that prevents RANKL from engaging its receptor; therefore, the level of the ratio of OPG to RANKL controls osteoclastogenesis. Once activated, osteoclasts adhere to the bone surface and secrete proteases and acid that degrades mineralized matrix. Growth factors including TGFβ and IGF-1 are released from the bone matrix, and this in turn stimulates new bone matrix formation by osteoblasts. This is a regenerating system that is in balance within the local environment; however, the rate of turnover and formation can be modulated by a series of endocrine hormones including PTH and calcitonin. Within the bone marrow, breast cancer cells produce a series of cytokines and growth factors including IL-11 and PTH-related protein (PTHrP) that increase the levels of RANKL relative to OPG leading to increased osteoclastogenesis. The increased bone resorption and resulting high level of growth factors enhance the survival of breast cancer cells, and also TGFβ increases gene expression of IL-11 and PTHrP, which begets more osteoclasts.

Profiling bone metastasis subclones of MDA-MB-231 cells resulted in an 11-gene signature (122). Several of the genes identified were factors like IL-11 that directly altered the RANKL/OPG ratio or connective tissue factor that enhanced osteoblast proliferation. Ectopic expression of a single gene from the profile had very little impact on the ability of modestly osteolytic 231 subclones to grow within in the bone of immunocompromised mice. However, the combination of 3 of the genes from the signature induced destructive growth in bone after intracardiac injection. Among the genes identified in the signature that produced increased osteolysis when overexpressed as part of a 3 gene cassette were the proteases, MMP1 and ADAMTS-1 (12). It was unclear what the role of these molecules would play in bone metastasis. Eventually, a careful evaluation of aggressively osteolytic MDA-MB-231 lines that were engineered to overexpress ADAMTS-1 and MMP1 were found to shed dramatically increased levels of AREG. Conditioned media from the ADAMTS-1 and MMP1 engineered MDA-MB-231 lines caused an increased RANKL/OPG ratio in primary murine bone cell cultures (12, 132). The conditioned media from the MDA-MB-231-ADAMTS-1 and MMP1 cells activated osteoclastogenesis in the primary bone cell cultures, and this could be inhibited by the EGFR inhibitors gefitinib or cetuximab. Remarkably, these agents (Gefitinib 100mg/kg daily or Cetuximab 100 mg/kg weekly) completely prevented the formation of osteolytic lesions by the MDA-MB-231 ADAMTS-1+MMP1 line delivered by either the intracardiac or intratibial injection method (12). These findings clearly support the notion that EGFR signaling on cells of the osteoblast is a major regulator of the RANKL/OPG ratio, but point out the requirement for appropriate protease expression to make EGFR ligands accessible to the bone microenvironment. These experiments provide an explanation of how bone resorbtion could be uncoupled from bone formation by breast cancer cells because stimulation of the EGFR should block osteoblast differentiation and matrix production.

To some extent, the identification of a role for AREG in bone metastasis is confounding given that its expression is associated with ERα+ breast cancers that generally have good prognosis (115). The MDA-MB-231 cells are ERα- and have a phenotype that is similar to basal cancers. So we interrogated the breast cancer transcriptome datasets GSE2034(133), GSE2603 (123), and GSE12276 (120) from the NCBI Gene Expression Omnibus to evaluate AREG expression in ERα- tumors. We found that AREG expression was lower in the ERα-negative tumors that ultimately metastasized to bone as compared to those that did not (134). A similar pattern of expression has been reported for the classical bone metastasis virulence factor PTHrP. Low expression of the peptide is observed in the primary tumors that ultimately metastasize to bone (135-137). PTHrP gene expression is thought to be activated by TGFβ when breast cancer cells enter the bone microenvironment (138). In contrast to PTHrP, the enhanced activity or expression of the proteases that cleave AREG would be sufficient to increase its expression in the bone microenvironment without activating gene expression. Consistent with this concept, high expression ADAMTS-1 and MMP1 protein have been observed in primary breast cancer tumors that ultimately metastasized to bone (12). Thus, the complex post-genomic regulation of EGFR ligand processing and receptor interactions provides mechanism beyond transcription where the amplitude of signaling of this system can be increased to contribute to colonization. Given that AREG appears to be the physiological mediator of EGFR signaling in the bone, it may be ideally suited to uncouple bone formation from bone resorbtion, which is a component of osteolytic predominant bone metastases that arise from breast cancers.

3.3 Conclusions: EGFR ligand function in breast cancer

EGFR ligands and receptors are frequently expressed together on epithelial cells and the cancers that are derived from these tissues, including the breast. Addition of exogenous EGFR ligands to breast epithelial or cancer cells typically has a profound impact on proliferation or migratory behavior, leading to the concept that autocrine receptor signaling would contribute to tumor progression. Despite this perspective, the unraveling of the developmental breast, heart and brain phenotypes of the various family member KOs suggest that EGFR, ligand and ADAM-17 function as part of a complex paracrine-signaling network. In addition, *in vitro and in vivo* models based on MDA-MB-231 cells where EGFR ligands have been found to function as metastasis genes, suggest they signal in a paracrine fashion to key elements of the microenvironment. On the basis of these conclusions, we speculate that TGFα expression in primary basal breast cancers may also be engaged in paracrine signaling with cells in the microenvironment. This conclusion suggests that the efficacy of EGFR targeted therapeutics will depend upon their uses in combination with other compounds that target the tumor microenvironment in primary basal tumors, as well as those that have metastasized to the lung, brain and bone.

4. References

Llombart-Cussac A. Improving decision-making in early breast cancer: who to treat and how? Breast Cancer Res Treat2008 Dec;112 Suppl 1:15-24.

Brufsky A. Trastuzumab-based therapy for patients with HER2-positive breast cancer: from early scientific development to foundation of care. Am J Clin Oncol2010 Apr;33(2):186-95.

Yarden Y, Sliwkowski MX. Untangling the ErbB signalling network. Nat Rev Mol Cell Biol2001 Feb;2(2):127-37.

Wilson KJ, Gilmore JL, Foley J, Lemmon MA, Riese DJ, 2nd. Functional selectivity of EGF family peptide growth factors: implications for cancer. Pharmacol Ther2009 Apr;122(1):1-8.

Daub H, Weiss FU, Wallasch C, Ullrich A. Role of transactivation of the EGF receptor in signalling by G-protein-coupled receptors. Nature1996 Feb 8;379(6565):557-60.

Iwamoto R, Mekada E. Heparin-binding EGF-like growth factor: a juxtacrine growth factor. Cytokine Growth Factor Rev2000 Dec;11(4):335-44.

Prince RN, Schreiter ER, Zou P, Wiley HS, Ting AY, Lee RT, Lauffenburger DA. The heparin-binding domain of HB-EGF mediates localization to sites of cell-cell contact and prevents HB-EGF proteolytic release. J Cell Sci2010 Jul 1;123(Pt 13):2308-18.

Sahin U, Weskamp G, Kelly K, Zhou HM, Higashiyama S, Peschon J, Hartmann D, Saftig P, Blobel CP. Distinct roles for ADAM10 and ADAM17 in ectodomain shedding of six EGFR ligands. J Cell Biol2004 Mar 1;164(5):769-79.

Tousseyn T, Jorissen E, Reiss K, Hartmann D. (Make) stick and cut loose--disintegrin metalloproteases in development and disease. Birth Defects Res C Embryo Today2006 Mar;78(1):24-46.

Zhang Q, Thomas SM, Lui VW, Xi S, Siegfried JM, Fan H, Smithgall TE, Mills GB, Grandis JR. Phosphorylation of TNF-alpha converting enzyme by gastrin-releasing peptide induces amphiregulin release and EGF receptor activation. Proc Natl Acad Sci U S A2006 May 2;103(18):6901-6.

Wagstaff L, Kelwick R, Decock J, Edwards DR. The roles of ADAMTS metalloproteinases in tumorigenesis and metastasis. Front Biosci2011;16:1861-72.

Lu X, Wang Q, Hu G, Van Poznak C, Fleisher M, Reiss M, Massague J, Kang Y. ADAMTS1 and MMP1 proteolytically engage EGF-like ligands in an osteolytic signaling cascade for bone metastasis. Genes Dev2009 Aug 15;23(16):1882-94.

Chokki M, Eguchi H, Hamamura I, Mitsuhashi H, Kamimura T. Human airway trypsin-like protease induces amphiregulin release through a mechanism involving protease-activated receptor-2-mediated ERK activation and TNF alpha-converting enzyme activity in airway epithelial cells. Febs J2005 Dec;272(24):6387-99.

Pawlowski V, Revillion F, Hebbar M, Hornez L, Peyrat JP. Prognostic value of the type I growth factor receptors in a large series of human primary breast cancers quantified with a real-time reverse transcription-polymerase chain reaction assay. Clin Cancer Res2000 Nov;6(11):4217-25.

McIntyre E, Blackburn E, Brown PJ, Johnson CG, Gullick WJ. The complete family of epidermal growth factor receptors and their ligands are co-ordinately expressed in breast cancer. Breast Cancer Res Treat2010 Jul;122(1):105-10.

Revillion F, Lhotellier V, Hornez L, Bonneterre J, Peyrat JP. ErbB/HER ligands in human breast cancer, and relationships with their receptors, the bio-pathological features and prognosis. Ann Oncol2008 Jan;19(1):73-80.

Edwin F, Wiepz GJ, Singh R, Peet CR, Chaturvedi D, Bertics PJ, Patel TB. A historical perspective of the EGF receptor and related systems. Methods Mol Biol2006;327:1- 24.

Riese DJ, 2nd, Stern DF. Specificity within the EGF family/ErbB receptor family signaling network. Bioessays1998 Jan;20(1):41-8.

Lemmon MA. Ligand-induced ErbB receptor dimerization. Exp Cell Res2009 Feb 15;315(4):638-48.

Riese DJ, 2nd, Gallo RM, Settleman J. Mutational activation of ErbB family receptor tyrosine kinases: insights into mechanisms of signal transduction and tumorigenesis. Bioessays2007 Jun;29(6):558-65.

Schulze WX, Deng L, Mann M. Phosphotyrosine interactome of the ErbB-receptor kinase family. Mol Syst Biol2005;1:2005 0008.

Roepstorff K, Grandal MV, Henriksen L, Knudsen SL, Lerdrup M, Grovdal L, Willumsen BM, van Deurs B. Differential effects of EGFR ligands on endocytic sorting of the receptor. Traffic2009 Aug;10(8):1115-27.

Avraham R, Yarden Y. Feedback regulation of EGFR signalling: decision making by early and delayed loops. Nat Rev Mol Cell Biol2011 Feb;12(2):104-17.

Bublil EM, Yarden Y. The EGF receptor family: spearheading a merger of signaling and therapeutics. Curr Opin Cell Biol2007 Apr;19(2):124-34.

Citri A, Yarden Y. EGF-ERBB signalling: towards the systems level. Nat Rev Mol Cell Biol2006 Jul;7(7):505-16.

Slamon DJ, Clark GM, Wong SG, Levin WJ, Ullrich A, McGuire WL. Human breast cancer: correlation of relapse and survival with amplification of the HER-2/ neu oncogene. Science1987 Jan 9;235(4785):177-82.

Salomon DS, Brandt R, Ciardiello F, Normanno N. Epidermal growth factor-related peptides and their receptors in human malignancies. Crit Rev Oncol Hematol1995 Jul;19(3):183-232.

Earp HS, Dawson TL, Li X, Yu H. Heterodimerization and functional interaction between EGF receptor family members: a new signaling paradigm with implications for breast cancer research. Breast Cancer Res Treat1995 Jul;35(1):115- 32.

Wada T, Qian XL, Greene MI. Intermolecular association of the p185neu protein and EGF receptor modulates EGF receptor function. Cell1990 Jun 29;61(7):1339-47.

Wang Z, Zhang L, Yeung TK, Chen X. Endocytosis deficiency of epidermal growth factor (EGF) receptor-ErbB2 heterodimers in response to EGF stimulation. Mol Biol Cell1999 May;10(5):1621-36.

Hendriks BS, Wiley HS, Lauffenburger D. HER2-mediated effects on EGFR endosomal sorting: analysis of biophysical mechanisms. Biophys J2003 Oct;85(4):2732-45.

Jones JT, Akita RW, Sliwkowski MX. Binding specificities and affinities of egf domains for ErbB receptors. FEBS Lett1999 Mar 26;447(2-3):227-31.

Liu W, Volpe MA, Zscheppang K, Nielsen HC, Dammann CE. ErbB4 regulates surfactant synthesis and proliferation in adult rat pulmonary epithelial cells. Exp Lung Res2009 Feb;35(1):29-47.

Zscheppang K, Korenbaum E, Bueter W, Ramadurai SM, Nielsen HC, Dammann CE. ErbB receptor dimerization, localization, and co-localization in mouse lung type II epithelial cells. Pediatr Pulmonol2006 Dec;41(12):1205-12.

Hatakeyama M, Yumoto N, Yu X, Shirouzu M, Yokoyama S, Konagaya A. Transformation potency of ErbB heterodimer signaling is determined by B-Raf kinase. Oncogene2004 Jun 24;23(29):5023-31.

Frolov A, Schuller K, Tzeng CW, Cannon EE, Ku BC, Howard JH, Vickers SM, Heslin MJ, Buchsbaum DJ, Arnoletti JP. ErbB3 expression and dimerization with EGFR influence pancreatic cancer cell sensitivity to erlotinib. Cancer Biol Ther2007 Apr;6(4):548-54.

Liles JS, Arnoletti JP, Tzeng CW, Howard JH, Kossenkov AV, Kulesza P, Heslin MJ, Frolov A. ErbB3 expression promotes tumorigenesis in pancreatic adenocarcinoma. Cancer Biol Ther2010 Sep;10(6):555-63.

Waterman H, Sabanai I, Geiger B, Yarden Y. Alternative intracellular routing of ErbB receptors may determine signaling potency. J Biol Chem1998 May 29;273(22):13819- 27.

French AR, Sudlow GP, Wiley HS, Lauffenburger DA. Postendocytic trafficking of epidermal growth factor-receptor complexes is mediated through saturable and specific endosomal interactions. J Biol Chem1994 Jun 3;269(22):15749-55.

Reddy CC, Niyogi SK, Wells A, Wiley HS, Lauffenburger DA. Engineering epidermal growth factor for enhanced mitogenic potency. Nat Biotechnol1996 Dec;14(13):1696-9.

Willmarth NE, Ethier SP. Autocrine and juxtacrine effects of amphiregulin on the proliferative, invasive, and migratory properties of normal and neoplastic human mammary epithelial cells. J Biol Chem2006 Dec 8;281(49):37728-37.

Streicher KL, Willmarth NE, Garcia J, Boerner JL, Dewey TG, Ethier SP. Activation of a nuclear factor kappaB/interleukin-1 positive feedback loop by amphiregulin in human breast cancer cells. Mol Cancer Res2007 Aug;5(8):847-61.

Willmarth NE, Baillo A, Dziubinski ML, Wilson K, Riese DJ, 2nd, Ethier SP. Altered EGFR localization and degradation in human breast cancer cells with an amphiregulin/EGFR autocrine loop. Cell Signal2009 Feb;21(2):212-9.

Shoyab M, McDonald VL, Bradley JG, Todaro GJ. Amphiregulin: a bifunctional growth-modulating glycoprotein produced by the phorbol 12-myristate 13-acetate-treated human breast adenocarcinoma cell line MCF-7. Proc Natl Acad Sci U S A1988 Sep;85(17):6528-32.

Shoyab M, Plowman GD, McDonald VL, Bradley JG, Todaro GJ. Structure and function of human amphiregulin: a member of the epidermal growth factor family. Science1989 Feb 24;243(4894 Pt 1):1074-6.

Stoll SW, Johnson JL, Bhasin A, Johnston A, Gudjonsson JE, Rittie L, Elder JT. Metalloproteinase-mediated, context-dependent function of amphiregulin and HB- EGF in human keratinocytes and skin. J Invest Dermatol2010 Jan;130(1):295-304.

Barnard JA, Graves-Deal R, Pittelkow MR, DuBois R, Cook P, Ramsey GW, Bishop PR, Damstrup L, Coffey RJ. Auto- and cross-induction within the mammalian epidermal growth factor-related peptide family. J Biol Chem1994 Sep 9;269(36):22817-22.

Cook PW, Mattox PA, Keeble WW, Pittelkow MR, Plowman GD, Shoyab M, Adelman JP, Shipley GD. A heparin sulfate-regulated human keratinocyte autocrine factor is similar or identical to amphiregulin. Mol Cell Biol1991 May;11(5):2547-57.

Neelam B, Richter A, Chamberlin SG, Puddicombe SM, Wood L, Murray MB, Nandagopal K, Niyogi SK, Davies DE. Structure-function studies of ligand-induced epidermal growth factor receptor dimerization. Biochemistry1998 Apr 7;37(14):4884-91.

Adam R, Drummond DR, Solic N, Holt SJ, Sharma RP, Chamberlin SG, Davies DE. Modulation of the receptor binding affinity of amphiregulin by modification of its carboxyl terminal tail. Biochim Biophys Acta1995 Apr 6;1266(1):83-90.

Gilmore JL, Scott JA, Bouizar Z, Robling A, Pitfield SE, Riese DJ, 2nd, Foley J. Amphiregulin-EGFR signaling regulates PTHrP gene expression in breast cancer cells. Breast Cancer Res Treat2007 Sep 20.

Stern KA, Place TL, Lill NL. EGF and amphiregulin differentially regulate Cbl recruitment to endosomes and EGF receptor fate. Biochem J2008 Mar 15;410(3):585- 94.

Chung E, Graves-Deal R, Franklin JL, Coffey RJ. Differential effects of amphiregulin and TGF-alpha on the morphology of MDCK cells. Exp Cell Res2005 Sep 10;309(1):149-60.

Kochupurakkal BS, Harari D, Di-Segni A, Maik-Rachline G, Lyass L, Gur G, Kerber G, Citri A, Lavi S, Eilam R, Chalifa-Caspi V, Eshhar Z, Pikarsky E, Pinkas-Kramarski R, Bacus SS, Yarden Y. Epigen, the last ligand of ErbB receptors, reveals intricate relationships between affinity and mitogenicity. J Biol Chem2005 Mar 4;280(9):8503- 12.

Strachan L, Murison JG, Prestidge RL, Sleeman MA, Watson JD, Kumble KD. Cloning and biological activity of epigen, a novel member of the epidermal growth factor superfamily. J Biol Chem2001 May 25;276(21):18265-71.

Elenius K, Paul S, Allison G, Sun J, Klagsbrun M. Activation of HER4 by heparin-binding EGF-like growth factor stimulates chemotaxis but not proliferation. Embo J1997 Mar 17;16(6):1268-78.

Higashiyama S, Abraham JA, Miller J, Fiddes JC, Klagsbrun M. A heparin-binding growth factor secreted by macrophage-like cells that is related to EGF. Science1991 Feb 22;251(4996):936-9.

Nishi E, Klagsbrun M. Heparin-binding epidermal growth factor-like growth factor (HB-EGF) is a mediator of multiple physiological and pathological pathways. Growth Factors2004 Dec;22(4):253-60.

Shing Y, Christofori G, Hanahan D, Ono Y, Sasada R, Igarashi K, Folkman J. Betacellulin: a mitogen from pancreatic beta cell tumors. Science1993 Mar 12;259(5101):1604-7.

Sweeney C, Lai C, Riese DJ, 2nd, Diamonti AJ, Cantley LC, Carraway KL, 3rd. Ligand discrimination in signaling through an ErbB4 receptor homodimer. J Biol Chem2000 Jun 30;275(26):19803-7.

Tada H, Sasada R, Kawaguchi Y, Kojima I, Gullick WJ, Salomon DS, Igarashi K, Seno M, Yamada H. Processing and juxtacrine activity of membrane-anchored betacellulin. J Cell Biochem1999 Mar 1;72(3):423-34.

Komurasaki T, Toyoda H, Uchida D, Morimoto S. Epiregulin binds to epidermal growth factor receptor and ErbB-4 and induces tyrosine phosphorylation of epidermal growth factor receptor, ErbB-2, ErbB-3 and ErbB-4. Oncogene1997 Dec 4;15(23):2841-8.

Sasaki E, Arakawa T, Fujiwara Y, Kawada N, Fukuda T, Higuchi K, Komurasaki T, Kobayashi K. Epiregulin stimulates proliferation of rabbit gastric cells in primary culture through autophosphorylation of the epidermal growth factor receptor. Eur J Pharmacol1997 Nov 12;338(3):253-8.

Riese DJ, 2nd, Komurasaki T, Plowman GD, Stern DF. Activation of ErbB4 by the bifunctional epidermal growth factor family hormone epiregulin is regulated by ErbB2. J Biol Chem1998 May 1;273(18):11288-94.

Shelly M, Pinkas-Kramarski R, Guarino BC, Waterman H, Wang LM, Lyass L, Alimandi M, Kuo A, Bacus SS, Pierce JH, Andrews GC, Yarden Y. Epiregulin is a potent pan-ErbB ligand that preferentially activates heterodimeric receptor complexes. J Biol Chem1998 Apr 24;273(17):10496-505.

Cardiff RD, Wellings SR. The comparative pathology of human and mouse mammary glands. J Mammary Gland Biol Neoplasia1999 Jan;4(1):105-22.

Hens JR, Wysolmerski JJ. Key stages of mammary gland development: molecular mechanisms involved in the formation of the embryonic mammary gland. Breast Cancer Res2005;7(5):220-4.

Fendrick JL, Raafat AM, Haslam SZ. Mammary gland growth and development from the postnatal period to postmenopause: ovarian steroid receptor ontogeny and regulation in the mouse. J Mammary Gland Biol Neoplasia1998 Jan;3(1):7-22.

Nandi S. Endocrine control of mammarygland development and function in the C3H/ He Crgl mouse. J Natl Cancer Inst1958 Dec;21(6):1039-63.

Snedeker SM, Brown CF, DiAugustine RP. Expression and functional properties of transforming growth factor alpha and epidermal growth factor during mouse mammary gland ductal morphogenesis. Proc Natl Acad Sci U S A1991 Jan 1;88(1):276-80.

Watson CJ, Khaled WT. Mammary development in the embryo and adult: a journey of morphogenesis and commitment. Development2008 Mar;135(6):995-1003.

Brisken C, Kaur S, Chavarria TE, Binart N, Sutherland RL, Weinberg RA, Kelly PA, Ormandy CJ. Prolactin controls mammary gland development via direct and indirect mechanisms. Dev Biol1999 Jun 1;210(1):96-106.

Brisken C, Park S, Vass T, Lydon JP, O'Malley BW, Weinberg RA. A paracrine role for the epithelial progesterone receptor in mammary gland development. Proc Natl Acad Sci U S A1998 Apr 28;95(9):5076-81.

Schroeder JA, Lee DC. Dynamic expression and activation of ERBB receptors in the developing mouse mammary gland. Cell Growth Differ1998 Jun;9(6):451-64.

Sebastian J, Richards RG, Walker MP, Wiesen JF, Werb Z, Derynck R, Hom YK, Cunha GR, DiAugustine RP. Activation and function of the epidermal growth factor receptor and erbB-2 during mammary gland morphogenesis. Cell Growth Differ1998 Sep;9(9):777-85.

Wiesen JF, Young P, Werb Z, Cunha GR. Signaling through the stromal epidermal growth factor receptor is necessary for mammary ductal development. Development1999 Jan;126(2):335-44.

Kenney NJ, Huang RP, Johnson GR, Wu JX, Okamura D, Matheny W, Kordon E, Gullick WJ, Plowman G, Smith GH, et al. Detection and location of amphiregulin and Cripto-1 expression in the developing postnatal mouse mammary gland. Mol Reprod Dev1995 Jul;41(3):277-86.

Luetteke NC, Qiu TH, Fenton SE, Troyer KL, Riedel RF, Chang A, Lee DC. Targeted inactivation of the EGF and amphiregulin genes reveals distinct roles for EGF receptor ligands in mouse mammary gland development. Development1999 Jun;126(12):2739-50.

Ciarloni L, Mallepell S, Brisken C. Amphiregulin is an essential mediator of estrogen receptor alpha function in mammary gland development. Proc Natl Acad Sci U S A2007 Mar 27;104(13):5455-60.

Rho JY, Wada-Kiyama Y, Onishi Y, Kiyama R, Sakuma Y. Expressional regulation of neuronal and cancer-related genes by estrogen in adult female rats. Endocr Res2004 May;30(2):257-67.

Britton DJ, Hutcheson IR, Knowlden JM, Barrow D, Giles M, McClelland RA, Gee JM, Nicholson RI. Bidirectional cross talk between ERalpha and EGFR signalling pathways regulates tamoxifen-resistant growth. Breast Cancer Res Treat2006 Mar;96(2):131-46.

Sternlicht MD, Sunnarborg SW, Kouros-Mehr H, Yu Y, Lee DC, Werb Z. Mammary ductal morphogenesis requires paracrine activation of stromal EGFR via ADAM17- dependent shedding of epithelial amphiregulin. Development2005 Sep;132(17):3923-33.

Asselin-Labat ML, Vaillant F, Shackleton M, Bouras T, Lindeman GJ, Visvader JE. Delineating the epithelial hierarchy in the mouse mammary gland. Cold Spring Harb Symp Quant Biol2008;73:469-78.

Eirew P, Stingl J, Raouf A, Turashvili G, Aparicio S, Emerman JT, Eaves CJ. A method for quantifying normal human mammary epithelial stem cells with in vivo regenerative ability. Nat Med2008 Dec;14(12):1384-9.

Lim E, Vaillant F, Wu D, Forrest NC, Pal B, Hart AH, Asselin-Labat ML, Gyorki DE, Ward T, Partanen A, Feleppa F, Huschtscha LI, Thorne HJ, Fox SB, Yan M, French JD, Brown MA, Smyth GK, Visvader JE, Lindeman GJ. Aberrant luminal progenitors as the candidate target population for basal tumor development in BRCA1 mutation carriers. Nat Med2009 Aug;15(8):907-13.

Asselin-Labat ML, Sutherland KD, Barker H, Thomas R, Shackleton M, Forrest NC, Hartley L, Robb L, Grosveld FG, van der Wees J, Lindeman GJ, Visvader JE. Gata-3 is an essential regulator of mammary-gland morphogenesis and luminal-cell differentiation. Nat Cell Biol2007 Feb;9(2):201-9.

Jackson-Fisher AJ, Bellinger G, Breindel JL, Tavassoli FA, Booth CJ, Duong JK, Stern DF. ErbB3 is required for ductal morphogenesis in the mouse mammary gland. Breast Cancer Res2008;10(6):R96.

Jackson-Fisher AJ, Bellinger G, Ramabhadran R, Morris JK, Lee KF, Stern DF. ErbB2 is required for ductal morphogenesis of the mammary gland. Proc Natl Acad Sci U S A2004 Dec 7;101(49):17138-43.

Tidcombe H, Jackson-Fisher A, Mathers K, Stern DF, Gassmann M, Golding JP. Neural and mammary gland defects in ErbB4 knockout mice genetically rescued from embryonic lethality. Proc Natl Acad Sci U S A2003 Jul 8;100(14):8281-6.

Lee KF, Simon H, Chen H, Bates B, Hung MC, Hauser C. Requirement for neuregulin receptor erbB2 in neural and cardiac development. Nature1995 Nov 23;378(6555):394-8.

Erickson SL, O'Shea KS, Ghaboosi N, Loverro L, Frantz G, Bauer M, Lu LH, Moore MW. ErbB3 is required for normal cerebellar and cardiac development: a comparison with ErbB2-and heregulin-deficient mice. Development1997 Dec;124(24):4999-5011.

Kramer R, Bucay N, Kane DJ, Martin LE, Tarpley JE, Theill LE. Neuregulins with an Ig- like domain are essential for mouse myocardial and neuronal development. Proc Natl Acad Sci U S A1996 May 14;93(10):4833-8.

Gassmann M, Casagranda F, Orioli D, Simon H, Lai C, Klein R, Lemke G. Aberrant neural and cardiac development in mice lacking the ErbB4 neuregulin receptor. Nature1995 Nov 23;378(6555):390-4.

Sanchez-Soria P, Camenisch TD. ErbB signaling in cardiac development and disease.
Semin Cell Dev Biol2010 Dec;21(9):929-35.

Schroeder JA, Jackson LF, Lee DC, Camenisch TD. Form and function of developing heart valves: coordination by extracellular matrix and growth factor signaling. J Mol Med2003 Jul;81(7):392-403.

Sibilia M, Wagner EF. Strain-dependent epithelial defects in mice lacking the EGF receptor. Science1995 Jul 14;269(5221):234-8.

Jackson LF, Qiu TH, Sunnarborg SW, Chang A, Zhang C, Patterson C, Lee DC. Defective valvulogenesis in HB-EGF and TACE-null mice is associated with aberrant BMP signaling. Embo J2003 Jun 2;22(11):2704-16.

Kornblum HI, Hussain R, Wiesen J, Miettinen P, Zurcher SD, Chow K, Derynck R, Werb Z. Abnormal astrocyte development and neuronal death in mice lacking the epidermal growth factor receptor. J Neurosci Res1998 Sep 15;53(6):697-717.

Kornblum HI, Zurcher SD, Werb Z, Derynck R, Seroogy KB. Multiple trophic actions of heparin-binding epidermal growth factor (HB-EGF) in the central nervous system. Eur J Neurosci1999 Sep;11(9):3236-46.

Kornblum HI, Hussain RJ, Bronstein JM, Gall CM, Lee DC, Seroogy KB. Prenatal ontogeny of the epidermal growth factor receptor and its ligand, transforming growth factor alpha, in the rat brain. J Comp Neurol1997 Apr 7;380(2):243-61.

Liu B, Neufeld AH. Activation of epidermal growth factor receptors in astrocytes: from development to neural injury. J Neurosci Res2007 Dec;85(16):3523-9.

Kang W, Hebert JM. Signaling pathways in reactive astrocytes, a genetic perspective. Mol Neurobiol2011 Jun;43(3):147-54.

Ibbotson KJ, D'Souza SM, Ng KW, Osborne CK, Niall M, Martin TJ, Mundy GR. Tumor-derived growth factor increases bone resorption in a tumor associated with humoral hypercalcemia of malignancy. Science1983 Sep 23;221(4617):1292-4.

Ibbotson KJ, D'Souza SM, Smith DD, Carpenter G, Mundy GR. EGF receptor antiserum inhibits bone resorbing activity produced by a rat Leydig cell tumor associated with the humoral hypercalcemia of malignancy. Endocrinology1985 Jan;116(1):469-71.

Shupnik MA, Ip NY, Tashjian AH, Jr. Characterization and regulation of receptors for epidermal growth factor in mouse calvaria. Endocrinology1980 Dec;107(6):1738-46.

Sibilia M, Wagner B, Hoebertz A, Elliott C, Marino S, Jochum W, Wagner EF. Mice humanised for the EGF receptor display hypomorphic phenotypes in skin, bone and heart. Development2003 Oct;130(19):4515-25.

Qin L, Partridge NC. Stimulation of amphiregulin expression in osteoblastic cells by parathyroid hormone requires the protein kinase A and cAMP response element-binding protein signaling pathway. J Cell Biochem2005 Oct 15;96(3):632-40.

Qin L, Qiu P, Wang L, Li X, Swarthout JT, Soteropoulos P, Tolias P, Partridge NC. Gene expression profiles and transcription factors involved in parathyroid hormone signaling in osteoblasts revealed by microarray and bioinformatics. J Biol Chem2003 May 30;278(22):19723-31.

Cole JA. Parathyroid hormone activates mitogen-activated protein kinase in opossum kidney cells. Endocrinology1999 Dec;140(12):5771-9.

van 't Veer LJ, Dai H, van de Vijver MJ, He YD, Hart AA, Mao M, Peterse HL, van der Kooy K, Marton MJ, Witteveen AT, Schreiber GJ, Kerkhoven RM, Roberts C, Linsley PS, Bernards R, Friend SH. Gene expression profiling predicts clinical outcome of breast cancer. Nature2002 Jan 31;415(6871):530-6.

van de Vijver MJ, He YD, van't Veer LJ, Dai H, Hart AA, Voskuil DW, Schreiber GJ, Peterse JL, Roberts C, Marton MJ, Parrish M, Atsma D, Witteveen A, Glas A, Delahaye L, van der Velde T, Bartelink H, Rodenhuis S, Rutgers ET, Friend SH, Bernards R. A gene-expression signature as a predictor of survival in breast cancer. N Engl J Med2002 Dec 19;347(25):1999-2009.

Sorlie T, Perou CM, Tibshirani R, Aas T, Geisler S, Johnsen H, Hastie T, Eisen MB, van de Rijn M, Jeffrey SS, Thorsen T, Quist H, Matese JC, Brown PO, Botstein D, Eystein Lonning P, Borresen-Dale AL. Gene expression patterns of breast carcinomas distinguish tumor subclasses with clinical implications. Proc Natl Acad Sci U S A2001 Sep 11;98(19):10869-74.

Wiseman SM, Makretsov N, Nielsen TO, Gilks B, Yorida E, Cheang M, Turbin D, Gelmon K, Huntsman DG. Coexpression of the type 1 growth factor receptor family members HER-1, HER-2, and HER-3 has a synergistic negative prognostic effect on breast carcinoma survival. Cancer2005 May 1;103(9):1770-7.

Zhu Y, Sullivan LL, Nair SS, Williams CC, Pandey AK, Marrero L, Vadlamudi RK, Jones FE. Coregulation of estrogen receptor by ERBB4/HER4 establishes a growth- promoting autocrine signal in breast tumor cells. Cancer Res2006 Aug 15;66(16):7991-8.

McGowan PM, McKiernan E, Bolster F, Ryan BM, Hill AD, McDermott EW, Evoy D, O'Higgins N, Crown J, Duffy MJ. ADAM-17 predicts adverse outcome in patients with breast cancer. Ann Oncol2008 Jun;19(6):1075-81.

Burness ML, Grushko TA, Olopade OI. Epidermal growth factor receptor in triple-negative and basal-like breast cancer: promising clinical target or only a marker? Cancer J2010 Jan-Feb;16(1):23-32.

Viale G, Rotmensz N, Maisonneuve P, Bottiglieri L, Montagna E, Luini A, Veronesi P, Intra M, Torrisi R, Cardillo A, Campagnoli E, Goldhirsch A, Colleoni M. Invasive ductal carcinoma of the breast with the "triple-negative" phenotype: prognostic implications of EGFR immunoreactivity. Breast Cancer Res Treat2009 Jul;116(2):317-28.

Chaffer CL, Weinberg RA. A perspective on cancer cell metastasis. Science2011 Mar 25;331(6024):1559-64.

Nguyen DX, Bos PD, Massague J. Metastasis: from dissemination to organ-specific colonization. Nat Rev Cancer2009 Apr;9(4):274-84.

Bos PD, Zhang XH, Nadal C, Shu W, Gomis RR, Nguyen DX, Minn AJ, van de Vijver MJ, Gerald WL, Foekens JA, Massague J. Genes that mediate breast cancer metastasis to the brain. Nature2009 Jun 18;459(7249):1005-9.

Gupta GP, Nguyen DX, Chiang AC, Bos PD, Kim JY, Nadal C, Gomis RR, Manova-Todorova K, Massague J. Mediators of vascular remodelling co-opted for sequential steps in lung metastasis. Nature2007 Apr 12;446(7137):765-70.

Kang Y, Siegel PM, Shu W, Drobnjak M, Kakonen SM, Cordon-Cardo C, Guise TA, Massague J. A multigenic program mediating breast cancer metastasis to bone. Cancer Cell2003 Jun;3(6):537-49.

Minn AJ, Gupta GP, Siegel PM, Bos PD, Shu W, Giri DD, Viale A, Olshen AB, Gerald WL, Massague J. Genes that mediate breast cancer metastasis to lung. Nature2005 Jul 28;436(7050):518-24.

Amin DN, Hida K, Bielenberg DR, Klagsbrun M. Tumor endothelial cells express epidermal growth factor receptor (EGFR) but not ErbB3 and are responsive to EGF and to EGFR kinase inhibitors. Cancer Res2006 Feb 15;66(4):2173-80.

Iivanainen E, Nelimarkka L, Elenius V, Heikkinen SM, Junttila TT, Sihombing L, Sundvall M, Maatta JA, Laine VJ, Yla-Herttuala S, Higashiyama S, Alitalo K, Elenius K. Angiopoietin-regulated recruitment of vascular smooth muscle cells by endothelial-derived heparin binding EGF-like growth factor. FASEB J2003 Sep;17(12):1609-21.

Russell KS, Stern DF, Polverini PJ, Bender JR. Neuregulin activation of ErbB receptors in vascular endothelium leads to angiogenesis. Am J Physiol1999 Dec;277(6 Pt 2):H2205-11.

Chen F, Hori T, Ohashi N, Baine AM, Eckman CB, Nguyen JH. Occludin is regulated by epidermal growth factor receptor activation in brain endothelial cells and brains of mice with acute liver failure. Hepatology2011 Apr;53(4):1294-305.

Yoneda T, Williams PJ, Hiraga T, Niewolna M, Nishimura R. A bone-seeking clone exhibits different biological properties from the MDA-MB-231 parental human breast cancer cells and a brain-seeking clone in vivo and in vitro. J Bone Miner Res2001 Aug;16(8):1486-95.

Fitzgerald DP, Palmieri D, Hua E, Hargrave E, Herring JM, Qian Y, Vega-Valle E, Weil RJ, Stark AM, Vortmeyer AO, Steeg PS. Reactive glia are recruited by highly proliferative brain metastases of breast cancer and promote tumor cell colonization. Clin Exp Metastasis2008;25(7):799-810.

Guise TA, Mohammad KS, Clines G, Stebbins EG, Wong DH, Higgins LS, Vessella R, Corey E, Padalecki S, Suva L, Chirgwin JM. Basic mechanisms responsible for osteolytic and osteoblastic bone metastases. Clin Cancer Res2006 Oct 15;12(20 Pt 2):6213s-6s.

Guise TA, Mundy GR. Cancer and bone. Endocr Rev1998 Feb;19(1):18-54.

Zhu J, Jia X, Xiao G, Kang Y, Partridge NC, Qin L. EGF-like ligands stimulate osteoclastogenesis by regulating expression of osteoclast regulatory factors by osteoblasts: implications for osteolytic bone metastases. J Biol Chem2007 Sep 14;282(37):26656-64.

Wang Y, Klijn JG, Zhang Y, Sieuwerts AM, Look MP, Yang F, Talantov D, Timmermans M, Meijer-van Gelder ME, Yu J, Jatkoe T, Berns EM, Atkins D, Foekens JA. Gene-expression profiles to predict distant metastasis of lymph-node- negative primary breast cancer. Lancet2005 Feb 19-25;365(9460):671-9.

Foley J, Nickerson NK, Nam S, Allen KT, Gilmore JL, Nephew KP, Riese DJ, 2nd. EGFR signaling in breast cancer: bad to the bone. Semin Cell Dev Biol2010 Dec;21(9):951-60.

Henderson M, Danks J, Moseley J, Slavin J, Harris T, McKinlay M, Hopper J, Martin T. Parathyroid hormone-related protein production by breast cancers, improved survival, and reduced bone metastases. J Natl Cancer Inst2001 Feb 7;93(3):234-7.

Powell GJ, Southby J, Danks JA, Stillwell RG, Hayman JA, Henderson MA, Bennett RC, Martin TJ. Localization of parathyroid hormone-related protein in breast cancer metastases: increased incidence in bone compared with other sites. Cancer Res1991 Jun 1;51(11):3059-61.

Southby J, Kissin MW, Danks JA, Hayman JA, Moseley JM, Henderson MA, Bennett RC, Martin TJ. Immunohistochemical localization of parathyroid hormone-related protein in human breast cancer. Cancer Res1990 Dec 1;50(23):7710-6.

Yin JJ, Selander K, Chirgwin JM, Dallas M, Grubbs BG, Wieser R, Massague J, Mundy GR, Guise TA. TGF-beta signaling blockade inhibits PTHrP secretion by breast cancer cells and bone metastases development. J Clin Invest1999 Jan;103(2):197-206.

9

Signal Transduction Pathways in Breast Cancer – Drug Targets and Challenges

Samar Azab[1] and Ayman Al-Hendy[2]
[1]*Pharmacology and Toxicology Department, Faculty of Pharmacy, Ain Shams University, Cairo,*
[2]*Center for Women Health Research, Department of Obstetrics and Gynecology, Meharry Medical College, Nashville, Tennessee,*
[1]*Egypt*
[2]*USA*

1. Introduction

Breast cancer is the most frequently diagnosed cancer and the leading cause of cancer death in females worldwide **[1]**. Over 1.1 million cases of breast cancer are diagnosed across the world each year, compared with about 500,000 cases in 1975. This represents about 10% of all new cancer cases and 23% of all female cancers **[2-3]**. An annual prevalence of more than 4.4 million cases of breast cancer is expected worldwide by the year 2012 **[4]**.

In the past years, our knowledge of the genetic changes that contribute to breast cancer development & progression has tremendously changed **[5]**. Our knowledge of alterations in the cancer cell have allowed us to identify the signaling pathways that when disrupted allow a cancer cell to escape from normal control mechanisms **[6]**. On the other hand, these aberrant processes have also provided many therapeutic points for intervention, which is the major topic of this chapter. Following the successful introduction of trastuzumab, the first human epidermal growth factor receptor (HER) targeted therapy to become widely used in breast cancer patients, other agents have been developed **[7]**. Other potential hallmarks of malignancy that represent a new opportunity for therapeutic targeting include abrogation of apoptosis, lack of senescence, angiogenesis, tumor invasion and metastasis **[8]**. Therefore, new compounds are being developed that may interfere with these hallmarks and that may prove to be effective in monotherapy or in combination with cytotoxic therapy or other targeted therapies. Novel agents are needed because many of the current therapies have limitations. These include drug resistance, lack of target receptor expression in tumors and relatively small improvements in survival **[9-12]**.

Thus, this chapter provides an updated overview of the several signaling transduction pathways involved in development of breast cancer. In addition, it focuses on recent progress with the therapeutic strategies targeting these pathways contributing to their promising success in the clinical setting. Furthermore, molecular signals of its resistance phenotype and breast cancer stem cells & their therapeutic targeting are discussed briefly. Finally, the challenges facing the significant contribution of targeted therapeutics in breast cancer chemotherapy are also extensively discussed. Wherever possible, advances in drug analogs, accepted or controversial mechanisms described for their antitumor activity will be discussed within the framework of the current chapter.

Section A describes a reported panel of potential signal transduction pathways (STPs) that are altered in breast cancer and are undergoing research as targeted therapeutics. Some of these have yielded therapeutics that already had clinical success, while others are still in the experimental stages (**Fig. 1 & Tab.1**). Though many of the underlying mechanisms of the multi-drug resistance (MDR) phenotype are still not clearly identified, several potential molecular targets and pathways of activation have been suggested. The advances in this field provide an emerging picture of how MDR arises and how it could be therapeutically targeted. In **Section B**, we review the potential role of cancer stem cells molecular signaling in development of breast cancer & its resistance phenotype. It also discusses their putative modulation contributing to the success of targeted therapeutics in breast cancer chemotherapy.

	STP	STI	Mechanism
1	**Receptor tyrosine Kinase: I- HER2 receptor**	-Trastuzumab -Lapatinib, Erlotinib, Gefitinib and Neratinib	-Extracellular Targeted Therapeutic: Monoclonal Antibody inhibiting ligand binding to receptor -Intracellular Targeted Therapeutic: HER Receptor tyrosine kinase catalytic inhibitor
	Receptor tyrosine Kinase: II- Src receptor	Dasatinib	Intracellular Targeted Therapeutic: Src Receptor tyrosine kinase catalytic inhibitor
2	**MAPK Signaling Pathway**	Tipifarnib	Farnesyl transferase inhibitor
3	**PI3K/Akt/mTOR pathway**	-Perifosine -Temsirolimus and Everolimus -Octreotide	-Inhibitor of Akt phosphorylation -mTOR inhibitors -Inhibitor of IGF-1R signaling
4	**HSP90 signaling pathway**	Tanespimycin and Alvespimycin	Potent inhibitiors of HSP90 function
5	**PARP signaling pathway**	Olapraib Veliparib	PARP inhibitors
6	**Apoptosis & Autophagy pathways**		Inhibitors of the components of apoptotic & autophagic pathways
7	**Angiogenesis**	Bevacizumab	Extracellular Targeted Therapeutic: Monoclonal Antibody inhibiting ligand binding to receptor
8	**Multi-Target Therapeutics**	Sunitinib, Pazopanib, Sorafenib and Axitinib	Intracellular Targeted Therapeutic: Receptor tyrosine kinase catalytic inhibitors
9	**Estrogen signaling transduction**	-Tamoxifen -Letrozole	-Anti-estrogen -Aromatase inhibitor
10	**UPS signaling pathway**	Bortezomib	Proteasome inhibitor

Table 1. A list of the action site for signal transduction inhibitors (STIs) in breast cancer.

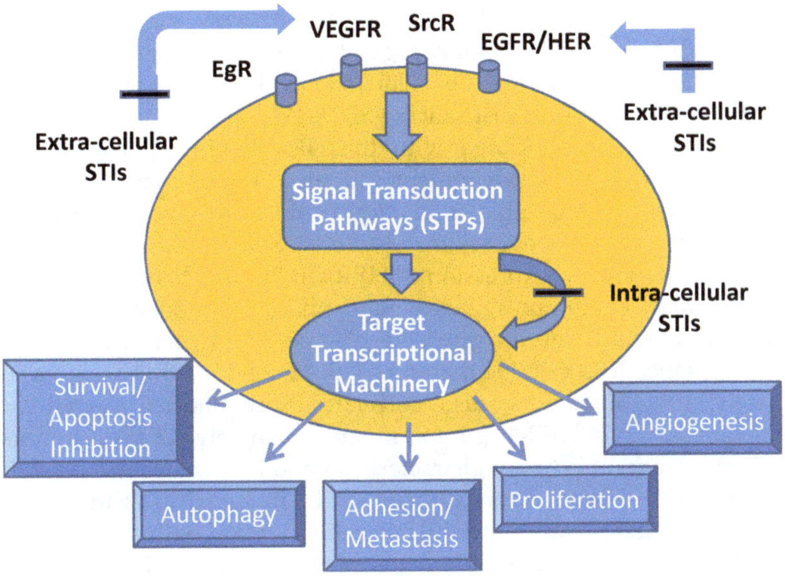

Fig. 1. Simplified schematic illustration of the multiple signal transduction pathways (STPs) in breast cancer.

2. Targeting signal transduction pathways in breast cancer

The mechanisms underlying the development of breast cancer are complex and vary among individual tumors **[13]**. Altered patterns of gene expression are associated with corresponding variations in growth rates, cellular composition and different prognoses **[14]**. Given the complex and varied factors that influence the development of breast cancer, and the use of increasingly sophisticated genetic analysis techniques, it is likely that more refined tumor subtypes and their associated prognoses will be identified**[13, 15]**. Advances in the understanding the etiology and biology of breast cancer have identified key targets among multiple signaling pathways involved in the development and survival of breast cancer cells. Thus, targeted therapies are among the most promising new agents for the treatment of breast cancer. Some of these reported breast cancer signaling transduction pathways (STPs) & their signal transduction inhibitors (STIs) are classified as follows:

2.1 STPs-1: Receptor Tyrosine Kinase (RTKs)

Altered patterns of gene expression can influence the activity of specific signaling pathways. For example, receptor tyrosine kinases (RTKs) are often aberrantly over-expressed or activated in human cancers. The epidermal growth factor receptor (EGFR) family is composed of cell surface tyrosine kinase receptors that are involved in the regulation of cellular proliferation and survival of epithelial cells. The EGFR (or also called HER) family includes four closely related receptors: EGFR/HER1/ErbB1, HER2 neu /ErbB2, HER3/ErbB3 and HER4/ErbB4 **[16]**.

2.1.1 HER2 receptor

Members of the HER family are encoded by genes on different chromosomes and regulate normal breast growth and development. The HER family couples to multiple signaling pathways that impact on all aspect of breast cancer biology. Through their interconnected cellular signaling network, the HER family regulates diverse biological processes, including cell proliferation, differentiation, and survival **[16-17].** Thus, they play a key role in the development and progression of breast cancer [16, 18-19].

Variations in the pathways associated with the HER family appear to be particularly important, not only in tumor development but also in treatment efficacy [20-21]. For example, in breast cancer, constitutive activation of the epidermal growth factor receptor (EGFR) and HER2 is found in approximately 16%–48% and 25%–30% of breast cancer tumors, respectively. Moreover, expression of HER family members in breast cancer tumors has a significant impact on tumor aggressiveness and patient survival. Importantly, their expression correlates with a more aggressive disease course, shorter survival time, and higher risk for resistance to endocrine therapies [10, 12, 22-27]. HER-3 expression, observed in approximately 18% of tumors, also correlates with shorter overall survival **[28].** Interestingly, expression of HER-4 (found in approximately 12% of tumors) has been associated with more favorable tumor characteristics and longer survival [27-28].

Each HER receptor has an extracellular domain (ECD) involved in ligand binding, a helical transmembrane segment, and an intracellular protein domain with tyrosine kinase activity. On ligand binding, the extracellular domains of the receptors undergo conformational changes, which allows them to form homodimers (consisting of two identical receptors) or heterodimers (consisting of two different receptors) of the HER family [16, 29]. Dimerization of HER receptors induces phosphorylation of their intracellular tyrosine kinase domains, which provide docking sites for adaptor proteins and signaling enzymes **[29]**.These molecules act as a link between membrane receptor kinases and "downstream" intracellular protein kinases, which results in the activation of multiple signaling pathways, of which the MAPK and PI3K pathways are probably the best studied **[29]**.

HER-2 is the preferred dimerization and signaling partner for all other members of the HER family, and it appears to function mainly as a co-receptor, increasing the affinity of ligand binding to dimerized receptor complexes [29-30]. With their multiple ligands, many dimerization combinations, and large number of downstream effectors, the HER family mediates an extensive range of signals, controlling a variety of cellular processes, including cellular proliferation, apoptosis, and angiogenesis [29, 31]. For example, HER2 receptor activation leads to the phosphorylation of the intracellular catalytic domains, and ultimately activation of signal transduction pathways that promote proliferation and survival, including the phosphatidylinositol 30-kinase (PI3K)/Akt/mTOR, the Erk1/2 mitogenactivated protein kinase (MAPK) and the Jak/Stat pathway **[32]**.

2.1.2 Src-family tyrosine kinases

The v-Src (Rous sarcoma virus) tyrosine kinase was the first oncogenic gene discovered **[33]**. The corresponding cellular gene, c-Src, is a non-receptor signaling kinase that functions as a hub of a vast array of signal transduction pathways that influence cellular proliferation, differentiation, motility and survival **[34]**. Several mechanisms lead to increased Src activity in tumors. Src is downstream in signaling from a number of growth factor receptors including PDGF receptor (PDGFR), epidermal growth factor receptor (EGFR) and insulin-like growth factor- 1 receptor (IGF-1R) **[35]**.

In many tumor types, over-expression of these receptors, their ligands or both is frequent **[36]**. For example, reported studies suggest an association between Src tyrosine kinase and the development, progression and metastasis of breast cancer [37-38]. In addition, it is described that mice over-expressing the HER2 oncogene develop highly metastatic mammary tumors with elevated Src activity **[37].** Further supporting the role of Src in breast cancer, it has been demonstrated that Src activity is profoundly increased in human breast cancer tissues compared with benign breast tumors or adjacent normal breast tissues[38-39] and that elevated c-Src tyrosine kinase activity is correlated with early systemic relapse **[40]**. Taken together, these results strongly indicate that the Src may play an important role in the development and progression of breast cancer **[41]**.

2.2 STIs-1: Receptor Tyrosine Kinase Inhibitors (RTKIs)

2.2.1 HER2 receptor inhibitors

Numerous agents targeting individual members of the HER family have been developed for use in the treatment of breast cancer. Existing therapeutic approaches have largely focused on two classes of agents:

2.2.1.1 Extracellular targeted therapies

Monoclonal antibodies

The first comprises monoclonal antibodies that bind to extracellular regions of HER to interfere with receptor function (e.g., trastuzumab, pertuzumab, and a number of pan-HER inhibitors). Trastuzumab binds to the juxtamembrane region of HER-2 with high specificity, but it is not currently known how it specifically interferes with HER-2 function **[42]**. Pertuzumab is the first in a class of HER-2 dimerization inhibitors. Binding to HER-2 inhibits its dimerization with other HER receptors and this is thought to result in slowed tumor growth [43].

Trastuzumab, an HER2 specific humanized monoclonal antibody was one of the first biologicals to be approved for metastatic breast cancer treatment [44]. In patients, HER2 is over-expressed and/or amplified in one-fourth of breast tumors and confers a more aggressive clinical course and a worse survival [25, 45]. The outcome of these highly aggressive tumors has markedly improved with the development of anti-HER2 therapies. Trastuzumab (Herceptin®) is a recombinant humanised monoclonal antibody that binds with high affinity to the extracellular juxtamembrane domain of HER2 and inhibits the proliferation of human tumor cells that over-express HER2 in vitro and in vivo [46-48].

Trastuzumab. Trastuzumab, administered as an i.v. infusion, is approved in the U.S. and Europe for the treatment of HER-2–over-expressing metastatic breast cancer (MBC) [7]. It is standard-of-care treatment for MBC patients with HER-2–over-expressing tumors, both as first-line treatment in combination with chemotherapy and as a single agent in women who have HER-2–over-expressing breast cancer that has progressed after chemotherapy for metastatic disease[44, 49]. Trastuzumab is approved for the adjuvant treatment of HER-2+, node negative (ER-/progesterone receptor [PgR-]) or node-positive breast cancer, either in combination with chemotherapy or as a single agent following multi-modality anthracycline-based treatment.

In patients with HER2 amplified tumors, trastuzumab has single agent activity and improves survival in the first-line setting when combined with chemotherapy in patients with advanced disease [44, 50]. Recently, a number of well powered clinical trials have demonstrated that administration of trastuzumab in the adjuvant setting, in combination and/or sequentially after chemotherapy, results in an improvement in disease-free survival as well as overall survival **[51-54].**

Trastuzumab efficacy in the metastatic setting has provided the rationale for several studies investigating the use of trastuzumab plus chemotherapy as adjuvant treatment for patients with earlystage HER-2+ breast cancer [52-53, 55-56]. Studies have evaluated a range of different trastuzumab-based combination regimens for the first-line treatment of MBC [50, 57]. Additionally, a number of trials are ongoing investigating trastuzumab in combination with hormonal therapy in MBC patients [58-59]. When administered as a single agent, trastuzumab has documented efficacy as a first-line therapy, with response rates typically in the range of 23%–33% [60-62]. Of those patients with MBC who do achieve an initial response, many experience disease progression within 12 months as a result of the high proportion of HER-2–over-expressing tumors that have intrinsic resistance to this agent **[63]**. Given the absence of known specific ligands for HER-2, thus there is no alternative approach to blocking this pathway except by trastuzumab. This has clinical implications as this may be related to the development of resistance to HER-2 blockade **[64]**.

On the other hand, changing the traditional treatment paradigm in patients progressing on trastuzumab and administering further trastuzumab-based therapy beyond disease progression may have clinical benefit [65-66].This "treatment beyond progression" approach is increasingly being studied in clinical trials by combining trastuzumab either with chemotherapy [67-68] or with another targeted agent, such as the RTKI lapatinib [69].

Trastuzumab-DM1 (T-DM1) is an anti–HER-2 antibody drug conjugate comprising trastuzumab linked to the maytansine derivative DM1. Combining these two agents facilitates anti–HER-2 activity as well as targeted intracellular delivery of a potent cytotoxic agent. Single-agent TDM1 as well tolerated, active and no dose-limiting cardiotoxicity was observed in a phase II study of 112 patients with pretreated MBC [7].

Limitations of Trastuzumab therapy

1. Trastuzumab is an effective treatment for patients with HER-2+ disease, yet its use is limited to this group (approximately 25%) [25]. Thus, accurate patient selection for treatment is important, using an appropriate method, such as immunohistochemistry or fluorescence in situ hybridization, to detect HER-2 over-expression.
2. Not all HER-2+ patients respond to treatment with trastuzumab, and the development of resistance is an issue. In the future, it may be possible to overcome resistance by combining trastuzumab with new therapies such as pertuzumab, by switching to an agent such as lapatinib that inhibits both HER-1 and HER-2 activity, or, if proven effective, the use of one of the pan-HER inhibitors currently in development.
3. Trastuzumab is unable to penetrate the blood– brain barrier (Guy et al., 1994) and over-expression of HER-2 is known to be associated with a greater risk for central nervous system (CNS) metastases [70]. Patients with HER-2+ MBC treated with trastuzumab appear to be at greater risk for developing CNS metastases than those who do not receive trastuzumab therapy [71]. However, HER-2+ patients with CNS metastases who are treated with trastuzumab appear to have a longer overall survival duration than those who are HER-2- or those unselected for HER-2 status. This may reflect greater control of extra-cranial disease as a result of trastuzumab therapy [72].
4. Treatment with trastuzumab is associated with a higher risk for cardiomyopathy (left ventricular dysfunction and congestive heart failure), particularly when used in combination with paclitaxel or anthracyclines [73]. However, these cardiotoxic effects appear to be reversible once trastuzumab treatment is discontinued or if they are managed with appropriate medical therapy [74-75]. The cellular mechanisms contributing to the cardiotoxicity observed with trastuzumab are still being explored. It

is known that HER-2 plays an important role in cardiomyocyte development and function, and trastuzumab- induced inhibition of HER-2 signaling in cardiomyocytes may be a central mechanism underlying the observed cardiomyopathy. However, the full explanation is likely to be more complex. Cardiotoxicity does not appear to be an issue with the RTKI lapatinib, which inhibits both HER-1 and HER- 2 [76]

5. Although cardiotoxicity is the primary safety concern with trastuzumab, potentially severe hypersensitivity reactions to infusion have also been reported [7].

Other example of novel anti-HER2 agents include antibodies that interfere with HER2 dimerisation. Pertuzumab is a recombinant, humanised MAb that targets an epitope within the HER2 dimerisation domain [77]. Once bound, pertuzumab inhibits ligand-activated HER dimerisation with HER2 and thereby inhibiting activation of intracellular signaling [78].

2.2.1.2 Intracellular targeted therapies

Receptor tyrosine kinase inhibitors (RKIs)

The second class of HER-targeted agents comprises the small molecule receptor tyrosine kinase inhibitors (RTKIs) that inhibit enzyme function of HER family members intracellularly. Oral RTKIs include lapatinib, neratinib (both inhibit HER-1 and HER-2), erlotinib and gefitinib that target the intracellular domain of HER-1, and the irreversible pan-HER inhibitors PF-00299804 and canertinib, which inhibit the kinase signaling of multiple HER family members [79].

Another strategy to target HER2 is with low molecular weight tyrosine kinase inhibitors. Lapatinib (Tykerb®) is a dual EGFR and HER2 inhibitor that has been studied extensively in multiple clinical settings. Lapatinib is approved in the U.S. (March 2007) and European Union (EU) (June 2008) for use (oral administration) in combination with capecitabine for the treatment of patients with advanced breast cancer or MBC whose tumors over-express HER-2 and who have received prior therapy including an anthracycline, a taxane, and trastuzumab [7].

Lapatinib increases survival in patients with advanced HER2-over-expressing breast cancer when given in combination with the chemotherapeutic agent capecitabine compared to capecitabine alone in patients that had previously failed anthracyclines and taxanes [80]. The incidences of adverse events (including those leading to treatment discontinuation) and symptomatic cardiac events were similar in both treatment groups. The observation that fewer patients in the lapatinib group developed central nervous system (CNS) metastases together with lapatinib's low molecular weight and capacity to cross the blood-brain barrier has led to a clinical trial to study the role of lapatinib in the treatment of brain metastasis in patients with HER2-over-expressing breast cancer [25, 28]. Thus, contrary to trastuzumab, lapatinib has a putative activity against CNS metastases in patients with HER-2+ breast cancer [81]. These data suggest that, as a small molecule RTKI, it may be able to cross the blood- brain barrier to provide effective therapeutic concentrations in cerebrospinal fluid (unlike monoclonal antibodies such as trastuzumab).

Lapatinib appears to be associated with less cardiotoxicity than trastuzumab [82]. However, as lapatinib development is extended to include the treatment of patients with lower-risk primary breast cancer, it will be increasingly important to monitor cardiotoxic effects. The most common adverse effects associated with lapatinib treatment are gastrointestinal; lapatinib-related diarrhea generally occurs early in the course of treatment, is mild to moderate, and does not require treatment, although monitoring is important to identify patients who may need intervention **[7]**.

Other examples of RTKIs include Erlotinib and Gefitinib. Recent clinical studies have not demonstrated any significant clinical benefit for erlotinib or gefitinib either as single agents or in combination with other agents in MBC [68, 83-85]. Given their lack of activity as monotherapy in MBC, studies continue to investigate the efficacy of erlotinib and gefitinib in combination with other targeted therapies, chemotherapy, or hormonal agents; however, tolerability issues may limit this approach.

Other anti-HER tyrosine kinase inhibitors in clinical development include HKI-272. Neratinib (HKI-272) is an orally administered, irreversible, pan-erbB kinase inhibitor [86] that covalently bind to the intracellular kinase domain. The observation that some patients with chronic myelogenous leukemia were developing resistance to the RTKI imatinib led to the development of neratinib. In preclinical models, neratinib has been shown to have promising antiproliferative activity in both HER-2–dependent cell lines and tumor xenografts.

Phase I/II data have confirmed that neratinib has antitumor activity in patients with HER-2+ MBC, either as a single agent in trastuzumab refractory patients or in combination with trastuzumab, and the safety profile of this agent has been manageable [87].

2.2.2 Src-family tyrosine kinases inhibitors

Currently, small-molecule Src inhibitors are in early phases of clinical development either as single agents, in combination with cytotoxic agents, biological therapies or in combination with hormonal treatment. Originally, dasatinib (BMS-354825) was selected as a synthetic small-molecule inhibitor of Src-family kinases; then, it was found to inhibit at least four other protein tyrosine kinases: bcr-abl, c-Kit, EphA2, PDGF-beta. Dasatinib is currently studied in clinical trials for the treatment of solid tumors, including breast cancer. Preclinical evidence suggests that dasatinib could be effective in breast cancer cell lines of basal-like subtype **[88]**. These findings provide scientific rationale for the clinical development of dasatinib in the treatment of patients with 'triple-negative' breast cancer, a tumor subtype that is categorised as being aggressive and lacking effective targeted treatments, such as endocrine therapies and anti- HER2 strategies. More recently, AZD-0530 a highly selective, dual-specific, orally available small-molecule inhibitor of Src kinase and Bcr-Abl has entered clinical trials **[89]**. In healthy volunteers, AZD-0530 has shown only mild adverse events.

Targeting downstream effector molecules

Targeting HER receptors with extracellular monoclonal antibodies and intracellular RTKIs has shown promising clinical activity. There is, however, a need for better treatment of MBC patients because many of these current therapies are restricted to a subset of the MBC patient population. Targeting cellular signaling pathways, such as the MAPK and PI3K pathways, downstream of HER receptors may be an attractive avenue for novel treatments. Additionally, there is some evidence that targeting heat shock proteins (Hsps) and the apoptotic pathway may be viable options for future therapeutic strategies in MBC. Recent developments in this field are briefly discussed in the following sections.

2.3 STPs-2: Targeting downstream MAPK signaling pathway

The MAPK pathway, also termed the extracellular signal-regulated kinase (ERK) pathway, contains downstream effectorsof the HER family and other tyrosine kinases, and is a central part of the signaling networks that control fundamental cellular processes, including cell proliferation, differentiation, and survival **[90]**.

2.4 STIs-2: Targeted therapies directed at the MAPK signaling pathway

The farnesyl transferase inhibitor tipifarnib (R115777) was evaluated in phase III trials for the treatment of breast cancer, although further development has now been terminated [91-93]. AZD6244 (ARRY-142886) is an inhibitor of the enzyme MEK, a component of the MAPK pathway. AZD6244 is currently in phase I clinical studies in several cancer types, including breast cancer.

2.5 STPs-3: Targeting downstream PI3K/Akt/mTOR pathway signaling pathway

The PI3K/Akt pathway plays a central role in diverse cellular functions including proliferation, growth, survival and metabolism. In addition to their physiological role, several isoforms of the PI3K family are implicated in tumor development, including cell proliferation, cell growth, cell motility, cell survival, and angiogenesis [29]. The relationship between dysregulated PI3K activity and the onset of cancer is well documented [94]. In particular, members of class 1A PI3Ks are often mutated in human cancer [95-100]. As a result of receptor tyrosine kinase RTK activation and phosphorylation, PI3K interacts with the intracellular domain of the receptors. Subsequent phosphorylation event by the mammalian target of rapamycin (mTOR)-complex is required for maximal Akt activity [101-102]. Akt is the central effector of the pathway. Akt reduces cell cycle inhibitors p27 and p21, and promotes cell cycle proteins c-Myc and cyclin D1, resulting in enhanced cellular proliferation. Its influence extends to a host of pro- and antiapoptotic proteins, such as the Bcl-2 family member Bad, limiting programmed cell death and boosting cellular survival. mTOR is a central regulator of cellular responses to multiple stimuli including amino acid availability and growth factor receptor signaling. In cells with sufficient nutrients, mTOR relays a signal to the translational machinery leading to an enhanced translation of mRNAs encoding proteins essential for cell growth and cell cycle progression [103-104].

There is growing evidence that uncontrolled activation of the phosphatidylinositol 3-kinase (PI3K)/Akt/mammalian target of rapamycin (mTOR) pathway, achieved via numerous genetic and epigenetic alterations, contributes to the development and progression of human cancers, including breast cancer [105]. In breast tumors, activating mutations in PIK3A, encoding the catalytic subunit of PI3K, or loss of PTEN, the negative regulator of PI3K activity, are very frequent and contribute to constitutive pathway activation and mTOR activity. Further, they may result in resistance to upstream anti-receptor agents. For example, trastuzumab depends on intact PTEN for its action in HER2-over-expressing breast cell lines, and PTEN loss predicts for trastuzumab resistance [106]. Therefore, this pathway is an attractive target for novel anticancer agents. Clinical trials are currently underway with mTOR, PI3K and Akt inhibitors.

2.6 STIs-3: Inhibitors of the PI3K/Akt/mTOR pathway

Therapies targeting the PI3K pathway include perifosine (KRX-0401), which inhibits Akt phosphorylation [107] and mTOR inhibitors are also further ahead in development within this class of agents. The rapamycin analogs that target mammalian target of rapamycin include temsirolimus (CCl-779) [108-109]. Rapamycin derivatives such as everolimus, temsirolimus and deforolimus are potent inhibitors of mTOR and do not share the problems of poor solubility and chemical stability of rapamycin.

Recent data from two phase I trials suggest that everolimus can help overcome resistance to trastuzumab in women with HER-2+ MBC. Everolimus plus trastuzumab and weekly paclitaxel was shown to slow tumor growth in 77% of patients, and the combination of everolimus with trastuzumab and vinorelbine halted tumor growth in 62% of patients [110-111]. Although early indications suggest that targeting components of the PI3K pathway may have some activity in the treatment of MBC, additional data, including an understanding of combinations and patient selection, are required.

However, in unselected patients with breast cancer these agents have modest anti-tumor activity in the range of around 10% **[112]**. There is therefore a need to identify the subset of patients that may benefit from it, and PI3K/Akt/mTOR-dependency genetic signatures are being developed. In this direction, it has been recently observed that a majority of locally advanced and inflammatory breast cancers over-express the translation regulatory protein4E-BP1 and the initiation factor eIF4G, both of them are mTOR downstream targets. While additional studies are planned to further dissect this interaction, it does seem reasonable to explore the benefits of mTOR inhibitors in the treatment of locally advanced breast cancer [113].

Another potential explanation for the limited activity of mTOR inhibitors in breast cancer and other tumor types may be related to a 'collateral effect' of mTOR blockade. mTOR inhibition blocks the natural negative feed-back on IGF-1R signaling exerted on PI3K [114]. The result is an increase in PI3K and Akt activations which could potentially counteract the inhibition of mTOR. Thus, dual inhibition of both IGF-1 signaling, with either MAbs against the receptor or tyrosine kinase inhibitors, and mTOR results in superior anti-proliferative effect over each single strategy.

In the clinic there is indirect evidence that this approach may be fruitful as well. Octreotide has been shown to inhibit IGF-1R signaling. Although octreotide has limited activity in patients with refractory neuroendocrine tumors, it has been shown to that the combination of everolimus and octreotide has resulted in an impressive activity **[115]**.

2.7 STPs-4: HSP90 signaling pathway

Heat shock protein 90 (HSP90) is a molecular chaperone required for the stability and function of several conditionally activated and/or expressed signaling proteins ([116-117]. Many of these client proteins such as Akt, HER2, Bcr-Abl, c-Kit, EGFR and PDGFR-a are oncoproteins and important cell-signaling proteins [118-119]. As signal transducers and molecular switches, these client proteins are inherently unstable. HSP90 keeps unstable signaling proteins poised for activation until they are stabilised by conformational changes associated with the formation of signal transduction complexes. As such, it is a single molecular target that is a central integrator of multiple pathways important to cancer. Activation of HSP90-dependent client proteins proceeds through an ordered sequence of events linked to the ATPase activity of HSP90 and involves a variety of co-chaperone complexes **[120]**.

HER2 is among the most sensitive client proteins of HSP90, demonstrating degradation within 2 h of HSP90 inhibition in cell culture experiments **[121]**. Geldanamycin analogues (17-allylamino- 17-demethoxygeldanamycin [17-AAG] and 17-dimethylaminoethylamino-

17-demethoxygeldanamycin [17-DMAG]) have demonstrated potent inhibition of HSP90 function in HER2-over-expressing cell lines, demonstrating significant anti-tumor activity in both cell culture and animal studies [121-122].

2.8 STIs-4: HSP90 inhibitors

(HSP90) is an exciting new therapeutic target, inhibition of which delivers a combinatorial attack on multiple oncogenic targets and pathways and on all of the hallmark traits of malignancy **[123]**. In the clinic, initial studies with the HSP90 inhibitor have demonstrated safety and anti-tumor activity and tolerability in combination with trastuzumab in patients with trastuzumab-refractory HER2- positive metastatic breast cancer patients **[120]**. It will be important to determine whether HSP90 inhibitors will have clinical activity as single agents in breast cancer patients.

2.9 STPs-5: PARP signaling pathway

Poly (ADP-ribose) polymerase 1 (PARP-1) is the initial and best characterised member of a family of enzymes largely associated with the maintenance of genomic stability. Activation of PARP-1 is part of the immediate cellular response to DNA strand breaks, converting them into an intracellular signal via poly (ADP-ribosylation) of nuclear proteins [124-125]. This results in a highly negatively charged target, which in turn leads to the unwinding and repair of the damaged DNA through the base excision repair pathway. In addition, PARP-1 is also known to bind dsDNA breaks (DSB) preventing accidental recombination of homologous DNA [126]. Upon binding DNA breaks, the catalytic activity of PARP-1 is stimulated >500- fold [127]. Enhanced PARP-1 expression or activity has been also observed in a number of different tumor cell lines and could provide a greater level of resistance to both endogenous genotoxic stress and to DNA damage-inducing therapeutic agents.

Studies of PARP expression in various tumor types identified that breast cancers with negative estrogen receptor, progesterone receptor and HER2 expression were much more likely to over-express PARP [128]. Additionally, it has been recently shown that BRCA1 and BRCA2 dysfunction sensitises cells to the inhibition of PARP enzymatic activity, resulting in chromosomal instability, cell cycle arrest and subsequent apoptosis. This seems to develop because the inhibition of PARP leads to the persistence of DNA lesions normally repaired by homologous recombination **[128].**

2.10 STIs-5: PARP inhibitors

PARP inhibitors have been developed to investigate the role of PARP-1 in cell biology and to overcome DNA repair-mediated resistance of cancer cells to genotoxic agents [129]. These novel PARP inhibitors have been shown to enhance the anti-tumor activity of DNA-methylating agents, such as temozolomide, topoisomerase poisons and ionising radiation in preclinical studies [130], and to restore sensitivity of resistant tumors to methylating agents or topoisomerase I inhibitors, agents presently used for the treatment of breast cancer.

2.11 STPs-6: Apoptosis & autophagy signaling pathways

Apoptosis, the process of programmed cell death, is governed by complex, gene-directed pathways [131-133]. Dysregulation of apoptosis plays a key role in tumorigenesis and can allow tumor cells to become resistant to anticancer treatments [132-133]. Rationale for targeting apoptosis in the treatment of breast cancer includes the over-expression of the Bcl-2 protein in 40%–80% of human breast tumors, which is associated with both resistance to chemotherapy **[134]** and a better prognosis after chemotherapy **[135].** Additionally, the association of Bcl-2 with ER and/or PgR, loss of expression of the gene for the pro-apoptotic protein Bax, and differential expression of tumor necrosis factor-related apoptosis-inducing ligand-receptor 2 have all been correlated with prognosis in breast cancer patients [134-137].

On the other hand, autophagy is an evolutionarily conserved lysosomal pathway for degrading cytoplasmic proteins, macromolecules, and organelles [138]. Many studies have described the role of autophagy as a protective mechanism for cell survival that is initiated in response to metabolic or therapeutic stress. Furthermore, autophagy may delay apoptotic cell death caused by DNA damaging agents and hormonal therapies [139-141].

2.12 STIs-6: Targeted therapies directed at the apoptotic & autophagic pathways

Anticancer agents targeting the components of apoptotic pathways are in the early stages of development, and no agent specifically targeting apoptosis has yet been approved for use in cancer treatment. A range of approaches is being tested, including antisense DNA oligonucleotides and antibody and small molecule inhibitors of the components of apoptotic pathways. Few clinical data are currently available in breast cancer; however, preclinical studies show that such agents do have anticancer activity, suggesting that this may be a promising approach, particularly when used in combination with chemotherapy [7].

On the other hand, recent studies have demonstrated that the inhibition of autophagy in cancer cells may be therapeutically beneficial in some circumstances, as it can sensitize cancer cells to different therapies, including DNA-damaging agents, antihormone therapies (e.g., tamoxifen), and radiation therapy. This supports the hypothesis that inhibiting autophagy can increase cell death when combined with anticancer agents, providing a therapeutic advantage against cancer proliferation & drug resistance [139-141].

2.13 STPs-7: Targeting the angiogenesis pathway

It is increasingly being accepted that tumor cell proliferation alone is insufficient to result in a substantial tumor mass. Angiogenesis is essential for tumors to develop into detectable localized masses, and for metastasis to occur [142-143]. The process of angiogenesis (the formation of new blood vessels from a pre-existing vascular bed) is complex and dynamic, and it is regulated by a range of pro- and anti-angiogenic molecules **[144].** The VEGF and platelet-derived growth factor (PDGF) families of proteins and their receptors (VEGFR-1, VEGFR-2, VEGFR-3, PDGFR-α, and PDGFR-β) appear central to the process **[144].** Activation of VEGFRs and PDGFRs initiates signaling that results in numerous cellular responses, including survival, mitogenesis, migration, proliferation, and differentiation [144-145]. Activation of the VEGF pathway also increases vascular permeability and the movement of endothelial progenitor cells from the bone marrow into the peripheral circulation [144]. Primary breast tumors express a variety of different angiogenic factors, with VEGF being the most abundant.

High VEGF expression appears to be correlated with poor clinical prognosis and response **[146]**. Levels of VEGF in breast cancer tumors are a prognostic factor for relapse-free and overall survival in patients with both lymph node-negative and lymph node-positive disease [147-148], and they predict response to both tamoxifen and chemotherapy in advanced disease **[149]**. Similarly, a proportion of invasive breast cancers that over-express PDGFR-α have been associated with greater biological aggressiveness and a higher likelihood of lymph node metastasis [150].

Given their central roles in tumor angiogenesis and growth, the VEGF and PDGF signaling pathways are key targets for breast cancer therapy. However, with considerable redundancy in angiogenic signaling pathways, the inhibition of more than one receptor is likely necessary to block angiogenesis. It has been hypothesized that anti-VEGF agents may prevent the development of new tumor vasculature and induce normalization of existing, inefficient tumor vasculature (resulting from over-expression of VEGF) **[151]**. These agents, then, may allow better delivery of cytotoxic therapies to the tumor, suggesting a potential role for anti-VEGF therapy in conjunction with chemotherapy [151-152].

2.14 STIs-7: Targeted therapies directed at angiogenesis

Several therapies targeting angiogenesis are in development for breast cancer. These include monoclonal antibodies that act extracellularly by binding to receptors or their ligands, such as bevacizumab (Avastin®), and RTKIs that act intracellularly, such as sunitinib (Sutent®). Intracellular VEGF targeting therapeutics will be discussed later as they were proven to be targeting multiple sites.

Monoclonal antibodies: Bevacizumab

Bevacizumab is an anti-VEGF humanized monoclonal antibody administered as an i.v. infusion. It acts by binding to all VEGF isoforms, thus removing VEGF from the circulation and preventing activation of VEGFRs **[153]**. In 2008, the U.S. Food and Drug Administration (FDA) approved bevacizumab in combination with paclitaxel for the first-line treatment of locally recurrent breast cancer or MBC **[7]**.

Although bevacizumab has shown little activity as a single agent in MBC patients, combination therapy with chemotherapeutic agents has been associated with clinical activity in this patient population. Several phase III studies have investigated bevacizumab combined with chemotherapy [154-155]. These data suggest that VEGF inhibition combined with chemotherapy is a promising treatment strategy in this setting. Further studies are under way to explore the use of bevacizumab with different chemotherapeutic regimens, hormonal treatments, and other targeted therapies (including lapatinib and trastuzumab) in patients with MBC. Additionally, trials of bevacizumab are ongoing in the adjuvant and neoadjuvant settings, and preliminary reports suggest that this approach may be feasible.

Hypertension, bleeding, and thrombosis remain potential safety concerns with a number of anti-VEGF therapies, and this area requires further study. Future trials should focus on identifying those patients who will derive the most benefit from bevacizumab- based regimens and how best to combine bevacizumab with other cancer therapies (which therapies should be combined and whether sequential or concurrent administration is most effective). Overall, growing clinical experience with agents targeting angiogenic processes, such as bevacizumab, has provided proof of concept for the use of these treatments in MBC patients **[7]**.

2.15 STPs-8: Multi-target therapeutics

There appears to be extensive crosstalk between the pathways driving tumorigenic processes, and this provides a good rationale for inhibiting multiple pathways and processes with multi-targeted agents, either as single agents or in combination [7]. A number of single-agent RTKIs with multiple molecular targets have been developed as an alternative to combining multiple agents. These were developed based on previous studies showing that combining agents that target different pathways may have synergistic activity and delay or reverse resistance [156-158].

2.16 STIs-8: Multi-target inhibitors

A range of oral, antiangiogenic RTKIs with multiple targets is currently in development for MBC. These include sunitinib, pazopanib, sorafenib (Nexavar®) and axitinib.

Sunitinib selectively inhibits several receptor tyrosine kinases (VEGFR-1, VEGFR-2, VEGFR-3, PDGFR- α, PDGFR-β, Kit, FMS-like tyrosine kinase [FLT]-3, and colony-stimulating factor 1 receptor). It has both anti-angiogenic and anti-tumor activities. Sunitinib has been shown to have antitumor activity in breast cancer preclinical studies, both as a single agent and in combination with chemotherapy [159-163].

Data from a phase II study of sunitinib monotherapy in patients with refractory MBC reported single-agent activity in heavily pretreated patients, previously exposed to an anthracycline and a taxane [164]. The toxicities were manageable [164]. Studies and case series evaluating sunitinib given in combination with taxane therapy for MBC have reported antitumor activity and a manageable and tolerable safety profile [165-166]. Phase III trials of sunitinib in combination with a variety of cytotoxic agents are under way in first- and second-line MBC therapy [7].

Pazopanib targets VEGFR, PDGFR, and Kit and is currently in development in a number of tumor types, including breast cancer. Although originally developed as a Raf inhibitor, sorafenib also inhibits the activity of VEGFR-2 and VEGFR-3, PDGFR-β, FLT-3, and Kit; thus, it may inhibit tumor growth both directly (through Raf and Kit) and indirectly, through inhibition of angiogenesis [167-168].

Sorafenib inhibited MAPK activity in breast cancer cell lines expressing mutations of K-Ras or B-Raf, and showed antitumor and antiangiogenic activity in a human breast cancer xenograft model [168]. Significant and sustained increases in blood pressure were reported in a study of sorafenib monotherapy in patients with metastatic solid tumors [169]. Current data suggest little activity for sorafenib as a single agent in MBC patients; ongoing studies are exploring combination treatment with paclitaxel and with anastrozole in MBC.

Axitinib inhibits all known VEGFRs, in addition to PDGFR-β and the stem cell factor receptor Kit, and is currently being investigated in a range of tumor types, including breast cancer. In preclinical studies, axitinib was shown to selectively block VEGF-stimulated receptor phosphorylation in vitro, resulting in the inhibition of endothelial cell proliferation and survival. In a human breast cancer xenograft model, it significantly inhibited tumor growth and disrupted tumor microvasculature as assessed by dynamic contrast-enhanced magnetic resonance imaging [170].

To date, the mult-itargeted RTKIs discussed have not been validated in phase III trials in MBC patients, although there is preliminary evidence of clinical activity. Of the four agents described above, three (pazopanib, sunitinib, and axitinib) appear to have the most clinical activity to date. Based on experience with other targeted agents in breast cancer, and with these RTKIs in other indications, combinations will hopefully show greater efficacy in the treatment of breast cancer [7].

2.17 STPs-9: Estrogen signaling transduction

Two of the genetic subtypes in breast cancer so far identified are those with gene expression characteristics typical of basal epithelial cells (which are predominantly estrogen receptor [ER-) and those with gene expression characteristics typical of luminal epithelial cells (which are predominantly ER+) [14, 171]. Typically, tumors of the ER-, basal subtype are associated with shorter relapse-free and overall survival times than those of the ER+, luminal subtype [171].

2.18 STIs-9: Estrogen signaling inhibitors

Endocrine therapy is widely used in the treatment of both early stage and recurrent/metastatic breast cancer. Tamoxifen and estrogen deprivation therapies such as aromatase inhibitors (AIs) and ovarian suppression have proved clinically effective and are generally well tolerated; they are the primary reason for the sustained improvement in survival for patients with early-stage [ER+] breast cancer [172]. Their long-term efficacy, however, is limited by relapse of disease and development of resistance following adjuvant endocrine therapy. This provides a strong rationale for using targeted agents against various growth factor and signaling pathways that are activated during endocrine resistance and for combining these targeted agents with ongoing endocrine therapy to either overcome endocrine resistance and enhance the efficacy of therapy for ER-positive breast cancer [173-174].

In this context, several selected targeted agents are being investigated in combination with endocrine therapy for patients with breast cancer in an attempt to overcome or prevent endocrine resistance. The role of EGFR/HER2 cross-talk with estrogen receptor (ER) signaling has been confirmed in preclinical studies [175] in which various inhibitors have yielded additive or synergistic effects when combined with endocrine agents. Recently, several results from clinical trials investigating this concept have been reported [59, 92].

2.19 STPs-10

Cancer progression is a multi-step process that enables tumor cells to invade through extracellular tissues and metastasize to distal organs **[8]**. Compelling recent evidence demonstrates that cooperation between signals from the extracellular matrix (ECM) and growth factors enhances malignant behaviors of aggressive cancer cells, such as proliferation, migration, survival, and invasion [176]. Examples of such cross talk signals include:

a. **The STATs** are a family of transcription factors that relay the interactions of cytokines and growth factors with their receptors at the cell surface to mediate changes in gene expression. In normal situations STATs are transiently activated; however, in many tumors tyrosine-phosphorylated STATs, mainly STAT3 and STAT5, can be detected, suggesting constitutive pathway activation [6].

b. **The NF-κB** pathway is triggered in response to microbial and viral infections and to pro-inflammatory cytokines. These agents activate the IκB kinase, which phosphoylates IκB allowing the liberated NF-κB family transcription factors to enter the nucleus. The pathway has an ever increasing interest for its role in human cancer [177]. The association of NF-κB pathway activity with inflammation-associated tumor progression is well documented in mouse tumor models [178] and in human cancer cells [179].

c. **The Notch network** in mammals consists of four Notch receptors and five ligands. Once activated, the receptor undergoes intramembrane proteolysis leading to release and nuclear translocation of the intracellular domain, which has transcriptional activity. The Notch-4 gene is frequently rearranged in mammary glands by MMTV proviral integration. This rearrangement leads to expression of the intracellular domain under MMTV promoter control [180] an early demonstration of Notch's ability to induce mammary cancer.
d. **The UPS pathway**: The ubiquitin proteasome system (UPS) consists of several crucial enzymes contributing to most, if not all, cellular events. During the past decade, progress in endocrine therapy and the use of trastuzumab has significantly contributed to the decline in breast cancer mortality for hormone receptor-positive and HER2-positive cases, respectively. As a result of these advances, a breast cancer cluster with poor prognosis that is negative for the estrogen receptor (ER1), the progesterone receptor (PRGR) and HER2 (triple negative; basal like phenotype) has come to the forefront of medical therapeutic attention. DNA microarray analyses have revealed that this cluster is phenotypically most like the basal-like breast cancer that is caused by deficiencies in the **BRCA1 pathways.** BRCA1 acts as a hub protein that coordinates a diverse range of cellular pathways to maintain genomic stability [181]. Indeed, BRCA1 dysfunction in sporadic basal-like cancers has been reported [182]. Thus, investigating the BRCA1 pathway could be an important approach for the treatment of basal-like breast cancer.

2.20 STIs-10

To gain further improvements in breast cancer survival, new types of drugs might be required, and small molecules targeting the ubiquitin proteasome system have moved into the spotlight. The success of bortezomib in the treatment of multiple myeloma has sent encouraging signals that proteasome inhibitors could be used to treat other types of cancers [183]. In addition, ubiquitin enzymes involved in ER1, HER2 or BRCA1 pathways could be ideal targets for therapeutic intervention. The therapeutic effect of proteasome inhibitors on breast cancer remains to be determined but is greatly anticipated [184].

3. Targeting molecular signal in breast cancer stem cells responsible for development of multi-drug resistance (MDR)

Success in Breast cancer chemotherapy is challenged by the development of tumors having a multi-drug resistance (MDR) phenotype **[185]**. It is one of the major causes of failures to cancer chemotherapy. This phenotype is most prevalent in aggressive carcinomas as breast and ovarian carcinomas. By definition, MDR is a term used to describe the resistance developed by some tumors to protect themselves against a number of structurally and functionally unrelated chemotherapeutic agents. MDR is not only referred to the drug with which the patient has been treated but also to a wide range of other drugs used in cancer chemotherapy **[186]**.

Acquired drug resistance arises from exposure of tumor cells to chemotherapeutic agents. Random spontaneous mutations, acceleration of proliferation rate and alteration of cell sensitivity to growth factors can occur in tumor cells under the influence of cytotoxic drugs. On the other hand, MDR does not only develop as the result of treatment of tumor cells by a drug. It may be intrinsic, i.e. connected with the type of cell differentiation or genetic profile of tumor cells **[187]**.

Studies of resistance of tumor cells to cytotoxic drugs are necessary for understanding the mechanisms for restoring back their sensitivity. Although, MDR is a multi-factorial problem i.e. multiple mechanisms were hypothesized to account for this phenomenon, some of them were frequently observed and their clinical significance was determined. These mechanisms are acting either alone or in concert with each other for the development of the MDR phenotype in breast cancer cells **[188]**. Over-expression of ABC transporters, detoxification enzymes (aldehyde dehydrogenase), low cell turn over rate and the ability to activate the DNA check point response are possibly all involved and previously described with other mechanisms **[189]**. Innovative therapies, based on a better understanding of cancer stem cells, should lead to enhanced and long-term cure rates in breast cancer.

Given that tumor resistance to chemotherapy is believed to account for the majority of treatment failure in breast cancer, research attention in the last two decades focused on developing agents to reverse MDR and enhance the response of tumors to chemotherapeutic agents. Although hundreds of compounds have been found in-vitro to be able to modulate the MDR phenotype, their clinical application was limited owing to their high toxicity in-vivo [190-191]. Accordingly, searching for compounds able to modulate the MDR phenotype and have low toxicity continues to be an important challenge for optimizing cancer chemotherapy. The development of several therapeutics targeting the MDR phenotype in breast cancer cells have been previously reviewed **[189]**.

Recently, the possible roles of cancer stem cells in carcinogenesis have become more obvious. Numerous investigations have recently provided evidence that the genetic alterations occurring in the multi-potent tissue-specific adult stem cells and/or their early progenies may lead to their malignant transformation into cancer progenitor cells also designated as cancer stem cells or cancer-initiating cells **[192]**. A small population of undifferentiated- or poorly differentiated cancer progenitor cells, which possesses the stem cell-like properties including their self-renewal ability and capacity to give rise to the bulk mass of further differentiated malignant cells, appears to represent the principal cancer cells that are responsible for tumor formation [193]. Accumulating genetic alterations in tumorigenic cancer progenitor cells occurring during cancer progression may also confer to them the invasive and resistant properties that are essential for their remission and migration to distant metastatic sites [194-195].

The role of cancer stem cells in breast cancer chemoresistance was recently reviewed [196]. One characteristic of cancer stem cells that differentiates them from other normal cells in the tumor is that they have high levels of ABC transporter proteins, in particular ABCG2 [197]. The ABC transporter molecules are responsible for protecting cells from drug damage via efflux pumping mechanisms. Thus, cancer stem cells, as a result of these biological properties, are rendered resistant to drug treatment, including chemotherapeutic drugs [198].

Since all the stem cell-like properties attributed to cancer progenitor cells may provide them with a higher resistance to current cancer therapies, thus they constitute a substantial obstacle to the successful treatment of cancer patients [196]. This finding underlines the critical importance of targeting the cancer progenitor cells and their early progenies as well as their local microenvironment in the earlier stages of cancer treatment to counteract the rapid progression of certain cancer types and prevent the metastatic spread at distant sites. The simultaneous blockade of several oncogenic cascades activated in cancer progenitor cells during cancer progression may be essential for improving the current clinical treatments against high-risk, metastatic or relapsed breast cancers [189, 199].

Recent studies have revealed the possibility of using therapeutic agents targeting the EGFR, Wnt/β-catenin and/or Notch cascades to inhibit the ABC muli-drug efflux transporters and/or eliminate the cancer progenitor cells **[200]**. Moreover, one compound, salinomycin, reduces the proportion of cancer stem cells by >100-fold relative to paclitaxel, a commonly used breast cancer chemotherapeutic drug [201]. In addition, treatment of mice with salinomycin inhibits mammary tumor growth in vivo and induces increased epithelial differentiation of tumor cells **[199]**. What remains to be discovered is the extensive and in depth understanding of the molecular basis of cancer stem cell contribution to breast cancer development. Such extensive investigations enable the development of more effective and selective treatment strategies.

4. Concluding remarks and perspectives

Considerable progress has been made over the last several decades in understanding specific cellular, molecular and genetic mechanisms that contribute to cancer growth and progression **[202]**. In recent years, research efforts have focused on the signaling pathways involved in the growth and survival of breast cancer cells, leading to the development of a range of targeted agents with promising clinical activity. The encouraging success of trastuzumab, based on the identification of HER-2 as a molecular target, has provided the rationale for studying the array of targeted agents currently in clinical development for breast cancer **[7]**.

We have reviewed some of the most promising new targeted agents in breast cancer. This list, however, is far from complete. It should be pointed out that there are still many important additional classes of agents in clinical development in breast cancer. Examples include other tyrosine kinase inhibitors and also enhancers of apoptosis. We all hope that this list will keep developing. However, despite recent advances, there are still unanswered questions regarding the management of breast cancer with targeted agents.

With our knowledge of the molecular modifications in breast cancer and the increasing number of new targeted therapeutics, the current challenge is to select the best combinations of the so-called signal transduction inhibitors (STIs) for every patient [6]. The development of these targeted therapeutics will require a new set of challenging skills & investigations of unresolved issues **[120]**. These challenges are:

First, future studies are necessary to identify those patient subgroups likely to derive most benefit from a given therapy. Despite the temptation to use a targeted agent in all patients, identification of patient subgroups most likely to benefit must be a key goal and will be critical to the successful future use of these treatments **[7]**. These agents, unlike chemotherapy, will only work in the subset of tumors that show dependency on the target the therapy is being directed to.

If STI would have been developed in an unselected patient population, its anti-tumor activity would have been missed due to a dilutional effect brought in by the non-STPs-over-expressing population. This principle probably applies to the majority of classes of agents under study. The implication of this principle is that patient selection strategies will be of paramount importance in the development of these agents [120]. For example, accurate patient selection based on HER-2 over-expression is essential for trastuzumab-based treatment and is likely to be important for other agents in this class. However, identifying suitable patients may prove more difficult for RTKIs, because receptor over-expression alone does not seem to predict response to treatment [16].

Second, future studies are necessary to determine the optimal combinations, doses, and schedules required to maximize clinical activity while minimizing toxicity. Also, in early clinical studies with these agents in addition to establishing their safety and optimal doses and schedules, it may prove to be instrumental to also check for the presence of the target in the studied tumors and to seek for indications of target engagement with the study agent using careful analysis of [120]**2007**). The need to determine target engagement is currently being taken into account with the majority of clinical trials with novel agents that are moved into the clinic.

Third, Predictive markers are factors that are associated with upfront response or resistance to a particular therapy. Predictive markers are important in oncology as tumors of the same tissue of origin vary widely in their response to most available systemic therapies. Currently recommended oncological predictive markers include both estrogen and progesterone receptors for identifying patients with breast cancers likely to benefit from hormone therapy, HER-2 for the identification of breast cancer patients likely to benefit from trastuzumab [203]. Thus, the drive to identify new biomarkers of target engagement and sensitivity with these novel agents is also promoting the search for new clinical study designs in a minimally pre-treated population **[120]**.

Fourth, future studies will need to address how best to incorporate these agents into existing treatment regimens and to determine when and in which combinations targeted therapy should be administered **[7]**. Some of these agents will have limited activity by themselves and yet have the capacity to markedly enhance the anti-tumor activity of conventional agents like chemotherapy or even other biological agents. For example, anti angiogenesis MAb bevacizumab that has no activity as a single agent and yet is clinically active when combined with chemotherapy. Furthermore, HER-targeted agents may need to be used in combination with chemotherapy to provide clinically relevant activity.

Fifth, the therapy end-points with these agents also need to be revisited. Some of these agents are not expected to result in tumor shrinkage (or response), and therefore we cannot propose a unified definition of clinical benefit as it has been done with chemotherapy in the past. Furthermore, genetic assay techniques used to provide information on clinical outcomes, including the risk for tumor recurrence and individual benefit from a particular chemotherapy also needs further critical development **[204]**.

Sixth, Targeting HER-2 is associated with cardiac toxicity, which is an especially important consideration in the adjuvant setting and when combining anti–HER-2 agents with cardiotoxic chemotherapeutic drugs. Targeting HER-1 in combination with HER-2, as with the RTKIs lapatinib and neratinib, appears to reduce the risk for cardiotoxicity, although the exact mechanisms underlying this observation remain unclear **[7]**.

Finally, with the increase in the number of available lines of therapy in breast cancer, there is a danger that novel agents will be tested in a heavily pre-treated patient population. While there is little debate if patients with advanced disease receiving multiple lines of therapy may be appropriate study participants in early clinical studies. There is also a growing concern that patients with advanced disease may not be the ideal population to detect the anti-tumor activity of novel agents since their tumors may have become highly resistant to any type of therapy **[120]**.

In summary, the contribution of STIs in cancer chemotherapy continues to be encouraging, and clinical trials are currently addressing whether the promising preclinical activities of STIs will translate into benefits for patients. Hopefully, the previously mentioned suggestions and mechanisms will ultimately be put into practice. Moreover, cellular responses to cancer chemotherapeutic agents are complex and several mechanisms are commonly associated with the resistance of laboratory human breast cancer cell lines. Clinical testing of breast cancer STIs like other modern day targeted therapeutics must be rationally developed with a firm basis in the lessons learned in the laboratory and with proper selection of patient populations in which the predictive power and the potential for benefit is greatest.

5. References

Jemal A., et al., Global Cancer Statistics. CANCER J CLIN, 2011. 61: p. 69–90.

Jemal, A., et al., Cancer statistics, 2009. CA Cancer J Clin, 2009. 59(4): p. 225-49.

Knutson, D. and E. Steiner, Screening for breast cancer: current recommendations and future directions. Am Fam Physician, 2007. 75(11): p. 1660-6.

Gonzalez-Angulo, A.M., F. Morales-Vasquez, and G.N. Hortobagyi, *Overview of resistance to systemic therapy in patients with breast cancer.* Adv Exp Med Biol, 2007. 608: p. 1-22.

Condeelis, J. and J.W. Pollard, *Macrophages: obligate partners for tumor cell migration, invasion, and metastasis.* Cell, 2006. 124(2): p. 263-6.

Hynes, N.E. and W. Gullick, *Therapeutic targeting of signal transduction pathways and proteins in breast cancer.* J Mammary Gland Biol Neoplasia, 2006. 11(1): p. 1-2.

Rosen, L.S., H.L. Ashurst, and L. Chap, *Targeting signal transduction pathways in metastatic breast cancer: a comprehensive review.* Oncologist, 2010. 15(3): p. 216-35.

Hanahan, D. and R.A. Weinberg, *The hallmarks of cancer.* Cell, 2000. 100(1): p. 57-70.

Bender, L.M. and R. Nahta, *Her2 cross talk and therapeutic resistance in breast cancer.* Front Biosci, 2008. 13: p. 3906-12.

Menard, S., et al., *HER2 as a prognostic factor in breast cancer.* Oncology, 2001. 61 Suppl 2: p. 67-72.

Milanezi, F., S. Carvalho, and F.C. Schmitt, *EGFR/HER2 in breast cancer*: a biological approach for molecular diagnosis and therapy. Expert Rev Mol Diagn, 2008. 8(4): p. 417- 34.

Slamon, D.J., et al., *Human breast cancer*: correlation of relapse and survival with amplification of the HER-2/neu oncogene. Science, 1987. 235(4785): p. 177-82.

Gasparini, G., et al., *Therapy of breast cancer with molecular targeting agents.* Ann Oncol, 2005. 16 Suppl 4: p. iv28-36.

Perou, C.M., et al., Molecular portraits of human breast tumours. Nature, 2000. 406(6797): p. 747-52.

Martin, M., Molecular biology of breast cancer. Clin Transl Oncol, 2006. 8(1): p. 7-14.

Lin, N.U. and E.P. Winer, New targets for therapy in breast cancer: small molecule tyrosine kinase inhibitors. Breast Cancer Res, 2004. 6(5): p. 204-10.

Riese, D.J., 2nd and D.F. Stern, Specificity within the EGF family/ErbB receptor family signaling network. Bioessays, 1998. 20(1): p. 41-8.

Mills, G.B., et al., The role of genetic abnormalities of PTEN and the phosphatidylinositol 3- kinase pathway in breast and ovarian tumorigenesis, prognosis, and therapy. Semin Oncol, 2001. 28(5 Suppl 16): p. 125-41.

Salomon, D.S., et al., Epidermal growth factor-related peptides and their receptors in human malignancies. Crit Rev Oncol Hematol, 1995. 19(3): p. 183-232.

Roskoski, R., Jr., The ErbB/HER receptor protein-tyrosine kinases and cancer. Biochem Biophys Res Commun, 2004. 319(1): p. 1-11.

Stern, D.F., Tyrosine kinase signalling in breast cancer: ErbB family receptor tyrosine kinases. Breast Cancer Res, 2000. 2(3): p. 176-83.

Barrett-Lee, P.J., Growth factor signalling in clinical breast cancer and its impact on response to conventional therapies: a review of chemotherapy. Endocr Relat Cancer, 2005. 12 Suppl 1: p. S125-33.

Normanno, N., et al., Mechanisms of endocrine resistance and novel therapeutic strategies in breast cancer. Endocr Relat Cancer, 2005. 12(4): p. 721-47.

Pawlowski, V., et al., A real-time one-step reverse transcriptase-polymerase chain reaction method to quantify c-erbB-2 expression in human breast cancer. Cancer Detect Prev, 2000. 24(3): p. 212-23.

Slamon, D.J., et al., Studies of the HER-2/neu proto-oncogene in human breast and ovarian cancer. Science, 1989. 244(4905): p. 707-12.

Tsutsui, S., et al., Prognostic value of epidermal growth factor receptor (EGFR) and its relationship to the estrogen receptor status in 1029 patients with breast cancer. Breast Cancer Res Treat, 2002. 71(1): p. 67-75.

Vogt, U., et al., Amplification of erbB-4 oncogene occurs less frequently than that of erbB-2 in primary human breast cancer. Gene, 1998. 223(1-2): p. 375-80.

Witton, C.J., Structure of HER receptors and intracellular localisation of downstream effector elements gives insight into mechanism of tumour growth promotion. Breast Cancer Res, 2003. 5(4): p. 206-7.

Atalay, G., et al., Novel therapeutic strategies targeting the epidermal growth factor receptor (EGFR) family and its downstream effectors in breast cancer. Ann Oncol, 2003. 14(9): p. 1346-63.

Graus-Porta, D., et al., ErbB-2, the preferred heterodimerization partner of all ErbB receptors, is a mediator of lateral signaling. EMBO J, 1997. 16(7): p. 1647-55.

Prenzel, N., et al., The epidermal growth factor receptor family as a central element for cellular signal transduction and diversification. Endocr Relat Cancer, 2001. 8(1): p. 11-31.

Schlessinger, J., Common and distinct elements in cellular signaling via EGF and FGF receptors. Science, 2004. 306(5701): p. 1506-7.

Martin, G.S., The hunting of the Src. Nat Rev Mol Cell Biol, 2001. 2(6): p. 467-75.

Thomas, S.M. and J.S. Brugge, Cellular functions regulated by Src family kinases. Annu Rev Cell Dev Biol, 1997. 13: p. 513-609.

Bromann, P.A., H. Korkaya, and S.A. Courtneidge, The interplay between Src family kinases and receptor tyrosine kinases. Oncogene, 2004. 23(48): p. 7957-68.

Blume-Jensen, P. and T. Hunter, Oncogenic kinase signalling. Nature, 2001. 411(6835): p. 355-65.

Muthuswamy, S.K., et al., Mammary tumors expressing the neu proto-oncogene possess elevated c-Src tyrosine kinase activity. Mol Cell Biol, 1994. 14(1): p. 735-43.

Verbeek, B.S., et al., c-Src protein expression is increased in human breast cancer. An immunohistochemical and biochemical analysis. J Pathol, 1996. 180(4): p. 383-8.

Rosen, N., et al., Analysis of pp60c-src protein kinase activity in human tumor cell lines and tissues. J Biol Chem, 1986. 261(29): p. 13754-9.

Ottenhoff-Kalff, A.E., et al., Characterization of protein tyrosine kinases from human breast cancer: involvement of the c-src oncogene product. Cancer Res, 1992. 52(17): p. 4773-8.

Hiscox, S., et al., Elevated Src activity promotes cellular invasion and motility in tamoxifen resistant breast cancer cells. Breast Cancer Res Treat, 2006. 97(3): p. 263-74.

Cho, H.S., et al., Structure of the extracellular region of HER2 alone and in complex with the Herceptin Fab. Nature, 2003. 421(6924): p. 756-60.

Albanell, J., et al., A phase I study of the safety and pharmacokinetics of the combination of pertuzumab (rhuMab 2C4) and capecitabine in patients with advanced solid tumors. Clin Cancer Res, 2008. 14(9): p. 2726-31.

Slamon, D.J., et al., Use of chemotherapy plus a monoclonal antibody against HER2 for metastatic breast cancer that overexpresses HER2. N Engl J Med, 2001. 344(11): p. 783- 92.

Yu, D. and M.C. Hung, Overexpression of ErbB2 in cancer and ErbB2-targeting strategies. Oncogene, 2000. 19(53): p. 6115-21.

Baselga, J., et al., Recombinant humanized anti-HER2 antibody (Herceptin) enhances the antitumor activity of paclitaxel and doxorubicin against HER2/neu overexpressing human breast cancer xenografts. Cancer Res, 1998. 58(13): p. 2825-31.

Carter, P., et al., Humanization of an anti-p185HER2 antibody for human cancer therapy. Proc Natl Acad Sci U S A, 1992. 89(10): p. 4285-9.

Tokuda, Y., et al., In vitro and in vivo anti-tumour effects of a humanised monoclonal antibody against c-erbB-2 product. Br J Cancer, 1996. 73(11): p. 1362-5.

Cobleigh, M.A., et al., *Multinational study of the efficacy and safety of humanized anti-HER2 monoclonal antibody in women who have HER2-overexpressing metastatic breast cancer that has progressed after chemotherapy for metastatic disease.* J Clin Oncol, 1999. 17(9): p. 2639-48.

Marty, M., et al., *Randomized phase II trial of the efficacy and safety of trastuzumab combined with docetaxel in patients with human epidermal growth factor receptor 2-positive metastatic breast cancer administered as first-line treatment: the M77001 study group.* J Clin Oncol, 2005. 23(19): p. 4265-74.

Joensuu, H., et al., *Adjuvant docetaxel or vinorelbine with or without trastuzumab for breast cancer.* N Engl J Med, 2006. 354(8): p. 809-20.

Piccart-Gebhart, M.J., et al., *Trastuzumab after adjuvant chemotherapy in* HER2-positive breast cancer. N Engl J Med, 2005. 353(16): p. 1659-72.

Romond, E.H., et al., Trastuzumab plus adjuvant chemotherapy for operable HER2-positive breast cancer. N Engl J Med, 2005. 353(16): p. 1673-84.

Smith, I., et al., 2-year follow-up of trastuzumab after adjuvant chemotherapy in HER2-positive breast cancer: a randomised controlled trial. Lancet, 2007. 369(9555): p. 29-36.

Spielmann, M., et al., Trastuzumab for patients with axillary-node-positive breast cancer: results of the FNCLCC-PACS 04 trial. J Clin Oncol, 2009. 27(36): p. 6129-34.

Untch, M. and C. Jackisch, *Optimal treatment strategies in hormone-responsive early breast cancer: the role of aromatase inhibitors*. Onkologie, 2007. 30(1-2): p. 55-64.

Chia, S., et al., Pegylated liposomal doxorubicin and trastuzumab in HER-2 overexpressing metastatic breast cancer: a multicenter phase II trial. J Clin Oncol, 2006. 24(18): p. 2773- 8.

Kaufman, B., et al., Trastuzumab plus anastrozole versus anastrozole alone for the treatment of postmenopausal women with human epidermal growth factor receptor 2-positive, hormone receptor-positive metastatic breast cancer: results from the randomized phase III TAnDEM study. J Clin Oncol, 2009. 27(33): p. 5529-37.

Marcom, P.K., et al., The combination of letrozole and trastuzumab as first or second-line biological therapy produces durable responses in a subset of HER2 positive and ER positive advanced breast cancers. Breast Cancer Res Treat, 2007. 102(1): p. 43-9.

Burris, H., 3rd, et al., Phase II trial of trastuzumab followed by weekly paclitaxel/ carboplatin as first-line treatment for patients with metastatic breast cancer. J Clin Oncol, 2004. 22(9): p. 1621-9.

Sawaki, M., et al., Efficacy and safety of trastuzumab as a single agent in heavily pretreated patients with HER-2/neu-overexpressing metastatic breast cancer. Tumori, 2004. 90(1): p. 40-3.

Vogel, C.L., et al., Efficacy and safety of trastuzumab as a single agent in first-line treatment of HER2-overexpressing metastatic breast cancer. J Clin Oncol, 2002. 20(3): p. 719-26.

Nahta, R., et al., Mechanisms of disease: understanding resistance to HER2-targeted therapy in human breast cancer. Nat Clin Pract Oncol, 2006. 3(5): p. 269-80.

Atalay, G., et al., Clinical outcome of breast cancer patients with liver metastases alone in the anthracycline-taxane era: a retrospective analysis of two prospective, randomised metastatic breast cancer trials. Eur J Cancer, 2003. 39(17): p. 2439-49.

Bartsch, R., et al., Analysis of trastuzumab and chemotherapy in advanced breast cancer after the failure of at least one earlier combination: an observational study. BMC Cancer, 2006. 6: p. 63.

Gelmon, K.A., et al., Use of trastuzumab beyond disease progression: observations from a retrospective review of case histories. Clin Breast Cancer, 2004. 5(1): p. 52-8; discussion 59-62.

Bartsch, R., et al., Capecitabine and trastuzumab in heavily pretreated metastatic breast cancer. J Clin Oncol, 2007. 25(25): p. 3853-8.

von Minckwitz, G., et al., A multicentre phase II study on gefitinib in taxane- and anthracycline-pretreated metastatic breast cancer. Breast Cancer Res Treat, 2005. 89(2): p. 165-72.

Storniolo, A.M., et al., Phase I dose escalation and pharmacokinetic study of lapatinib in combination with trastuzumab in patients with advanced ErbB2-positive breast cancer. J Clin Oncol, 2008. 26(20): p. 3317-23.

Kallioniemi, O.P., et al., Association of c-erbB-2 protein over-expression with high rate of cell proliferation, increased risk of visceral metastasis and poor long-term survival in breast cancer. Int J Cancer, 1991. 49(5): p. 650-5.

Weil, R.J., et al., Breast cancer metastasis to the central nervous system. Am J Pathol, 2005. 167(4): p. 913-20.

Gori, S., et al., Central nervous system metastases in HER-2 positive metastatic breast cancer patients treated with trastuzumab: incidence, survival, and risk factors. Oncologist, 2007. 12(7): p. 766-73.

Ng, R., N. Better, and M.D. Green, Anticancer agents and cardiotoxicity. Semin Oncol, 2006. 33(1): p. 2-14.

Ewer, M.S., et al., Reversibility of trastuzumab-related cardiotoxicity: new insights based on clinical course and response to medical treatment. J Clin Oncol, 2005. 23(31): p. 7820-6.

Guarneri, V., et al., Long-term cardiac tolerability of trastuzumab in metastatic breast cancer: the M.D. Anderson Cancer Center experience. J Clin Oncol, 2006. 24(25): p. 4107-15.

Force, T., D.S. Krause, and R.A. Van Etten, Molecular mechanisms of cardiotoxicity of tyrosine kinase inhibition. Nat Rev Cancer, 2007. 7(5): p. 332-44.

Agus, D.B., et al., Targeting ligand-activated ErbB2 signaling inhibits breast and prostate tumor growth. Cancer Cell, 2002. 2(2): p. 127-37.

Franklin, M.C., et al., Insights into ErbB signaling from the structure of the ErbB2-pertuzumab complex. Cancer Cell, 2004. 5(4): p. 317-28.

Nemunaitis, J., et al., Phase 1 clinical and pharmacokinetics evaluation of oral CI-1033 in patients with refractory cancer. Clin Cancer Res, 2005. 11(10): p. 3846-53.

Geyer, C.E., et al., Lapatinib plus capecitabine for HER2-positive advanced breast cancer. N Engl J Med, 2006. 355(26): p. 2733-43.

Lin, N.U., et al., Multicenter phase II study of lapatinib in patients with brain metastases from HER2-positive breast cancer. Clin Cancer Res, 2009. 15(4): p. 1452-9.

Perez, E.A., et al., Cardiac safety of lapatinib: pooled analysis of 3689 patients enrolled in clinical trials. Mayo Clin Proc, 2008. 83(6): p. 679-86.

Arteaga, C.L., et al., A phase I-II study of combined blockade of the ErbB receptor network with trastuzumab and gefitinib in patients with HER2 (ErbB2)-overexpressing metastatic breast cancer. Clin Cancer Res, 2008. 14(19): p. 6277-83.

Britten, C.D., et al., A phase I/II trial of trastuzumab plus erlotinib in metastatic HER2-positive breast cancer: a dual ErbB targeted approach. Clin Breast Cancer, 2009. 9(1): p. 16-22.

Green, M.D., et al., Gefitinib treatment in hormone-resistant and hormone receptor-negative advanced breast cancer. Ann Oncol, 2009. 20(11): p. 1813-7.

Bose, P. and H. Ozer, Neratinib: an oral, irreversible dual EGFR/HER2 inhibitor for breast and non-small cell lung cancer. Expert Opin Investig Drugs, 2009. 18(11): p. 1735-51.

Chow, B.H., et al., Increased expression of annexin I is associated with drug-resistance in nasopharyngeal carcinoma and other solid tumors. Proteomics Clin Appl, 2009. 3(6): p. 654-62.

Huang, F., et al., Identification of candidate molecular markers predicting sensitivity in solid tumors to dasatinib: rationale for patient selection. Cancer Res, 2007. 67(5): p. 2226-38.

Hennequin, L.F., et al., N-(5-chloro-1,3-benzodioxol-4-yl)-7-[2-(4-methylpiperazin-1-yl)ethoxy]-5-(tetrahydro-2H-pyran-4-yloxy)quinazolin-4-amine, a novel, highly selective, orally available, dual-specific c-Src/Abl kinase inhibitor. J Med Chem, 2006. 49(22): p. 6465-88.

Kolch, W., Meaningful relationships: the regulation of the Ras/Raf/MEK/ERK pathway by protein interactions. Biochem J, 2000. 351 Pt 2: p. 289-305.

Johnston, S.R., et al., Phase II study of the efficacy and tolerability of two dosing regimens of the farnesyl transferase inhibitor, R115777, in advanced breast cancer. J Clin Oncol, 2003. 21(13): p. 2492-9.

Johnston, S.R., et al., A phase II, randomized, blinded study of the farnesyltransferase inhibitor tipifarnib combined with letrozole in the treatment of advanced breast cancer after antiestrogen therapy. Breast Cancer Res Treat, 2008. 110(2): p. 327-35.

Sparano, J.A., et al., Targeted inhibition of farnesyltransferase in locally advanced breast cancer: a phase I and II trial of tipifarnib plus dose-dense doxorubicin and cyclophosphamide. J Clin Oncol, 2006. 24(19): p. 3013-8.

McCubrey, J.A., et al., Roles of the Raf/MEK/ERK pathway in cell growth, malignant transformation and drug resistance. Biochim Biophys Acta, 2007. 1773(8): p. 1263-84.

Bachman, K.E., et al., The PIK3CA gene is mutated with high frequency in human breast cancers. Cancer Biol Ther, 2004. 3(8): p. 772-5.

Campbell, I.G., et al., Mutation of the PIK3CA gene in ovarian and breast cancer. Cancer Res, 2004. 64(21): p. 7678-81.

Lee, J.W., et al., PIK3CA gene is frequently mutated in breast carcinomas and hepatocellular carcinomas. Oncogene, 2005. 24(8): p. 1477-80.

Levine, D.A., et al., Frequent mutation of the PIK3CA gene in ovarian and breast cancers. Clin Cancer Res, 2005. 11(8): p. 2875-8.

Philp, A.J., et al., The phosphatidylinositol 3′-kinase p85alpha gene is an oncogene in human ovarian and colon tumors. Cancer Res, 2001. 61(20): p. 7426-9.

Samuels, Y., et al., High frequency of mutations of the PIK3CA gene in human cancers. Science, 2004. 304(5670): p. 554.

Cantley, L.C., The phosphoinositide 3-kinase pathway. Science, 2002. 296(5573): p. 1655-7. Sarbassov, D.D., et al., Phosphorylation and regulation of Akt/PKB by the rictor-mTOR *complex.* **Science, 2005. 307(5712): p. 1098-101.**

Inoki, K., et al., TSC2 is phosphorylated and inhibited by Akt and suppresses mTOR signalling. Nat Cell Biol, 2002. 4(9): p. 648-57.

Wullschleger, S., R. Loewith, and M.N. Hall, TOR signaling in growth and metabolism. Cell, 2006. 124(3): p. 471-84.

Hennessy, B.T., et al., Exploiting the PI3K/AKT pathway for cancer drug discovery. Nat Rev Drug Discov, 2005. 4(12): p. 988-1004.

Nagata, Y., et al., PTEN activation contributes to tumor inhibition by trastuzumab, and loss of PTEN predicts trastuzumab resistance in patients. Cancer Cell, 2004. 6(2): p. 117-27.

Kondapaka, S.B., et al., Perifosine, a novel alkylphospholipid, inhibits protein kinase B activation. Mol Cancer Ther, 2003. 2(11): p. 1093-103.

Baselga, J., et al., Phase II and tumor pharmacodynamic study of gefitinib in patients with advanced breast cancer. J Clin Oncol, 2005. 23(23): p. 5323-33.

Chan, S., et al., Phase II study of temsirolimus (CCI-779), a novel inhibitor of mTOR, in heavily pretreated patients with locally advanced or metastatic breast cancer. J Clin Oncol, 2005. 23(23): p. 5314-22.

Andre, F., et al., Phase I study of everolimus plus weekly paclitaxel and trastuzumab in patients with metastatic breast cancer pretreated with trastuzumab. J Clin Oncol, 2010. 28(34): p. 5110-5.

Mariani, G., et al., Trastuzumab as adjuvant systemic therapy for HER2-positive breast cancer. Nat Clin Pract Oncol, 2009. 6(2): p. 93-104.

Raymond, E., et al., Safety and pharmacokinetics of escalated doses of weekly intravenous infusion of CCI-779, a novel mTOR inhibitor, in patients with cancer. J Clin Oncol, 2004. 22(12): p. 2336-47.

Braunstein, S., et al., A hypoxia-controlled cap-dependent to cap-independent translation switch in breast cancer. Mol Cell, 2007. 28(3): p. 501-12.

O'Reilly, K.E., et al., mTOR inhibition induces upstream receptor tyrosine kinase signaling and activates Akt. Cancer Res, 2006. 66(3): p. 1500-8.

Yao, J.C., et al., Efficacy of RAD001 (everolimus) and octreotide LAR in advanced low- to intermediate-grade neuroendocrine tumors: results of a phase II study. J Clin Oncol, 2008. 26(26): p. 4311-8.

Neckers, L., A. Kern, and S. Tsutsumi, Hsp90 inhibitors disrupt mitochondrial homeostasis in cancer cells. Chem Biol, 2007. 14(11): p. 1204-6.

Neckers, L., Heat shock protein 90: the cancer chaperone. J Biosci, 2007. 32(3): p. 517-30. Maloney, A. and P. Workman, HSP90 as a new therapeutic target for cancer therapy: the *story unfolds*. Expert Opin Biol Ther, 2002. 2(1): p. 3-24.

Zhang, H. and F. Burrows, Targeting multiple signal transduction pathways through inhibition of Hsp90. J Mol Med, 2004. 82(8): p. 488-99.

Di Cosimo, S. and J. Baselga, Targeted therapies in breast cancer: where are we now? Eur J Cancer, 2008. 44(18): p. 2781-90.

Basso, A.D., et al., Ansamycin antibiotics inhibit Akt activation and cyclin D expression in breast cancer cells that overexpress HER2. Oncogene, 2002. 21(8): p. 1159-66.

Neckers, L., Effects of geldanamycin and other naturally occurring small molecule antagonists of heat shock protein 90 on HER2 protein expression. Breast Dis, 2000. 11: p. 49-59.

Powers, M.V. and P. Workman, Targeting of multiple signalling pathways by heat shock protein 90 molecular chaperone inhibitors. Endocr Relat Cancer, 2006. 13 Suppl 1: p. S125-35.

Ame, J.C., et al., PARP-2, A novel mammalian DNA damage-dependent poly(ADP-ribose) polymerase. J Biol Chem, 1999. 274(25): p. 17860-8.

Schreiber, V., et al., Poly(ADP-ribose) polymerase-2 (PARP-2) is required for efficient base excision DNA repair in association with PARP-1 and XRCC1. J Biol Chem, 2002. 277(25): p. 23028-36.

Yang, Y.G., et al., Ablation of PARP-1 does not interfere with the repair of DNA double-strand breaks, but compromises the reactivation of stalled replication forks. Oncogene, 2004. 23(21): p. 3872-82.

Schreiber, V., et al., Poly(ADP-ribose): novel functions for an old molecule. Nat Rev Mol Cell Biol, 2006. 7(7): p. 517-28.

Farmer, H., et al., Targeting the DNA repair defect in BRCA mutant cells as a therapeutic strategy. Nature, 2005. 434(7035): p. 917-21.

Ratnam, K. and J.A. Low, Current development of clinical inhibitors of poly(ADP-ribose) polymerase in oncology. Clin Cancer Res, 2007. 13(5): p. 1383-8.

Graziani, G. and C. Szabo, Clinical perspectives of PARP inhibitors. Pharmacol Res, 2005. 52(1): p. 109-18.

Lowe, S.W. and A.W. Lin, Apoptosis in cancer. Carcinogenesis, 2000. 21(3): p. 485-95. Reed, J.C., Dysregulation of apoptosis in cancer. J Clin Oncol, 1999. 17(9): p. 2941-53. Reed, J.C., Apoptosis-targeted therapies for cancer. Cancer Cell, 2003. 3(1): p. 17-22.

Nahta, R. and F.J. Esteva, Bcl-2 antisense oligonucleotides: a potential novel strategy for the *treatment of breast cancer*. Semin Oncol, 2003. 30(5 Suppl 16): p. 143-9.

Sjostrom, J., et al., The predictive value of bcl-2, bax, bcl-xL, bag-1, fas, and fasL for chemotherapy response in advanced breast cancer. Clin Cancer Res, 2002. 8(3): p. 811-6.

Krajewski, S., et al., Prognostic significance of apoptosis regulators in breast cancer. Endocr Relat Cancer, 1999. 6(1): p. 29-40.

McCarthy, M.M., et al., Evaluating the expression and prognostic value of TRAIL-R1 and TRAIL-R2 in breast cancer. Clin Cancer Res, 2005. 11(14): p. 5188-94.

Dalby, K.N., et al., Targeting the prodeath and prosurvival functions of autophagy as novel therapeutic strategies in cancer. Autophagy, 2010. 6(3): p. 322-9.

Abedin, M.J., et al., Autophagy delays apoptotic death in breast cancer cells following DNA damage. Cell Death Differ, 2007. 14(3): p. 500-10.

Boya, P., et al., Inhibition of macroautophagy triggers apoptosis. Mol Cell Biol, 2005. 25(3): p. 1025-40.

Qadir, M.A., et al., Macroautophagy inhibition sensitizes tamoxifen-resistant breast cancer cells and enhances mitochondrial depolarization. Breast Cancer Res Treat, 2008. 112(3): p. 389-403.

Folkman, J., Role of angiogenesis in tumor growth and metastasis. Semin Oncol, 2002. 29(6 Suppl 16): p. 15-8.

Folkman, J., Angiogenesis. Annu Rev Med, 2006. 57: p. 1-18.

Board, R. and G.C. Jayson, Platelet-derived growth factor receptor (PDGFR): a target for anticancer therapeutics. Drug Resist Updat, 2005. 8(1-2): p. 75-83.

Hicklin, D.J. and L.M. Ellis, Role of the vascular endothelial growth factor pathway in tumor growth and angiogenesis. J Clin Oncol, 2005. 23(5): p. 1011-27.

Relf, M., et al., Expression of the angiogenic factors vascular endothelial cell growth factor, acidic and basic fibroblast growth factor, tumor growth factor beta-1, platelet-derived endothelial cell growth factor, placenta growth factor, and pleiotrophin in human primary breast cancer and its relation to angiogenesis. Cancer Res, 1997. 57(5): p. 963-9.

Gasparini, G., et al., Prognostic significance of vascular endothelial growth factor protein in node-negative breast carcinoma. J Natl Cancer Inst, 1997. 89(2): p. 139-47.

Gasparini, G., et al., Clinical relevance of vascular endothelial growth factor and thymidine phosphorylase in patients with node-positive breast cancer treated with either adjuvant chemotherapy or hormone therapy. Cancer J Sci Am, 1999. 5(2): p. 101-11.

Foekens, J.A., et al., High tumor levels of vascular endothelial growth factor predict poor response to systemic therapy in advanced breast cancer. Cancer Res, 2001. 61(14): p. 5407-14.

Carvalho, I., et al., Overexpression of platelet-derived growth factor receptor alpha in breast cancer is associated with tumour progression. Breast Cancer Res, 2005. 7(5): p. R788-95.

Jain, R.K., Normalization of tumor vasculature: an emerging concept in antiangiogenic therapy. Science, 2005. 307(5706): p. 58-62.

Rosen, L.S., VEGF-targeted therapy: therapeutic potential and recent advances. Oncologist, 2005. 10(6): p. 382-91.

Presta, L.G., et al., Humanization of an anti-vascular endothelial growth factor monoclonal antibody for the therapy of solid tumors and other disorders. Cancer Res, 1997. 57(20): p. 4593-9.

Miller, K., et al., Paclitaxel plus bevacizumab versus paclitaxel alone for metastatic breast cancer. N Engl J Med, 2007. 357(26): p. 2666-76.

Miller, K.D., et al., Randomized phase III trial of capecitabine compared with bevacizumab plus capecitabine in patients with previously treated metastatic breast cancer. J Clin Oncol, 2005. 23(4): p. 792-9.

Carraway, H. and M. Hidalgo, New targets for therapy in breast cancer: mammalian target of rapamycin (mTOR) antagonists. Breast Cancer Res, 2004. 6(5): p. 219-24.

Chu, I., et al., The dual ErbB1/ErbB2 inhibitor, lapatinib (GW572016), cooperates with tamoxifen to inhibit both cell proliferation- and estrogen-dependent gene expression in antiestrogen-resistant breast cancer. Cancer Res, 2005. 65(1): p. 18-25.

Konecny, G.E., et al., Activity of the dual kinase inhibitor lapatinib (GW572016) against HER-2-overexpressing and trastuzumab-treated breast cancer cells. Cancer Res, 2006. 66(3): p. 1630-9.

Abrams, T.J., et al., SU11248 inhibits KIT and platelet-derived growth factor receptor beta in preclinical models of human small cell lung cancer. Mol Cancer Ther, 2003. 2(5): p. 471- 8.

Abrams, T.J., et al., Preclinical evaluation of the tyrosine kinase inhibitor SU11248 as a single agent and in combination with "standard of care" therapeutic agents for the treatment of breast cancer. Mol Cancer Ther, 2003. 2(10): p. 1011-21.

Mendel, D.B., et al., In vivo antitumor activity of SU11248, a novel tyrosine kinase inhibitor targeting vascular endothelial growth factor and platelet-derived growth factor receptors: determination of a pharmacokinetic/pharmacodynamic relationship. Clin Cancer Res, 2003. 9(1): p. 327-37.

Murray, L.J., et al., SU11248 inhibits tumor growth and CSF-1R-dependent osteolysis in an experimental breast cancer bone metastasis model. Clin Exp Metastasis, 2003. 20(8): p. 757-66.

Sapi, E., The role of CSF-1 in normal physiology of mammary gland and breast cancer: an update. Exp Biol Med (Maywood), 2004. 229(1): p. 1-11.

Burstein, H.J., et al., Phase II study of sunitinib malate, an oral multitargeted tyrosine kinase inhibitor, in patients with metastatic breast cancer previously treated with an anthracycline and a taxane. J Clin Oncol, 2008. 26(11): p. 1810-6.

Kozloff, M., et al., An exploratory study of sunitinib plus paclitaxel as first-line treatment for patients with advanced breast cancer. Ann Oncol, 2010. 21(7): p. 1436-41.

Liljegren, A., J. Bergh, and R. Castany, Early experience with sunitinib, combined with docetaxel, in patients with metastatic breast cancer. Breast, 2009. 18(4): p. 259-62.

Adnane, L., et al., Sorafenib (BAY 43-9006, Nexavar), a dual-action inhibitor that targets RAF/MEK/ERK pathway in tumor cells and tyrosine kinases VEGFR/PDGFR in tumor vasculature. Methods Enzymol, 2006. 407: p. 597-612.

Wilhelm, S.M., et al., BAY 43-9006 exhibits broad spectrum oral antitumor activity and targets the RAF/MEK/ERK pathway and receptor tyrosine kinases involved in tumor progression and angiogenesis. Cancer Res, 2004. 64(19): p. 7099-109.

Veronese, M.L., et al., Mechanisms of hypertension associated with BAY 43-9006. J Clin Oncol, 2006. 24(9): p. 1363-9.

Wilmes, L.J., et al., AG-013736, a novel inhibitor of VEGF receptor tyrosine kinases, inhibits breast cancer growth and decreases vascular permeability as detected by dynamic contrast- enhanced magnetic resonance imaging. Magn Reson Imaging, 2007. 25(3): p. 319-27.

Sotiriou, C., et al., Breast cancer classification and prognosis based on gene expression profiles from a population-based study. Proc Natl Acad Sci U S A, 2003. 100(18): p. 10393-8.

Sevelda, P., [Tamoxifen in the treatment of patients with breast cancer: results of the latest meta-analysis of prospective randomized clinical trials]. Gynakol Geburtshilfliche Rundsch, 1998. 38(2): p. 81-4.

Ali, S. and R.C. Coombes, Endocrine-responsive breast cancer and strategies for combating resistance. Nat Rev Cancer, 2002. 2(2): p. 101-12.

Osborne, C.K. and R. Schiff, Estrogen-receptor biology: continuing progress and therapeutic implications. J Clin Oncol, 2005. 23(8): p. 1616-22.

Shou, J., et al., Mechanisms of tamoxifen resistance: increased estrogen receptor-HER2/ neu cross-talk in ER/HER2-positive breast cancer. J Natl Cancer Inst, 2004. 96(12): p. 926-35.

Larsen, M., et al., The matrix reorganized: extracellular matrix remodeling and integrin signaling. Curr Opin Cell Biol, 2006. 18(5): p. 463-71.

Karin, M., et al., NF-kappaB in cancer: from innocent bystander to major culprit. Nat Rev Cancer, 2002. 2(4): p. 301-10.

Greten, F.R., et al., IKKbeta links inflammation and tumorigenesis in a mouse model of colitis-associated cancer. Cell, 2004. 118(3): p. 285-96.

Wiener, Z., et al., Synergistic induction of the Fas (CD95) ligand promoter by Max and NFkappaB in human non-small lung cancer cells. Exp Cell Res, 2004. 299(1): p. 227-35.

Robbins, J., et al., Mouse mammary tumor gene int-3: a member of the notch gene family transforms mammary epithelial cells. J Virol, 1992. 66(4): p. 2594-9.

Zheng, L., et al., Lessons learned from BRCA1 and BRCA2. Oncogene, 2000. 19(53): p. 6159-75.

Turner, N.C., et al., BRCA1 dysfunction in sporadic basal-like breast cancer. Oncogene, 2007. 26(14): p. 2126-32.

Richardson, P.G., et al., A phase 2 study of bortezomib in relapsed, refractory myeloma. N Engl J Med, 2003. 348(26): p. 2609-17.

Sato, K., E. Rajendra, and T. Ohta, The UPS: a promising target for breast cancer treatment. BMC Biochem, 2008. 9 Suppl 1: p. S2.

Kuwano, M., et al., Multidrug resistance-associated protein subfamily transporters and drug resistance. Anticancer Drug Des, 1999. 14(2): p. 123-31.

Dantzig, A.H., D.P. de Alwis, and M. Burgess, Considerations in the design and development of transport inhibitors as adjuncts to drug therapy. Adv Drug Deliv Rev, 2003. 55(1): p. 133-50.

Nielsen, D., C. Maare, and T. Skovsgaard, Cellular resistance to anthracyclines. Gen Pharmacol, 1996. 27(2): p. 251-5.

Stavrovskaya, A.A., Cellular mechanisms of multidrug resistance of tumor cells. Biochemistry (Mosc), 2000. 65(1): p. 95-106.

Azab, S.S.E.-D., E. and Al-Hendy, A., Multi-drug resistance as a problem challenging breast cancer chemotherapy in Aggressive Breast Cancer, R.H.D. ed., Editor. 2010. p. pp. 53-100.

Kerb, R., S. Hoffmeyer, and U. Brinkmann, ABC drug transporters: hereditary polymorphisms and pharmacological impact in MDR1, MRP1 and MRP2. Pharmacogenomics, 2001. 2(1): p. 51-64.

Ling, V., Multidrug resistance: molecular mechanisms and clinical relevance. Cancer Chemother Pharmacol, 1997. 40 Suppl: p. S3-8.

Mimeault, M. and S.K. Batra, Recent advances on multiple tumorigenic cascades involved in prostatic cancer progression and targeting therapies. Carcinogenesis, 2006. 27(1): p. 1-22.

Rubin, L.L. and F.J. de Sauvage, Targeting the Hedgehog pathway in cancer. Nat Rev Drug Discov, 2006. 5(12): p. 1026-33.

Mimeault, M., et al., Recent advances in cancer stem/progenitor cell research: therapeutic implications for overcoming resistance to the most aggressive cancers. J Cell Mol Med, 2007. 11(5): p. 981-1011.

Nicolis, S.K., Cancer stem cells and "stemness" genes in neuro-oncology. Neurobiol Dis, 2007. 25(2): p. 217-29.

Chuthapisith, S., et al., Breast cancer chemoresistance: emerging importance of cancer stem cells. Surg Oncol, 2010. 19(1): p. 27-32.

Hirschmann-Jax, C., et al., A distinct "side population" of cells with high drug efflux capacity in human tumor cells. Proc Natl Acad Sci U S A, 2004. 101(39): p. 14228-33.

Dean, M., T. Fojo, and S. Bates, Tumour stem cells and drug resistance. Nat Rev Cancer, 2005. 5(4): p. 275-84.

Gupta, P.B., et al., Identification of selective inhibitors of cancer stem cells by high-throughput screening. Cell, 2009. 138(4): p. 645-59.

Mimeault, M., R. Hauke, and S.K. Batra, Recent advances on the molecular mechanisms involved in the drug resistance of cancer cells and novel targeting therapies. Clin Pharmacol Ther, 2008. 83(5): p. 673-91.

Al-Hajj, M., et al., *Prospective identification of tumorigenic breast cancer cells*. Proc Natl Acad Sci U S A, 2003. 100(7): p. 3983-8.

Harari, P.M., *Epidermal growth factor receptor inhibition strategies in oncology*. Endocr Relat Cancer, 2004. 11(4): p. 689-708.

Duffy, M.J., N. O'Donovan, and J. Crown, Use *of molecular markers for predicting therapy response in cancer patients*. Cancer Treat Rev, 2011. 37(2): p. 151-9.

Paik, S., *Molecular profiling of breast cancer*. Curr Opin Obstet Gynecol, 2006. 18(1): p. 59-63.

10

ErbB2/HER2: Its Contribution to Basic Cancer Biology and the Development of Molecular Targeted Therapy

Tadashi Yamamoto et al.*
The Institute of Medical Science, The University of Tokyo, Japan

1. Introduction

ErbB2, one of the receptor tyrosine kinase superfamily has attracted the attention of cancer researchers since its discovery. Thirty years ago, *ErbB2* was discovered as an oncogene that transforms NIH3T3 cells. The first decade of ErbB2 research revealed that it is a member of the ErbB receptor family and is deregulated in various types of human cancer. In the second decade, one significant discovery came from the crystallography with the rational theory that explains why no ligands specific for ErbB2 have been identified so far, and the other breakthrough came from the clinical field with the appearance of ErbB-targeted therapeutics. Today, cancer researchers strive to describe the elaborate signaling network of ErbB receptors by proteomic analysis, and our knowledge of their function, which is far from complete, is being applied to develop more efficient ErbB-targeted therapeutics for cancer patients.

We will begin the story of *ErbB2* with its discovery as an oncogene called *neu*. In the dawn of oncogene research, this gene, derived from a rat tumor, was classified as one of the most pivotal genes in human cancer, along with the oncogenes Ras and Myc and the tumor suppressor gene p53. This is because *ErbB2* is frequently amplified and overexpressed in certain human cancers, such as breast carcinoma. Similar to other oncogenes, subsequent research demonstrated its indispensable role in development. Now, our interest is whether ErbB2 acts on the same target proteins in cancer and in normal development.

The signaling networks downstream of ErbB receptors are complex because there are various ligands for each receptor, except ErbB2, and the composition of the ErbB dimer seems to define downstream signaling targets. For example, EGFR (epidermal growth factor receptor)-containing heterodimers prefer to stimulate the mitogen-activated protein kinase (MAPK) cascade, while ErbB3-containing dimers preferably activate phosphatidylinositol 3-kinase (PI3K). This characteristic is reflected in the difficulty in choosing the best therapeutics corresponding to each case in the clinic.

---

* Makoto Saito[1], Kentaro Kumazawa[1], Ayano Doi[1], Atsuka Matsui[1], Shiori Takebe[1], Takuya Amari[1], Masaaki Oyama[2] and Kentaro Semba[1]
[1]*Department of Life Science and Medical Bioscience, Waseda University, Japan*
[2]*The Institute of Medical Science, The University of Tokyo, Japan*

Our passion for determining the function of ErbB2 in cancer has inspired us to develop experimental methods to reveal mechanisms of tumorigenesis in humans. One such method is the MCF10A morphogenesis assay, which will be useful for identifying new oncogenes.

2. Discovery of *ErbB2*

This section describes the history of the discovery of *ErbB2/HER2/neu*. The *ErbB2* gene was initially identified as an oncogene named *neu* in NIH3T3 cells. Soon after, several groups, including our laboratory revealed that this gene was the second member of the EGFR family. Initial studies showed that this gene was amplified in human cancer cell lines and tissues, indicating its importance in human cancer. This finding prompted the extensive studies of ErbB2 in human cancer. By the way, official NCBI gene symbol is ERBB2 (human), however, for simplicity, we will use one term "ErbB2" in this article.

2.1 *Neu*, an oncogene cloned from murine brain tumors

The origin of *ErbB2/HER2/neu* research can be traced back to the 1980s, when virtually all cancer researchers were hunting for novel oncogenes. Cancer researchers, using the tools for introducing foreign DNA into mammalian cells, were seeking genes that render normal cells cancerous, what we call "oncogenes." Scientists introduced genomic DNA that was isolated from mouse or human tumor cells into NIH3T3 mouse fibroblast cells (Shih et al., 1979) using the calcium-phosphate DNA precipitation technique (Graham & van der Eb, 1973) and examined their morphological changes, or their "transformation". This transformation assay described in detail in section 6 produced several fruitful discoveries. For us, the most significant was the discovery of *neu*.

The first report about *neu* came in 1981 when Shih et al. indicated that DNA prepared from rat neuro-/glioblastoma cell lines transformed NIH3T3 cells (Shih et al., 1981). In 1984, Schechter et al. demonstrated that several independently isolated transformed cells contained the same oncogene, based on resistance to inactivation by restriction enzyme cleavage, and thus named the oncogene "*neu*" (Schechter et al., 1984). They also showed that the *neu* gene encoded a protein of relative molecular mass 185,000 (p185), and it was related to EGFR serologically. This finding was consistent with the fact that *neu* showed significant similarity to v-*erbB*, a retroviral oncogene of avian erythroblastosis virus (Vennstrom & Bishop, 1982; Yamamoto et al., 1983), and was homologous with the cellular gene (c-*erbB*) encoding EGFR (Downward et al., 1984).

2.2 A second member of the ErbB family, *c-erbB2/HER2*

After the initial discoveries regarding *neu*, *neu* blossomed out into one of the most famous oncogenes. In 1985, Schechter et al. demonstrated that the homology between *neu* and *erbB* was limited to the region of the kinase domain of EGFR and that *neu* mapped to human chromosome 17, distinct from c-*erbB* on chromosome 7 (Schechter et al., 1985). Semba et al. identified the human v-*erbB*-related sequence as distinct from the EGFR gene and its amplification in the human adenocarcinoma of the salivary gland (Semba et al., 1985), and they named the gene c-*erbB2*, as a separate gene from c-*erbB1*, encoding EGFR. Soon after, several groups cloned this human version of the *neu* oncogene and designated it c-*erbB2* or *HER2* (Bargmann et al., 1986b; Coussens et al., 1985; Yamamoto et al., 1986), and cDNA clones of the *neu* oncogene itself were also isolated (Hung et al., 1986). Subsequent studies revealed that *ErbB2* encodes a 185-kDa transmembrane glycoprotein that is highly similar to

EGFR (Akiyama et al., 1986; Bargmann et al., 1986b). To date, there are four ErbB family receptors: EGFR (also ErbB1, HER1), ErbB2(HER2, Neu), ErbB3(HER3) (Kraus et al., 1989), and ErbB4(HER4) (Plowman et al., 1993). We will describe their structural similarities and differences in section 3.

In what ways does the *neu* oncogene cause murine neuro-/glioblastoma? In the case of the v-*erbB* oncogene, encoding the truncated form of EGFR, we could assume that its aberrant protein, which has no ligand binding domain, phosphorylates its substrates independently of ligand binding, resulting in hyperproliferation (Khazaie et al., 1988). The *neu* proto-oncogene, however, is activated by a single point mutation, V664E, in the transmembrane domain (Bargmann et al., 1986a), and not by gross rearrangements as seen in v-*erbB*. Does this single point mutation, which causes neuro-/glioblastoma in rats, also occur in humans? Interestingly, such a single point mutation of c-*erbB2* has never been observed in cancer patients. Instead, gene amplification and overexpression of its protein product are frequently observed in various types of human cancer, especially breast cancer (Slamon et al., 1989), as described in section 4.

3. Regulation of ErbB receptors and downstream signaling pathways

The ErbB receptors are closely related, single-chain glycoproteins. ErbB receptors are activated by binding to their specific ligands. Activated ErbB receptors then transmit signals to downstream signal transducers. In this section, we describe structural features of ErbB receptors and focus on recent observations of ErbB2 signal transduction pathways.

3.1 ErbB ligands

ErbB ligands act in a paracrine or autocrine fashion. Whereas paracrine ErbB ligands are derived from stromal cells, autocrine ErbB ligands are produced as transmembrane precursors that are subsequently cleaved by proteases to be released as soluble ligands when cells are stimulated (Hynes & Lane, 2005).

At least ten ErbB ligands are known (Figure 1) and are divided into three groups with respect to binding specificity. The first group includes EGF, amphiregulin (AR) and transforming growth factor-α (TGF-α), which bind specifically to ErbB1. The second group includes betacellulin (BTC), heparin-binding EGF (HB-EGF) and epiregulin (EPR), which show dual specificity, binding to both ErbB1 and ErbB4. The third group includes neuregulins (NRGs). They are composed of two subgroups. NRG1 and NRG2 bind specifically to both ErbB3 and ErbB4, whereas NRG3 and NRG4 bind specifically to only ErbB4 (Hynes & Lane, 2005).

None of these ErbB ligands bind and activate ErbB2. However, the mucin MUC4, a transmembrane glycoprotein, modulates the ErbB2 signaling pathway. MUC4 is composed of two subunits, ASGP-1, an O-glycosylated mucin subunit, and ASGP-2, an N-glycosylated transmembrane subunit. ASGP-2 possesses two EGF-like domains, EGF-1 and EGF-2, and interacts specifically with ErbB2, inducing its phosphorylation. MUC4 retains ErbB2 and ErbB3 on the cell membrane by suppressing their ligand-induced internalization. However, the mechanisms of ErbB2 signaling activation by MUC4 are largely unknown (Singh et al., 2007).

3.2 ErbB receptors

3.2.1 Structures of ErbB receptors and their conformational changes on ligand binding

Each ErbB receptor comprises five functional domains, the extracellular domain for ligand binding (~620 residues), the α-helical transmembrane segment (~23 residues), and

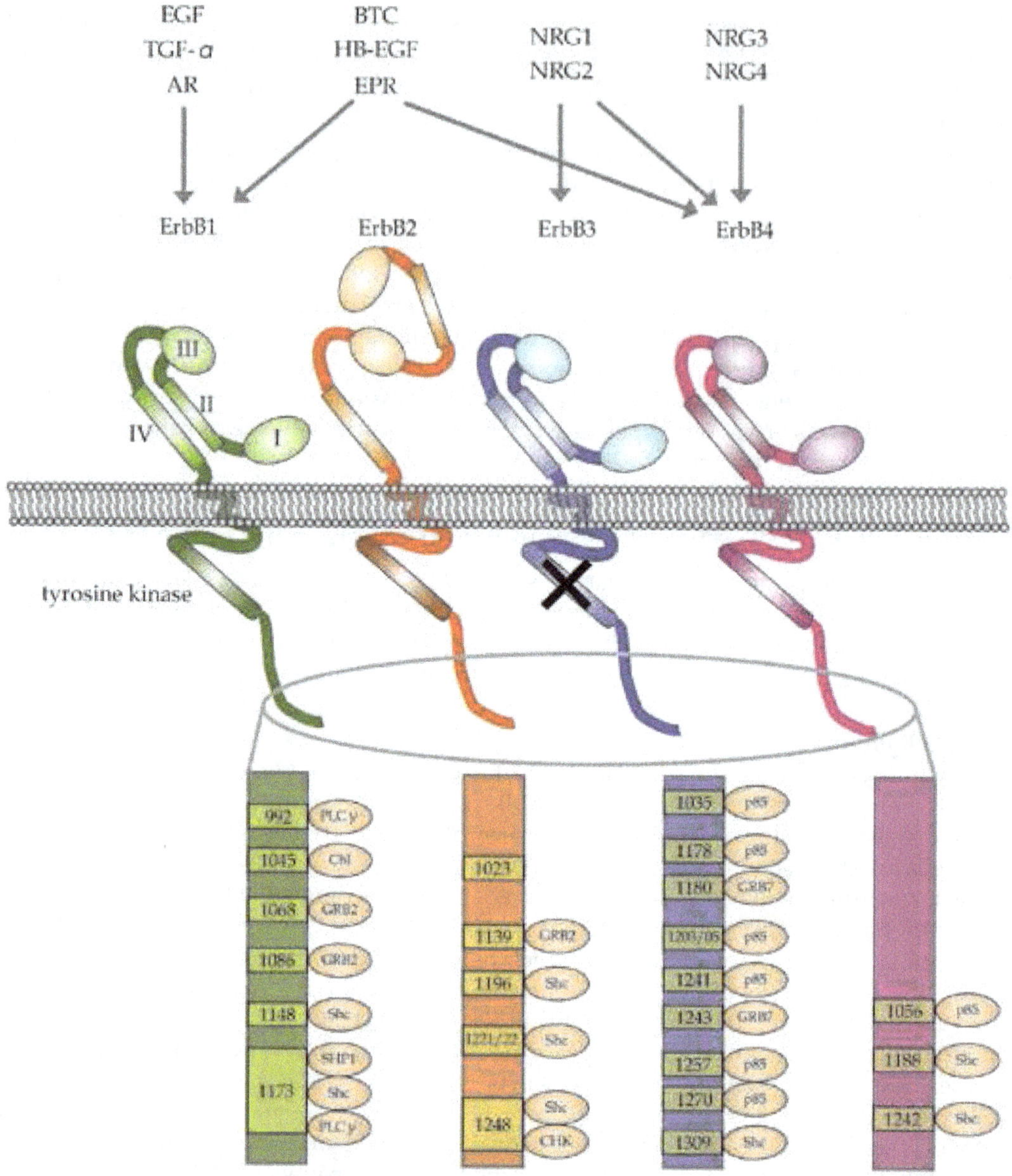

Fig. 1. ErbB ligands and receptors.
ErbB ligands, which act in an autocrine or paracrine fashion, are divided into three groups based on binding specificity. None of the ErbB ligands binds to ErbB2. However, MUC4 modulates ErbB2 signaling activity. Ligand binding to the extracellular domain of ErbB receptors changes the receptor's conformation and promotes homo- and heterodimerization. Its dimerization induces the tyrosine kinase activity of the intracellular domain, resulting in the cross-phosphorylation of specific tyrosine residues, which recruits and activates specific downstream signaling proteins. The intracellular domain of each ErbB receptor possesses unique docking sites for downstream signaling proteins, which consist of tyrosine residues and the surrounding amino acids (Baselga & Swain, 2009; Hynes & Lane, 2005; Olayioye et

al., 2000). ErbB1 has docking sites for growth factor receptor-bound 2 (GRB2) and Src homology 2-containing (Shc), which activate the MAPK and PI3K–Akt pathways though Ras activation, although it has no direct docking site for PI3K (Hynes & Lane, 2005). ErbB1 has a docking site for Cbl, an E3 ubiquitin ligase. ErbB1 dimerization induced by ligand binding induces receptor internalization into endosomes, which is followed by recycling. In the endosome, Cbl directly binds to tyrosine residues of ErbB1 and undergoes ubiquitylation, resulting in its degradation in lysosomes (Citri & Yarden, 2006). ErbB2 functions as the preferred partner of other ErbB receptors and possesses the strongest kinase activity. ErbB3 possesses six p85 docking sites, which effectively activate the PI3K–Akt pathway, although it lacks tyrosine kinase activity (Moasser, 2007). ErbB1, ErbB2 and ErbB3 are implicated in the progression of cancer. However, ErbB4 is associated with the inhibition of cell proliferation, although it has docking sites for p85 and Shc (Baselga & Swain, 2009).

a juxtamembranedomain (~40 residues), an intracellular tyrosine kinase domain (~260 residues), and a C-terminal regulatory region (~232residues) (Burgess et al., 2003). Intriguingly, the structures of ErbB2 and ErbB3 are unique among the ErbB family. ErbB2 is an orphan receptor, but it always has a ligand-activated conformation (Garrett et al., 2003), while ErbB3 has impaired intrinsic tyrosine kinase activity (P.M. Guy et al., 1994).

The ErbB family is conserved during evolution. Although we will not discuss the issue in detail, the biological significance of EGFR in the physiological state lies in its involvement in epithelial development in mammals (Miettinen et al., 1995; Sibilia & Wagner, 1995; Threadgill et al., 1995). EGFR has similar functions in invertebrates. For instance, both *Caenorhabditis elegans* and *Drosophila melanogaster* have a single EGFR homolog (Aroian et al., 1990; Livneh et al., 1985). EGFR regulates vulva development in *Caenorhabditis elegans* (Moghal & Sternberg, 2003) and the development of various organs in *Drosophila* (Shilo, 2003). In *Caenorhabditis elegans*, in parallel with the simplicity of the ErbB family of receptors, there are only one ligand for the receptors (Yarden & Sliwkowski, 2001), while humans have ten. The versatility of ErbB receptors and their ligands in mammals, which evolved from a simple cascade important for development in invertebrates, can endow signaling networks with not only robustness but also vulnerability, represented by tumorigenesis, a collapse of the regulatory circuit. The evolutional conservation of tumor-promoting ability of EGFR is well known, for instance, from the melanoma model of *Xiphophorus* (Gomez et al., 2004).

The extracellular domain consists of domains I–IV. Domain II promotes receptor dimerization. In the absence of ligand binding, ErbB exists in a tethered conformation in which intramolecular interaction between domains II and IV blocks the function of dimerization domain II. Ligand binding to ErbB receptors changes the tethered conformation into the extended conformation, which exposes domain II, allowing them to undergo homo- and heterodimerization (Hynes & Lane, 2005). However, ErbB3 lacks the ability to homodimerize (Baselga & Swain, 2009). ErbB2 has a unique structure of the ligand-activated conformation and is the most preferred partner for other ligand-bound ErbB receptors. This is because the structure of the ErbB2 extracellular domain originally resembles the extended conformation that exhibits no interaction between domain II and domain IV and exposes the dimerization domain II (Hynes & Lane, 2005). The intracellular domain possesses the protein tyrosine kinase activity and unique docking sites for specific downstream signaling proteins, which consist of tyrosine residues and surrounding amino acid side chains (Hynes & Lane, 2005). ErbB2 possesses the strongest tyrosine kinase activity among the ErbB receptors (Moasser, 2007). However, ErbB3 lacks the tyrosine kinase activity because it is unable to bind to ATP (Baselga & Swain, 2009).

3.2.2 HSP90–ErbB2 complex

Heat shock proteins (HSPs), a large family of highly conserved molecular chaperone proteins, mediate the conformational maturation and folding of target proteins. HSP90 protects the ErbB system from damage. Whereas other ErbB receptors are HSP90-independent, ErbB2 and several downstream signaling proteins are stabilized by HSP90. A ternary complex of HSP90, ErbB2 and a co-chaperone, CDC37, stabilizes ErbB2 at the cell membrane (Baselga & Swain, 2009; Citri & Yarden, 2006) . Inhibition of HSP90 function by specific drugs results in ubiquitylation and proteasomal degradation of ErbB2 and its downstream signaling proteins (Baselga & Swain, 2009). HSP90 also controls ErbB2 signaling activity. Binding of the complex of HSP90 and CDC37 to the tyrosine kinase domain of ErbB2 suppresses its tyrosine kinase activity and heterodimerization with other ligand-bound ErbB receptors.

3.3 Signaling pathways activated by ErbB receptors

Ligand-binding to the extracellular domain of ErbB receptors changes the tethered conformation into the extended conformation, inducing homo- and heterodimerization. Only ErbB2 is able to dimerize without ligand-binding. ErbB receptor dimerization results in phosphorylation on specific tyrosine residues of the intracellular domain. These phosphorylated tyrosine residues and surrounding amino acid side chains allow the recruitment and activation of downstream signaling proteins, which initiate multiple signaling pathways (Baselga & Swain, 2009).

The combination of ligands and heterodimer partners determines which downstream signaling proteins are recruited and which signaling pathways are activated. The heterodimer of ErbB2–ErbB3 is the most active in ErbB downstream signaling (Baselga & Swain, 2009).

Two main signaling pathways activated by ErbB receptors are the MAPK and the PI3K-Akt pathways. Other important ErbB signaling proteins are the signal transducers and activators of transcription (STATs) and the Src tyrosine kinase (Hynes & Lane, 2005). Although ErbB receptors are largely known as receptor tyrosine kinases (RTKs), recent studies indicate they can localize to the nucleus and act as transcription factors (S.-C. Wang et al., 2004).

3.3.1 MAPK pathway

GRB2, an adaptor protein, binds to ErbB receptors either indirectly through Shc or directly to the phosphorylated tyrosine residues. The GRB2–son of sevenless (Sos) complex, with or without Shc, recruits Ras and activates the MAPK pathway, inducing cell proliferation, migration, differentiation and angiogenesis (Baselga & Swain, 2009). Recent analysis using MCF10A cells showed that Shc is required for the inhibition of apoptosis and for paclitaxel resistance (see also section 6 for MCF10A system).

3.3.2 PI3K–Akt pathway

PI3K, a heterodimer composed of a p85 regulatory subunit and p110 catalytic subunit, is activated by at least two ErbB-related pathways. In the first pathway, p85 directly binds to phosphorylated tyrosine residues, triggering the activation of the p110 catalytic subunit. In the second pathway, GRB2 binds to ErbB either indirectly though Shc or directly to phosphorylated tyrosine residues and activates Ras, which also triggers the activation of p110 (Baselga & Swain, 2009; Cully et al., 2006). Activated PI3K phosphorylates phosphatidylinositol 4,5-bisphosphate (PIP2) into phosphatidylinositol 3,4,5-triphosphate (PIP3), which recruits Akt and phosphatidylinositol-dependent kinase 1 (PDK1) and activates PDK1. PDK1 phosphorylates and activates Akt. The tumor-suppressor phosphatase with tensin homology (PTEN) dephosphorylates PIP3 into PIP2 and inhibits PI3K–Akt pathway activation (Cully et al., 2006).

Activated Akt phosphorylates many target proteins associated with cell survival, proliferation (increased cell number), and growth (increased cell size). In addition, Akt promotes angiogenesis through vascular endothelial growth factor (VEGF) and hypoxia-inducible factor-1α (HIF-1α) (Vivanco & Sawyers, 2002).

3.3.2.1 Survival

Activated Akt directly phosphorylates several target proteins to suppress apoptosis. BAD, a pro-apoptotic member of the BCL2 family, antagonizes the survival protein BCL-X_L to promote cell death. Activated Akt phosphorylates BAD, which prevents it from interacting with BCL-X_L, allowing BCL-X_L to function as an anti-apoptotic protein. Caspase-9, a member of the cysteine-dependent aspartyl-specific protease family, cleaves and activates pro-caspase-3, resulting in apoptosis. Activated Akt phosphorylates caspase-9 and inhibits its catalytic activity. Forkhead box 1 (FOXO1), a member of the forkhead family of transcription factors, activates several pro-apoptotic proteins, including BIM and FAS ligand. Activated Akt phosphorylates FOXO1 and prevents its nuclear translocation. Nuclear factor κB (NF-κB), a transcription factor, is constantly inhibited by IκB. Activated Akt phosphorylates IκB kinase (IKK), which degrades IκB, allowing NF-κB to translocate to the nucleus and activate its target genes. Murine double minute (MDM2), a p53-binding protein, mediates proteasomal degradation of p53. Activated Akt phosphorylates and activates MDM2 (Vivanco & Sawyers, 2002).

3.3.2.2 Proliferation

Activated Akt directly phosphorylates several target proteins to regulate cell cycle control. Glycogen synthase kinase-3β (GSK-3β) phosphorylates cyclin D1 which mediates G1/S phase transition to induce its proteasomal degradation. Activated Akt directly phosphorylates and inhibits GSK-3β, which allows cyclin D1 to accumulate (Vivanco & Sawyers, 2002). Activated Akt phosphorylates and inhibits p27, a CDK inhibitor (CKI), promoting cell cycle entry. In addition, p27 expression is regulated by the transcription factor FOXO3A. FOXO3A activates p27 and BIM expression, and inhibit cyclin D1 expression. Activated Akt phosphorylates FOXO3A, which promotes its translocation from the nucleus. Activated Akt also modulates p21 activity by affecting its phosphorylation, presumably through other kinases (Cully et al., 2006).

3.3.2.3 Growth

Activated Akt directly phosphorylates tuberous sclerosis 2 (TSC2) to affect cell growth. TSC2 heterodimerizes with TSC1 to promote the GTPase activity of the Ras homolog enriched in brain (RHEB). Activated Akt phosphorylates TSC2 and inhibits the ability of the TSC1–TSC2 complex to act as RHEB-GTPase activating protein (RHEB-GAP), which allows GTP-bound RHEB to accumulate. Active GTP-bound RHEB promotes the kinase activity of the mammalian target of rapamycin (mTOR), a key regulator of cell growth. Activated mTOR, regulatory associated protein of TOR (raptor) and G-protein β-subunit-like (GβL) complex phosphorylates S6 kinase (S6K) and the eukaryotic translation-initiatin factor 4E (EIF4E)-inhibitory binding protein (4E-BP) to modulate the mRNA translation and protein synthesis (Cully et al., 2006).

3.3.3 ErB2–ErbB3 heterodimer and PI3K–Akt pathway

Several lines of evidence indicate that the heterodimer ErbB2–ErbB3 is the most important oncogenic signaling associated with the activation of the PI3K–Akt pathway. ErbB2, which lacks p85-binding sites, possesses strong kinase activity, and ErbB3, which lacks tyrosine kinase activity, possesses six p85-binding sites. Akt is frequently activated in ErbB2-overexpressing tumors, as well as in tumors generated in mouse mammary tumor virus (MMTV)-*neu* transgenic mice. Cell transformation by overexpressed ErbB2 *in vitro* is associated with increased ErbB3 phosphorylation and activation of the PI3K–Akt pathway. These results suggest the transactivation of ErbB3, and the PI3K–Akt pathway is strongly associated with the tumorigenic function of overexpressed ErbB2 (Moasser, 2007).

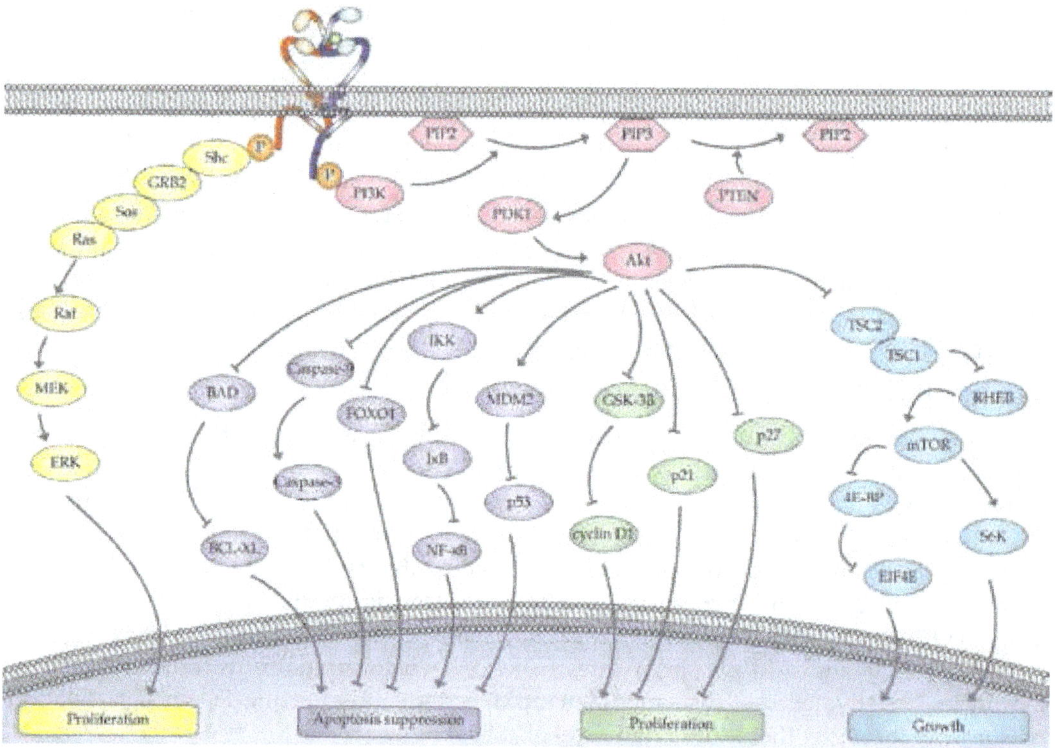

Fig. 2. Downstream signaling pathways of ErbB2–ErbB3 heterodimer.

The MAPK pathway and PI3K–Akt pathway are the two main pathways activated by ErbB receptors. GRB2–Sos complex, with or without Shc, recruits Ras and activates MAPK signaling, inducing cell proliferation, migration, differentiation and angiogenesis. PI3K is a heterodimer composed of a p85 regulatory subunit and a p110 catalytic subunit. p110 is activated by p85 directly binding to phosphorylated tyrosine residues or indirectly binding though the GRB2–Sos–Ras complex, with or without Shc, to phosphorylated tyrosine residues within RTKs. Activated PI3K phosphorylates PIP2 into PIP3, which recruits and activates PDK1. PDK1 phosphorylates and activates PI3K. PTEN dephosphorylates PIP3 into PIP2. Activated Akt phosphorylates many downstream proteins, inducing cell survival, proliferation, growth, and angiogenesis (Baselga & Swain, 2009; Cully et al., 2006; Vivanco & Sawyers, 2002). The heterodimer ErbB2–ErbB3 is the most oncogenic signaling activator of the PI3K–Akt pathway because ErbB2 possesses strong kinase activity, and ErbB3 possesses six p85-binding sites (Moasser, 2007).

3.3.4 Inhibition of PI3K–Akt signaling though PTEN by trastuzumab

Nagata et al. suggested the potency of trastuzumab (a humanized anti-ErbB2 monoclonal antibody, Herceptin®) is dependent on the ability to inhibit PI3K–Akt signaling pathway though activation of PTEN. PTEN dephosphorylates PIP3 into PIP2 and inhibits PI3K–Akt pathway activation. Overexpression of ErbB2 induces dimerization, resulting in phosphorylation on specific tyrosine residues of the intracellular domain. These phosphorylated tyrosine residues and surrounding amino acid side chains allow the recruitment and activation of downstream signaling proteins, including PI3K and Src. Activated PI3K activates PI3K–Akt pathway associated with cell survival, proliferation, growth and angiogenesis. Phosphorylated Src becomes activated and phosphorylates PTEN on tyrosine residues within the PTEN C2 domain, preventing PTEN from localizing to the cell membrane and dephosphorylating PI3K, and this also activates PI3K–Akt signaling. Treatment with trastuzumab keeps Src from binding ErbB2, leading to the dephosphorylation and inactivation of Src. PTEN is released from phosphorylation of Src and is localized to the cell membrane, which allows PTEN to antagonize PI3K function and negatively regulate the PI3K–Akt signaling pathway. However, Nagata et al. did not explore the mechanism that trastuzumab treatment rapidly keeps Src from ErbB2 (Crowder et al., 2004; Nagata et al., 2004).

3.3.5 The role of Src in the signaling pathway activated by ErbB2

Src, a non-receptor tyrosine kinase, is a critical component of multiple signaling pathways, leading to proliferation, survival, metastasis and angiogenesis. Several results indicate a functional and physical interaction between ErbB2 and Src. Src and ErbB receptors are overexpressed in ~70% of breast tumors (Ishizawar & Parsons, 2004). Src and Yes are activated in mammary tumors of MMTV-*neu* transgenic mice. Activation of Src is also observed in mammary epithelial cells transformed by ErbB2, but not by H-Ras, indicating that Src is a downstream signaling protein of ErbB2. Src directly interacts with the kinase domain of ErbB2. ErbB2 activates Src function by stabilizing Src and promoting increased Src expression or by directly phosphorylating Src in its SH2 domain. Src promotes ErbB2–ErbB3 dimerization, resulting in activation of their signaling activity. Src also phosphorylates the activation loop of the tyrosine kinase domain of ErbB2, which increases its kinase activity (Moasser, 2007).

3.3.6 The role of Cyclin D1 in ErbB2–induced tumorigenesis

Cyclin D1 is the key protein in ErbB2-induced tumorigenesis. ErbB2 overexpression in breast epithelial cells shows a short G1 phase and early S phase entry, mediated by the up-regulation of cyclin D1, cyclin E, and Cdk6 expression and enhanced degradation and relocalization of p21, leading to hyperproliferation (Timms et al., 2002). Cyclin D1-deficient mice show resistance to breast cancers induced by the *neu* oncogene, whereas they remain fully sensitive to other oncogenic pathways, such as c-myc or Wnt1 (Yu et al., 2001). Ectopic expression of *neu* or Wnt oncogene in the mammary glands of mice deficient in Cdk4, the partner of cyclin D1, shows Cdk4 expression is required for efficient *neu*-induced tumorigenesis, whereas it is not required for Wnt-induced tumorigenesis (Reddy, 2005). p16, a CKI, blocks Cdk4 and Cdk6 activity, and the MMTV-p16 transgene blocks ErbB2-induced tumorigenesis. These results suggest the importance of cyclin D1 in ErbB2-induced tumorigenesis and cell cycle control (Yang et al., 2004). Furthermore, cyclin D1 kinase activity is required for the self-renewal of mammary stem and progenitor cells that are targets of MMTV-ErbB2 tumorigenesis (Jeselsohn et al., 2010).

3.3.7 Cooperation of ErbB2 and α6β4 integrin to promote breast cancers

Integrins, heterodimeric cell surface proteins mediate adhesion between cells and the extracellular matrix (ECM) and also regulate signaling pathways. Guo et al. suggested β4 integrin amplifies ErbB2 signaling, promoting mammary tumorigenesis, by studying a targeted deletion of the β4 signaling domain in MMTV-*neu* mice. A complex of ErbB2, Src, and β4 integrin induces phosphorylation of the signaling domain of β4 integrin and the P loop kinase domain of ErbB2, which enhances ErbB2 kinase activity through activation of Src. Cooperative signaling by ErbB2 and α6β4 integrins activates Jun and STAT3. JNK-mediated phosphorylation of Jun promotes oncogenic hyperproliferation. STAT3 promotes the loss of epithelial adhesion and acquisition of an invasive phenotype (W. Guo et al., 2006; Muthuswamy, 2006).

3.3.8 The role of ErbB2 as a nuclear tyrosine kinase receptor

Although ErbB receptors have been considered strictly plasma membrane receptors, recent studies suggest that they can translocate to the nucleus and act as transcription factors. Full-length ErbB1 and ErbB3 translocate to the nucleus. Nuclear ErbB1 physically interacts with STAT3, leading to the transcriptional activation of inducible nitric oxide synthase (iNOS). An intracellular fragment of ErbB4 translocates to the nucleus. First, the extracellular domain of ErbB4 is cleaved by ADAM17/TACE. Second, the transmembrane domain is cleaved by γ-secretase, allowing the cytoplasmic fragment of ErbB4 to translocate to the nucleus (Citri & Yarden, 2006; S.-C. Wang et al., 2004). The study of Wang et al. suggested that ErbB2 acts as a nuclear tyrosine kinase receptor. Full-length ErbB2 is also localized in the nucleus in both cultured cells and primary tumor tissues, where it is recruited to several gene promoters. For example, ErbB2 is recruited to the cyclooxygenase-2 (COX-2) promoter and activates its transcription. The increased expression of COX-2 is associated with angiogenesis, invasiveness and anti-apoptotic effects (S.-C. Wang et al., 2004). Because it lacks a DNA-binding domain, however, ErbB2 may interact with other nuclear factors to indirectly bind to these promoters.

3.3.9 Mass spectrometry–based quantitative proteomics of ErbB2 signaling networks

Recent technological advances in mass spectrometry (MS) have enabled us to understand the whole signaling networks in combination of biological and mathematical analyses. Pioneering research investigated EGFR signaling with MS-based quantitative proteomics (Blagoev et al., 2004). In this report, three cell populations were labeled by stable isotopes using amino acids in a cell culture technique called SILAC, and each population was

stimulated by EGF for a variable length of time. Subsequently, tyrosine-phosphorylated proteins and associated proteins were purified by anti-phosphotyrosine antibodies and then quantified by MS. A large number of signaling proteins were identified, and the dynamics of their activation were revealed. Following this study, the ErbB2 signaling pathway was studied by similar methods (Bose, 2006). Three groups of cell lysates (ErbB2-overexpressing cells, cells transfected with empty vector, ErbB2-overexpressing cells with EGFR and the ErbB2 selective tyrosine kinase inhibitor PD168393) were affinity-purified. Phosphoproteins were separated by SDS-PAGE and subjected to liquid chromatography–tandem MS. In their study, 462 proteins were identified and quantified. There were four major patterns of dynamics in protein phosphorylation. For example, the adaptor protein Dok1 showed increased phosphorylation in ErbB2-overexpressing cells and decreased phosphorylation when treated with PD168393. Another adaptor protein, Fyn-binding protein (Fyb), showed increased phosphorylation in ErbB2-overexpressing cells, but under PD168393 treatment, there was no significant change in phosphorylation. Focal adhesion kinase (FAK) showed decreased phosphorylation in ErbB2-overexpressing cells, whereas Grb2 showed no significant changes in phosphorylation. Overall, 198 proteins showed remarkable (>1.5-fold) increases in phosphorylation, and 81 proteins showed remarkable (<0.66-fold) decreases.
Another report examined phosphorylation in the ErbB2 signaling pathway with MS (Wolf-Yadlin et al., 2006). In this report, ErbB2-overexpressing cells were stimulated by EGF or NRG. From this analysis, they identified 332 phosphorylated peptides from 175 proteins. Among these peptides, 289 were singly phosphorylated, 42 were doubly phosphorylated, and one was triply phosphorylated. Altogether, 20 phosphorylation sites were identified on EGFR, HER2, and HER3. These results show that EGF stimulation of ErbB2-overexpressing cells activates multiple signaling pathways to induce migration, while HRG stimulation of these cells leads to the amplification of a specific subset of proteins in the migratory signal pathway. Most of these novel phosphorylations have not been studied in detail, but these studies have definitely improved our understanding of ErbB2 signal transduction networks. Besides phosphorylation, EGF-induced ubiquitination network also has been studied (Argenzio et al., 2011).

4. ErbB2 in human cancer

ErbB2 amplification and overexpression have been reported in several human cancers, including breast, ovarian, lung and other cancers (Baselga & Swain, 2009; Santarius et al., 2010). In contrast, recent sequence analysis revealed that point mutation and internal deletion of *ErbB2* were rare (http://www.sanger.ac.uk/). ErbB2 overexpression is associated with poor prognosis in most cancers (Baselga & Swain, 2009; Santarius et al., 2010). ErbB2 is thus used as a tumor marker as well as a target for cancer therapy. ErbB2-targeted therapy uses the humanized monoclonal antibody trastuzumab or the ErbB kinase inhibitor lapatinib, pertuzumab, trastuzumab-DM1, or ertumaxomab (see section 5). However, resistance to trastuzumab is a critical issue for this therapy. As described above in section 3.3, PTEN and Src are the key modulators of trastuzumab resistance. PTEN function has been positively correlated with the clinical effect of trastuzumab (Baselga & Swain, 2009). A recent report showed that targeting Src in combination with trastuzumab sensitized trastuzumab-resistant cells to trastuzumab and eliminated trastuzumab-resistant tumors *in vivo* (Zhang et al., 2011). This section summarizes the current findings on *ErbB2* amplification and prognosis in each type of cancer (Table 1).

4.1 Breast cancer

In the initial study by Slamon et al., 28% of 189 breast tumors showed evidence of *ErbB2* gene amplification (Slamon et al., 1989). In other reports, amplification rates vary from 18 to 40% of breast cancers (Baselga & Swain, 2009; Santarius et al., 2010). ErbB2 is overexpressed in most amplified cases and in some non-amplified cases as well. *ErbB2* amplification and overexpression are associated with poor prognosis, namely overall survival and time to relapse (Baselga & Swain, 2009; Santarius et al., 2010; Sircoulomb et al., 2010). As described in section 6.2, various types of breast cancer models with enforced expression of ErbB2 have been developed. Intriguingly, the growth of both primary mammary tumors and pulmonary metastases depends on the continuous expression of ErbB2 (Moody et al., 2002).

Amplification of the *ErbB2* gene correlates with enhanced ErbB2 expression. One study of the transcriptional regulation of *ErbB2* demonstrated that the X-linked FOXP3, which is a member of the forkhead/winged helix transcription factor family, represses transcription of *ErbB2* (Zuo et al., 2007). X-linked tumor suppressor genes are relevant to tumorigenesis because several of such genes are subject to X inactivation, leading to the realization of Knudson's two-hit hypothesis. According to that report, FOXP3 binds to its consensus sequence in the 5′ promoter of the *ErbB2* gene and works as a transcriptional repressor. Moreover, somatic mutation of *FOXP3* was found in some breast cancer samples, and there was an inverse correlation between FOXP3 expression and that of ERBB2 among the samples, which is consistent with FOXP3's transcriptional activity. Finally, exogenous expression of FOXP3 inhibited the growth and tumorigenicity of various cancer cell lines. Recently, microRNAs (miRNAs) have attracted cancer researchers' attention because the relationships between deregulation of some miRNAs and tumorigenesis have been extensively reported. As expected, microarray analysis demonstrated that the expression level of each miRNA varied between types of cancer (Mattie et al., 2006). Interestingly, *miR-125b* and its homolog *miR-125a* were both downregulated in ErbB2-positive breast cancer. A subsequent study on the function of *miR-125* revealed that *miR-125* targeted the 3′-UTRs of *ErbB2* and *ErbB3*, and the overexpression of *miR-125* inhibited anchorage-dependent growth of SKBR3 and MCF10A cells. Interestingly, the migration and invasion of SKBR3 cells, which are derived from human ErbB2-positive breast cancer cells, was also inhibited by these miRNAs.

These results indicate that not only the amplification of the *ErbB2* gene but also regulation at the transcriptional level contributes to the overexpression of the gene, leading to human breast cancer.

4.2 Ovarian cancer

The initial study on ErbB2 in ovarian cancer was also conducted by Slamon et al., demonstrating that *ErbB2* is a reliable indicator of prognosis (Slamon et al., 1989). Among 73 ovarian cancers, 50 (68%) had staining similar to that of normal ovarian epithelium, while 23 (32%) showed strong staining (Berchuck et al., 1990). The prognosis of the 23 patients with ErbB2 overexpression was poorer than that of the 50 patients with normal ErbB2 expression (Berchuck et al., 1990). In ovarian cancer, therefore, ErbB2 is a predictor of prognosis. Recently, Zheng et al. showed that human immortalized ovarian epithelial cells with ErbB2 expression developed into papillary carcinoma in mice when injected intraperitoneally (Zheng et al., 2010).

cancer	amplification	mutation	prognosis	treatment	reference
breast cancer	18-40%	-	poor	trastuzumab, pertuzumab(phase III), trastuzumab-DM1(phase III), ertumaxomab(phase II), lapatinib	(Baselga & Swain, 2009; Santarius et al., 2010; Sircoulomb et al., 2010)
ovarian cancer	20%	-	poor	pertuzumab(phase II)	(Baselga & Swain, 2009; Berchuck et al., 1990; Santarius et al., 2010)
lung cancer	rare	10%	negative	lapatinib(phase II)	(Baselga & Swain, 2009; Hirsch et al., 2002; Santarius et al., 2010)
gastric cancer	10-30%	-	not clear	Trastuzumab(phase III), lapatinib(phase III)	(Baselga & Swain, 2009)
endometrial cancer	15-35%	-	poor	-	(Santarius et al., 2010)
oesophageal carcinoma	20%	-	poor	-	(Santarius et al., 2010)
bladder cancer	5-15%	-	poor	-	(Santarius et al., 2010)
medullo-blastoma	13%	-	poor	-	(Santarius et al., 2010)
glioma	-	-	poor	-	(Santarius et al., 2010)

Table 1. ErbB2 aberrations in human cancer.

4.3 Lung cancer

Ten percent of the adenocarcinoma subtype of lung cancer and a small proportion of non-small cell lung tumors show ErbB2-activating mutations in the kinase domain (Hirsch et al., 2002; Santarius et al., 2010). One important ErbB2 mutation is a G776 insertion in exon 20. *ErbB2* amplifications are rare in lung cancers (Hirsch et al., 2002). For example, among 238 non-small cell lung tumors, 39 (16%), including 35% of the adenocarcinomas, 20% of the large cell carcinomas and only 1% of the squamous cell carcinomas, were 2+ or 3+ overexpressed by immunohistochemistry using the HercepTest (S.E. Wang et al., 2006), whereas 3+ overexpression was rare (4%) (S.E. Wang et al., 2006). Inducible expression of ErbB2 mutations in lung epithelial cells causes invasive adenocarcinoma in mice (Perera et al., 2009). In contrast to EGFR, *ErbB2* mutations are not associated with prognosis (Tomizawa et al., 2011). In addition, one patient with the *ErbB2* mutation YVMA776–779ins responded to trastuzumab plus vinorelbine after failure of platinum-based chemotherapy and gefitinib.

4.4 Other cancers

10-30% of gastric cancers, 10–35% of endometrial cancers, 20% of Barrett's esophageal carcinomas, and 13% of medulloblastomas show *ErbB2* amplification and overexpression (Santarius et al., 2010). For example, in a panel of nine gastric cell lines, two of which showed *ErbB2* amplification and overexpression, were more sensitive to trastuzumab than cells without *ErbB2* amplification. In endometrial cancer and esophageal carcinomas, *ErbB2* amplifications are associated with poor prognosis.

5. ErbB2 as a therapeutic target

5.1 Antibody-based agents

Accumulating evidence demonstrating the significance of ErbB2 in human cancer has prompted researchers and pharmaceutical companies to develop ErbB2-targeting cancer therapies. Monoclonal antibody therapy has finally demonstrated significant benefits for patients with cancer and has been established as a standard of care. Antibodies can inhibit tumor growth by several mechanisms (Hansel et al., 2010). In contrast to other ErbB receptors, ErbB2 has no known ligand. Therefore, antibodies targeting ErbB2 suppress ErbB2 signaling by inhibiting receptor homo- or hetero-dimerization and/or internalization (Chen et al., 2003). Alternatively, tumor-bound antibodies can initiate an immunological assault against the cancer by activating antibody-dependent cellular cytotoxicity (ADCC) or complement-dependent cytotoxicity (CDC).

An important issue in the use of antibodies for therapy is the immunogenicity of the antibodies; antibodies derived from animals are easily recognized as foreign and cause strong immune responses (Khazaeli et al., 1994). This issue has been overcome by the generation of chimeric, humanized and fully human monoclonal antibodies, with a reduction in potentially immunogenic mouse components (Lonberg, 2005). The advances in antibody engineering have led to monoclonal antibodies with marked successes in the clinic (Adams & Weiner, 2005).

Trastuzumab, a humanized monoclonal antibody directed against the extracellular juxtamembrane (domain IV) of ErbB2, has had a major impact on the breast cancer therapy. In patients with breast cancer that overexpresses ErbB2, trastuzumab has anti-tumor activity and improves outcome and survival in combination with chemotherapy in patients with metastatic breast cancer (Slamon et al., 2001). Trastuzumab represents the standard of care in the adjuvant treatment of ErbB2-overexpressing breast cancers. The mechanisms through which trastuzumab exerts its effects are likely to include ADCC (Clynes et al., 2000), the inhibition of receptor dimerization and cleavage of the ErbB2 extracellular domain (Hudis, 2007).

However, the majority of patients with ErbB2-overexpressing tumors do not respond to trastuzumab or develop acquired resistance within a year. Several molecular mechanisms that could contribute to the development of trastuzumab resistance have been reported (Nahta & Esteva, 2006). In addition to alterations in ErbB2, other members of the ErbB family are thought to play roles in trastuzumab resistance by signaling downstream to the PI3K and MAPK pathways, bypassing trastuzumab's ErbB2-based inhibition of these pathways (Kruser & Wheeler, 2010). Loss of functionally of PTEN and mutations that activate PI3K are possible mechanisms of resistance to trastuzumab (see also 3.3.4 and Berns et al., 2007). Decreased interaction between trastuzumab and its target receptor ErbB2 due to steric hindrance of ErbB2 by MUC4 may prevent the actions of trastuzumab (Nagy et al., 2005). Because blocking ErbB2 to inhibit cancer cell growth can be circumvented through alternative signaling pathways, the combination of different agents that target molecules that contribute to anti-ErbB2 resistance may be a promising tool in the treatment of ErbB2-positive breast cancer.

Several other monoclonal antibodies that target ErbB2 are being tested in the clinic. Pertuzumab (developed by Genentech) is a humanized monoclonal antibody that binds to extracellular domain II of ErbB2, which is distinct from the binding site of trastuzumab. It sterically inhibits dimerization of ErbB2 with other ErbB proteins (Agus et al., 2002) and with IGF-1R (Nahta et al., 2005) and blocks the downstream signaling pathways of these dimers. The fact that pertuzumab and trastuzumab recognize different sites causes distinct downstream effects, and the combination of pertuzumab with trastuzumab synergistically inhibits the survival of breast tumor cells (Nahta et al., 2004).

Monoclonal antibodies are generally well tolerated in humans and are now established as targeted therapies. However, administration of mAbs carries the risk of immune and innate reactions (Presta, 2006). ErbB2-targeted therapies have been associated with cardiotoxicity because they can interrupt ErbB2 signaling, which is important for receptor signaling in the heart (Force et al., 2007). Fortunately, symptomatic cardiac toxicity frequently improves when trastuzumab therapy has been stopped (Romond et al., 2005).

The next generation of mAbs currently under development incorporates additional beneficial modifications, such as alterations in glycosylation and sequences that enhance ADCC (Lazar et al., 2006) or modifications in size and antigen-binding affinity that increase the ability of the mAb to penetrate solid tumors. Recombinant technology allows extensive modifications to be made to the structures of antibodies, including the production of recombinant antibody fragments. One advantage to this is that they are smaller and penetrate tissues and tumors more rapidly and deeply than whole antibodies (Jain, 1990). Bispecific and trispecific antibodies that target ErbB2 are also under investigation. These antibodies are designed to interact with other key proteins to facilitate, for example, the binding of a single antibody to all of the target antigens, to draw the immune cell into close proximity with the tumor cell that overexpresses ErbB2, with consequent recruitment of cytotoxic T cells to the T cell–antibody–tumor cell complex and immunological destruction of the tumor cell (Kiewe et al., 2006). Multifunctional mAbs will achieve more selective and effective cancer therapies.

5.2 Chemical compounds

In addition to antibodies targeting the extracellular domain of ErbR2, small-molecule tyrosine kinase inhibitors that directly inhibit the tyrosine kinase activity of ErbB2 have been developed. Among them, lapatinib (Tykerb®) is a dual tyrosine kinase inhibitor that targets both ErbB2 and EGFR. Lapatinib was developed as a safe and orally effective drug for the treatment of EGFR- or/and ErbB2-overexpressing breast cancer (Reid et al., 2007). It binds the ATP-binding pocket of the EGFR/ErbB2 protein kinase domain, preventing self-phosphorylation and the subsequent activation of the signaling cascade, leading to an increase in apoptosis and a decrease in cellular proliferation. In comparison to other tyrosine kinase inhibitors in clinical trials (for example, gefitinib and erlotinib), the interaction of lapatinib with EGFR and ErbB2 is reversible, but dissociation is much slower, allowing for prolonged downregulation of receptor tyrosine phosphorylation in tumor cells. Lapatinib in combination with trastuzumab exhibits a synergistic effect in ErbB2-overexpressing breast cancer cells, and it also has activity against trastuzumab-resistant cells (Konecny et al., 2006). Furthermore, due to the small size of lapatinib compared to antibodies, it can penetrate the blood–brain barrier and act against central nervous system (CNS) metastases. Moreover, clinical trials have demonstrated that lapatinib is a safe drug with no serious or symptomatic cardiotoxicity (Cameron & Stein, 2008).

5.3 Innovative materials for future drugs

Antibodies can also be used as a targeting device for other cytotoxic systems. The overexpression of ErbB2 on tumor cells and the accessibility of the extracellular domain of ErbB2 make it an ideal target for the targeted delivery of anti-tumor drugs as well as imaging agents (Colombo et al., 2010). Cytotoxic drugs, radioisotopes, toxins, enzymes or nano-scaled drug carriers can be conjugated with the antibody (Wu & Senter, 2005).

One successful application of such a complex is trastuzumab–DM1 (T–DM1), which consists of the trastuzumab antibody conjugated to the potent antimicrotubule drug DM1, a maytansine derivative. After binding to ErbB2, T–DM1 is internalized, and DM1 is subsequently released into the cell, thus delivering chemotherapy directly to cells that overexpress ErbB2. T-DM1 has antitumor activity in trastuzumab-sensitive and trastuzumab-resistant ErbB2-overexpressing breast cancer (Lewis Phillips et al., 2008).

Antibody-conjugated nano-scaled drug carriers offer major improvements in the therapeutic index of anticancer agents through the site-specific, efficient delivery of agents, which reduces side effects. Moreover, they can avoid multi-drug resistance (Peer et al., 2007). Many materials, such as liposomes, micelles, polymeric and metal nanoparticles, solid lipid particles, dendrimers and quantum dots, are used as nanocarriers. The material properties of each nanocarrier have been developed to enhance delivery to the tumor. These nano-scaled systems can be used to deliver small-molecule drugs as well as nucleic acid drugs. For example, anti-ErbB2 antibody fragment–conjugated, PEG-stabilized immunoliposomes display long-term circulation and selective delivery of the encapsulated drug into ErbB2-overexpressing cancer (Park et al., 2002). These anti-ErbB2 delivery systems greatly increase the therapeutic index by enhancing anti-tumor efficacy and reducing systemic toxicity. In part, this superior activity is attributed to the ability of the immunoliposomes to deliver their load inside the target cells via receptor-mediated endocytosis. The initial target accumulation could be achieved by passive targeting via the enhanced permeability and retention (EPR) effect (Maeda et al., 2009). Although antibody targeting is regarded as a promising strategy, some groups have reported that antibody targeting did not increase tumor localization but instead increased internalization (Kirpotin et al., 2006). Many pharmaceutical agents need to be delivered intracellularly to exert their therapeutic action in the cytoplasm or on individual organelles.

However, a problem with intracellular delivery is that any molecule/particle entering the cell via the endocytic pathway can become trapped in the endosome and eventually be degraded in the lysosome. As a result, only a small fraction of unaffected substance appears in the cytoplasm. Thus, even if efficient cellular uptake via endocytosis is observed, the delivery of intact agents is compromised by insufficient endosomal escape and subsequent lysosomal degradation (Lee et al., 2008). Improvement against lysosomal degradation is an important issue to be resolved.

6. Experimental methods to assesscellular transformation and tumorigenesis

This chapter focuses on representative experimental methods that have contributed to the studies of ErbB2 function, which include classical transformation assays using NIH3T3 cells, three-dimentional(3D) culture of MCF10A, transgenic and knock-in mice and recent techniques with non-germline genetically engineered mouse models.

6.1 Cell culture–based analysis

To analyze ErbB2 function, the transformation assay is the first choice because *ErbB2* was identified as an oncogene, as discussed above. We will review the classical transformation assay and introduce a novel, improved method we developed.

Transformation assays are usually carried out with NIH3T3 cells (Todaro & Green, 1963). The term "transformation assay" classically includes three representative assays: focus formation, colony formation, and tumor formation. Although they differ in detectable phenotype, the principle behind them is simple; if candidate genes introduced into NIH3T3 cells are oncogenic, they can confer cancerous phenotypes, such as the loss of contact inhibition, anchorage-independent growth, and tumorigenicity to the NIH3T3 cells.

The focus formation assay detects one of these oncogenic abilities, to cause the loss of contact inhibition. Contact inhibition is a phenotype usually present in NIH3T3 cells; NIH3T3 cells proliferate until they form a monolayer of cells. If oncogenes are introduced, then some of the cells might become transformed into cancer cells. Transformation can be quantified by the appearance of "foci" of transformants (Figure 3).

The colony formation assay detects another ability, to cause anchorage-independent growth. Anchorage-independent growth is a phenotype virtually all cancer cells have (Cifone & Fidler, 1980); cancer cells can multiply without attachment to the extracellular matrix or solid substrate, such as the bottom of the Petri dish. A transformant that can proliferate in soft agar in suspension forms a "colony", that is, amass of descendants from a single transformant. Thus, transformation activity can be quantified by the number of colonies formed.

The tumor formation assay detects the ability to generate tumors *in vivo*. In this assay, transformants are injected into a syngeneic host or immunocompromised mice, such as nude (*nu/nu*) mice, to examine whether they are able to grow and form tumors in their animal hosts.

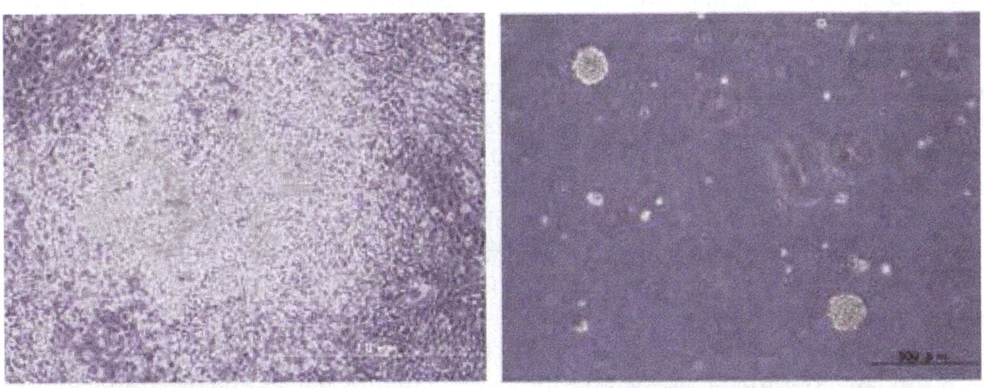

(a) ERBB2 V659E focus (b) H-RAS G12V colony

Fig. 3. Transformation assay with NIH3T3. (a)ERBB2 V659E has transformation activity. (b)H-RAS G12V, a mutant frequently observed in human cancer can also transform NIH3T3.

Rat *neu* transforms NIH3T3 cells, and the transformants are recognized as foci, which led to the discovery of *neu* itself (Schechter et al., 1984). Overexpression of wild-type ErbB2, as seen in human cancers, also transforms NIH3T3 cells (Di Fiore et al., 1987; Hudziak et al., 1987) by the colony formation and tumor formation assays. In contrast to human *ErbB2*, the rat *neu* proto-oncogene *ErbB2* does not transform cells when only expressed in NIH3T3 cells (Hung et al., 1986), but it transforms them when coexpressed with EGFR (Kokai et al., 1989). About ten years after its discovery, the *neu* oncogene was found not to transform the NIH3T3-7d cell line, which is devoid of detectable ErbB family members (Cohen et al., 1996). *ErbB2* itself probably does not have enough oncogenic activity to achieve the transformation of regular NIH3T3 cells but can transform them in the presence of EGFR. Our data also indicate that ErbB2 itself does not transform NIH3T3 cells (M.S., unpublished data), in contrast to DiFiore et al. (Di Fiore et al., 1987; Hudziak et al., 1987). This discrepancy probably results from the variations in the NIH3T3 cells used in these assays, as they have been passaged dozens of times since their early establishment. To detect a novel gene that transforms NIH3T3 cells in harmony with *ErbB2*, we established *ErbB2*-expressing NIH3T3 cells and introduced genes that are overexpressed in breast cancer using a retroviral expression vector. In fact, we demonstrated that one gene transforms NIH3T3 cells only in the presence of ErbB2 (M.S., unpublished data). This phenomenon seems to resemble the tumorigenesis of ErbB2-positive breast cancer *in vitro*.

Breast cancer can progress step by step along a continuum of changes from a normal phenotype to a malignant disease. The human mammary gland consists of multiple ducts and lobes (Vargo-Gogola & Rosen, 2007). Lobes are composed of multiple acinal structures with hollow lumens surrounded by layers of luminal epithelial cells, outer myoepithelial cells, and basement membranes. However, this well-organized structure is disrupted at early premalignant stages of breast cancer, such as ductal carcinoma *in situ* (DCIS). DCIS is the most common type of non-invasive breast cancer in women. DCIS can progress to malignant invasive breast cancer (IBC) and, subsequently, metastatic cancer (Espina & Liotta, 2010). The genetic events that cause progression to malignant stages are only partially understood.

A 3D culture of MCF10A cells within Matrigel, which are derived from the Englebreth-Holm Swarm (EHS) tumor (Kleinman et al., 1982), is an excellent *in vitro* model for understanding the biological processes and signaling pathways responsible for tissue morphogenesis *in vivo* and the disruption of epithelial architecture at early stages of tumorigenesis (Debnath & Brugge, 2005). MCF10A cells are a spontaneously immortalized but non-transformed human breast epithelial cell line (Soule et al., 1990). Following a reported method (Debnath, 2003b), MCF10A cells in Matrigel form acinar structures characterized by a hollow lumen surrounded by polarized, growth-arrested luminal epithelial cells, as shown in Figure 4. 3D cultures can provide a physiologically relevant context to the *in vivo* breast microenvironment, while monolayer cultures on plastic involve an environment that is considerably different from the *in vivo* environment (Vargo-Gogola & Rosen, 2007; Yamada & Cukierman, 2007). Certainly, both primary cultures of human tumor tissues and mouse models of cancer are practical to study carcinoma formation; however, they are relatively difficult to handle for understanding the biochemical and molecular biological pathways involved in the early stages of oncogenesis (Debnath, 2003b).

Madin-Darby canine kidney (MDCK) cells represent another widely used 3D culture model. When MDCK cells are embedded within collagen gels as single cells, they form polarized cysts with a central hollow lumen (Figure 5). During morphogenesis, intracellular vesicles containing apical membrane components are delivered to the cell surface between closely apposed cells, and membranes are separated, leading to the generation of several small lumens (Andrew & Ewald, 2010; Bryant & Mostov, 2008). Fusion of the lumens into a single large lumen subsequently occurs, and this phase requires apoptosis of luminal cells to clear

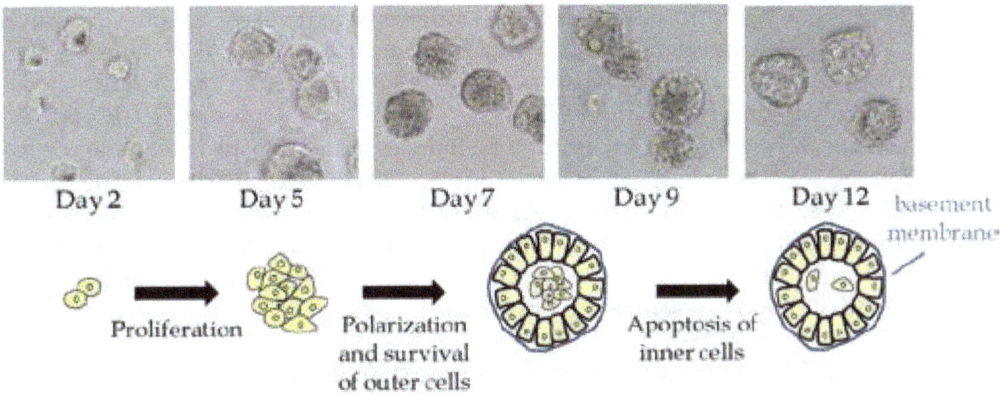

Fig. 4. MCF10A acinal structures constructed within Matrigel.
(1) Single cells embedded in Matrigel proliferate and form cell clusters. (2) At day 5-7, cells are distinguished between matrix-attached outer cells and matrix-deprived inner cells within each acinus. (3) After their fate has been determined, outer epithelial cells acquire apical-to-basal polarity and receive survival signals. (4) At day 8, however, non-polarized inner cells start to die via apoptosis. (5) Finally, replicated mammary acini with luminal spaces are constructed at day 14.

the lumen (Andrew & Ewald, 2010; Martin-Belmonte et al., 2008). Given that laminin is essential for initiating polarization mediated by the interaction between integrins and the ECM in the MDCK system, MDCK cells grown within the laminin-rich ECM, as within Matrigel, can polarize more efficiently than within collagen gels. The cells polarize and form clear lumens much faster, without the requirement of apoptosis (Martin-Belmonte et al., 2008).

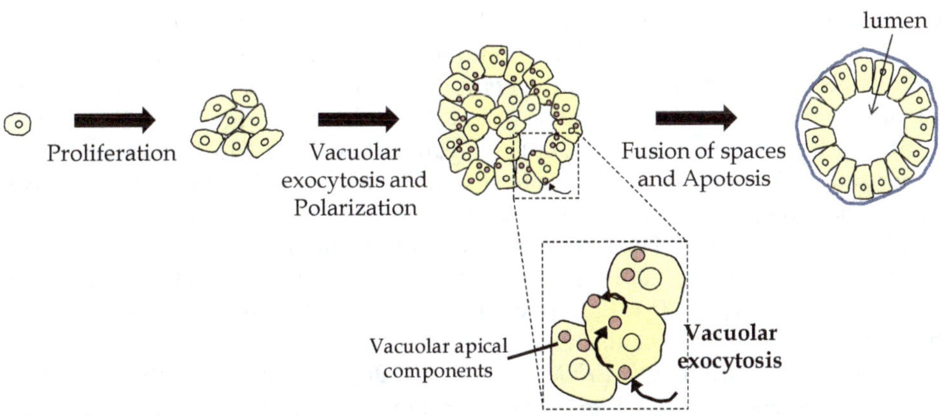

Fig. 5. Lumen formation by MDCK cells through vacuolar exocytosis of apical proteins.
(1) Single cells embedded in collagen gel or Matrigel proliferate to form groups of cells. (2) Intracellular vesicles containing apical membrane components are delivered to regions between cells and create luminal spaces via the fusion of vesicles and the plasma membrane. The surrounding cells now exhibit apical–basal polarity. (3) Several small lumens fuse with each other and generate one large lumen. Under the condition where cells are cultured within the laminin-lacking ECM, inner cell death by apoptosis is essential to clear the lumen (Andrew & Ewald, 2010; Bryant & Mostov, 2008).

Using the MCF10A 3D culture system, previous studies have revealed the effects of several oncogenes and viral oncoproteins on the process of acini formation (Debnath & Brugge, 2005; Shaw et al., 2004). For example, inactivation of the retinoblastoma protein (Rb) by HPV E7 facilitates proliferation (Debnath et al., 2002). Co-overexpression of CSF1-R and CSF1, both of which are elevated in mammary tumors, induces inner cell survival and loss of cell–cell adhesion, as well as hyperproliferation (Wrobel, 2004). Activated Akt leads to large, distorted, and filled-lumen structures (Debnath, 2003a). Each phenotype in these studies results from the biological activities of the introduced gene, suggesting that specific biological processes and pathways are modulated by the oncogene. Furthermore, these morphologies in 3D culture resemble the histological changes observed in human tumors *in vivo* (Debnath & Brugge, 2005).

Recently, the MCF10A 3D culture has been used to search for novel candidate oncogenes, such as the Yes kinase–associated protein (YAP) gene. *YAP* is included in the chromosome 11q22 amplicon that frequently appears in human tumors. Overexpression of YAP induces an anti-apoptotic and invasive morphology (Overholtzer, 2006). Further analysis has identified tumorigenic functions of generally non-tumorigenic proteins. For example, a study of MCF10A 3D structures suggested that not only oncogenes but also antioxidants could facilitate malignancy of carcinoma. In mammary acini, centrally located cells lack glucose transport and produce reactive oxygen species (ROS). Antioxidants could antagonize such metabolic stresses and promote the survival of cells detaching from the ECM by rescuing ATP production through fatty acid oxidation (FAO) (Schafer et al., 2009). Additionally, overexpression of a glycosyltransferase, N-acetylglucosaminyltransferase V (GnT-V) induces the disarrangement of mammary acinar morphogenesis, including increased cell proliferation, filled lumens, and disrupted polarity. Thus, altered expression of GnT-V, which catalyzes posttranslational modification, affects early stages of breast carcigenesis (H.B. Guo et al., 2010).

ERBB2 amplification in breast cancer is correlated with poor prognosis due to increased metastasis and resistance to chemotherapy. This gene is overexpressed in 50–60% of DCIS (Lu et al., 2009; Nofech-Mozes et al., 2005). Muthuswamy et al. showed that ErbB2-induced cells generate aberrant acini in 3D culture *in vitro*. To trigger homodimerization and activate ErbB2 signaling, they constructed chimeric receptors, as shown in Figure 6(a) (Muthuswamy et al., 1999; Muthuswamy et al., 2001). Treatment with AP1510 induced receptor homodimerization, leading to multi-acinar structures with filled lumens but no invasive phenotype. Therefore, additional genetic events as "second hits" may be required for invasion (Seton-Rogers, 2004). Those features are reminiscent of ErbB2-overexpressing DCIS *in vivo* (Muthuswamy et al., 2001). A recent analysis of ErbB2-mediated transformation indicated the significance of Tyr 1201 phosphorylation for the disruption of apical–basal polarity of MCF10A cells (Lucs et al., 2010).

Our laboratory uses a full-length *ErbB2* mutant, V659E, as a model of the constitutively activated ErbB2 receptor. It has higher intrinsic kinase activity and increased ability to induce transformation compared to wild-type ErbB2. This receptor can form a heterodimer with the other ErbB receptor family members as well as a homodimer, whereas chimeric receptors only form homodimers (Figure 6(b)). Thus our system may mimic physiological condition *in vivo* (A.D., unpublished data). We control the induction timing of ErbB2VE using the reverse tetracycline (Tet)-controlled transcriptional activator system, called "Tet-on". Induction of ErbB2VE leads to unregulated proliferation and filling of luminal spaces, whose structures are similar to "multi-acini" reported in a previous study (Muthuswamy et al., 2001).

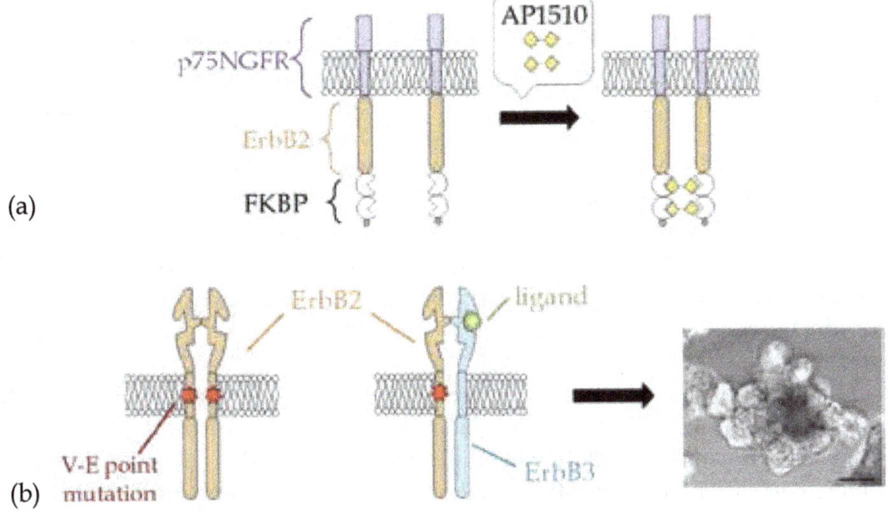

Fig. 6. Disruption of acinal structures due to ErbB2 signaling activation.
(a) Chimeric ErbB2 receptors induce homodimerization mediated by AP1510. MCF10A acini were treated with AP1510 at day 10 and cultured in Matrigel until day 20, resulting in the aberrant structure composed of multiple acini with filled lumens (Muthuswamy et al., 2001; Seton-Rogers, 2004). (b) In our laboratory, Tet-responsive ErbB2VE was expressed by treatment with Dox, forming both homo- and hetero-dimers. ErbB2VE activation from day 4 induces hyperproliferation and exhibits multi-acinar structures at day 12. This structure is similar to the phenotype previously reported (Muthuswamy et al., 2001). The scale bar represents 50 μm.

There is no evidence for how DCIS, which is a non-invasive and premalignant lesion, acquires invasive behavior. Given that DCIS with *ErbB2* amplification or overexpression frequently progresses to IBC, it is important to identify genes that collaborate with ErbB2 and induce tumor progression, including invasion and metastasis. Several investigators have been successful in detecting such factors using the MCF10A system. For example, either transforming growth factorβ (TGFβ) or prostate-derived Ets factor (PDEF) dramatically alters MCF10A spheroid-like acinal structures into protrusive cords invading the ECM in cooperation with ErbB2 (Gunawardane, 2005; Seton-Rogers, 2004). Additionally, co-overexpression of ErbB2 and 14-3-3γ, which shows increased expression in the early stages of breast cancer, results in larger acinar size, filled lumen, the gain of invasiveness, and disordered basal membrane protein laminin (Lu et al., 2009).

6.2 Animal models

Genetically engineered mouse (GEM) models have contributed broadly to the field of cancer research. First, we will review GEM models of breast cancer as a representative cancer related to the deregulation of ErbB2. The earliest model was generated by introducing *neu* oncogenes under the transcriptional control of the mouse mammary tumor virus (MMTV) LTR (Bouchard et al., 1989; C.T. Guy et al., 1992; Muller et al., 1988). MMTV LTR drives the expression of neu specifically in mammary gland intargeted mice. Tissue-specific expression is also achieved by using the whey acidic protein (WAP) promoter (Piechocki et al., 2003). The next useful development for GEM models was the Cre-loxP system (Wagner et al.,

1997). Cre-loxP models have genetic elements flanked by loxP sites that are processed by Cre recombinase, and its utility is widely known. Although *neu* under the strong viral LTR has questionable relevance to human breast cancers, mammary-specific expression of *neu* at endogenous levels had been desired. Thus, knock-in mice generated by interbreeding transgenic mice that have the *neu* promoter flanked by loxP sites with mice expressing Cre under the MMTV LTR (Andrechek et al., 2000) were developed, providing a valuable murine cancer model. *Neu* under the physiological promoter does not cause rapid tumor progression as seen in transgenic mice harboring MMTV-driven *neu*. However, they show amplification of the recombinant *neu* allele, as observed in human cancers (Andrechek et al., 2000). Furthermore, microarray profiling revealed that tumors arise in the knock-in mice, which demonstrated increased expression of GRB7 (Andrechek et al., 2003), as seen in human breast cancers.

More recently, several non-germline GEM models have been developed (Heyer et al., 2010). For example, generating chimeric mice is a novel way to increase the physiological relevance to human cancer, where cancer cells are surrounded by normal tissue, and it is also relatively cost-efficient. As in other models, chimeric mice carrying ErbB2 V659E in the lung, develop lung adenocarcinomas (Zhou et al., 2010). The necessity and desire to reproduce human cancers in mice will lead to more efficient translational research toward cancer therapies in the future.

7. Conclusion

We reviewed the history of the discovery of *ErbB2* with the recent progress on ErbB2 function. Thirty years have passed since the *neu* oncogene was discovered, and extensive research on ErbB proteins has been carried out since then. As long as tumor cell growth depends on ErbB2 expression, it is a rational target for therapy, and efforts will be made to develop more effective drugs than trastuzumab. In basic as well as clinical ErbB2 research, studies of cancer stem cells and the cells of origin (Visvader, 2011) of the ErbB2-induced tumors should be carried out. ErbB2 expression increases the population of stem/progenitor cells (Korkaya et al., 2008). Two distinct mammary progenitors have been identified, one of which is a target of MMTV-ErbB2 tumorigenesis and requires cyclin D1 kinase activity for its self-renewal (Jeselsohn et al., 2010). This suggests a combinational therapy with trastuzumab and cyclin D1 inhibitors may be more effective at treating ErbB2-mediated tumorigenesis than trastuzumab alone. The recent notion of non-oncogene addiction also needs to be considered (Luo et al., 2009). Identification of such genes will enable us to develop more effective targeted therapies as well as to understand the mechanism of ErbB2-mediated tumorigenesis itself.

8. Acknowledgement

We thank all the members of our laboratories, especially Jiro Fujimoto, Kosuke Ishikawa and Takaomi Ishida for valuable discussions.

9. References

Adams, G. P., & Weiner, L. M. (2005). Monoclonal antibody therapy of cancer. *Nat Biotechnol*, Vol.23, No.9, pp.1147-1157.

Agus, D. B., Akita, R. W., Fox, W. D., Lewis, G. D., Higgins, B., Pisacane, P. I., Lofgren, J. A., Tindell, C., Evans, D. P., Maiese, K., Scher, H. I., & Sliwkowski, M. X. (2002). Targeting ligand-activated ErbB2 signaling inhibits breast and prostate tumor growth. *Cancer Cell,* Vol.2, No.2, pp.127-137.

Akiyama, T., Sudo, C., Ogawara, H., Toyoshima, K., & Yamamoto, T. (1986). The product of the human c-erbB-2 gene: a 185-kilodalton glycoprotein with tyrosine kinase activity. *Science,* Vol.232, No.4758, pp.1644-1646.

Andrechek, E. R., Hardy, W. R., Siegel, P. M., Rudnicki, M. A., Cardiff, R. D., & Muller, W. J. (2000). Amplification of the neu/erbB-2 oncogene in a mouse model of mammary tumorigenesis. *Proc Natl Acad Sci USA,* Vol.97, No.7, pp.3444-3449.

Andrechek, E. R., Laing, M. A., Girgis-Gabardo, A. A., Siegel, P. M., Cardiff, R. D., & Muller, W. J. (2003). Gene expression profiling of neu-induced mammary tumors from transgenic mice reveals genetic and morphological similarities to ErbB2-expressing human breast cancers. *Cancer Res,* Vol.63, No.16, pp.4920-4926.

Andrew, D. J., & Ewald, A. J. (2010). Morphogenesis of epithelial tubes: Insights into tube formation, elongation, and elaboration. *Dev Biol,* Vol.341, No.1, pp.34-55.

Argenzio, E., Bange, T., Oldrini, B., Bianchi, F., Peesari, R., Mari, S., Di Fiore, P. P., Mann, M., Polo, S. (2011). Proteomic snapshot of the EGF-induced ubiquitin network. *Mol Syst Biol,* Vol.7.

Aroian, R. V., Koga, M., Mendel, J. E., Ohshima, Y., & Sternberg, P. W. (1990). The let-23 gene necessary for Caenorhabditis elegans vulval induction encodes a tyrosine kinase of the EGF receptor subfamily. *Nature,* Vol.348, No.6303, pp.693-699.

Bargmann, C. I., Hung, M. C., & Weinberg, R. A. (1986a). Multiple independent activations of the neu oncogene by a point mutation altering the transmembrane domain of p185. *Cell,* Vol.45, No.5, pp.649-657.

---. (1986b). The neu oncogene encodes an epidermal growth factor receptor-related protein. *Nature,* Vol.319, No.6050, pp.226-230.

Baselga, J., & Swain, S. M. (2009). Novel anticancer targets: revisiting ERBB2 and discovering ERBB3. *Nat Rev Cancer,* Vol.9, No.7, pp.463-475.

Berchuck, A., Kamel, A., Whitaker, R., Kerns, B., Olt, G., Kinney, R., Soper, J. T., Dodge, R., Clarke-Pearson, D. L., Marks, P., & et al. (1990). Overexpression of HER-2/neu is associated with poor survival in advanced epithelial ovarian cancer. *Cancer Res,* Vol.50, No.13, pp.4087-4091.

Berns, K., Horlings, H. M., Hennessy, B. T., Madiredjo, M., Hijmans, E. M., Beelen, K., Linn, S. C., Gonzalez-Angulo, A. M., Stemke-Hale, K., Hauptmann, M., Beijersbergen, R. L., Mills, G. B., van de Vijver, M. J., & Bernards, R. (2007). A functional genetic approach identifies the PI3K pathway as a major determinant of trastuzumab resistance in breast cancer. *Cancer Cell,* Vol.12, No.4, pp.395-402.

Blagoev, B., Ong, S-E., Kratchmarova, I., & Mann, M. (2004). Temporal analysis of phosphotyrosine-dependent signaling networks by quantitative proteomics. *Nat Biotechnol,* Vol.22, No.9, pp.1139-1145.

Bose, R. (2006). Phosphoproteomic analysis of Her2/neu signaling and inhibition. *Proc Natl Acad Sci USA,* Vol.103, No.26, pp.9773-9778.

Bouchard, L., Lamarre, L., Tremblay, P. J., & Jolicoeur, P. (1989). Stochastic appearance of mammary tumors in transgenic mice carrying the MMTV/c-neu oncogene. *Cell,* Vol.57, No.6, pp.931-936.

Bryant, D. M., & Mostov, K. E. (2008). From cells to organs: building polarized tissue. *Nat Rev Mol Cell Biol,* Vol.9, No.11, pp.887-901.

Burgess, A. W., Cho, H. S., Eigenbrot, C., Ferguson, K. M., Garrett, T. P., Leahy, D. J., Lemmon, M. A., Sliwkowski, M. X., Ward, C. W., & Yokoyama, S. (2003). An open-and-shut case? Recent insights into the activation of EGF/ErbB receptors. *Mol Cell,* Vol.12, No.3, pp.541-552.

Cameron, D. A., & Stein, S. (2008). Drug Insight: intracellular inhibitors of HER2--clinical development of lapatinib in breast cancer. *Nat Clin Pract Oncol,* Vol.5, No.9, pp.512-520.

Chen, J. S., Lan, K., & Hung, M. C. (2003). Strategies to target HER2/neu overexpression for cancer therapy. *Drug Resist Updat,* Vol.6, No.3, pp.129-136.

Cifone, M. A., & Fidler, I. J. (1980). Correlation of patterns of anchorage-independent growth with in vivo behavior of cells from a murine fibrosarcoma. *Proc Natl Acad Sci USA,* Vol.77, No.2, pp.1039-1043.

Citri, A., & Yarden, Y. (2006). EGF–ERBB signalling: towards the systems level. *Nat Rev Mol Cell Biol,* Vol.7, No.7, pp.505-516.

Clynes, R. A., Towers, T. L., Presta, L. G., & Ravetch, J. V. (2000). Inhibitory Fc receptors modulate in vivo cytoxicity against tumor targets. *Nat Med,* Vol.6, No.4, pp.443-446.

Cohen, B. D., Kiener, P. A., Green, J. M., Foy, L., Fell, H. P., & Zhang, K. (1996). The relationship between human epidermal growth-like factor receptor expression and cellular transformation in NIH3T3 cells. *J Biol Chem,* Vol.271, No.48, pp.30897-30903.

Colombo, M., Corsi, F., Foschi, D., Mazzantini, E., Mazzucchelli, S., Morasso, C., Occhipinti, E., Polito, L., Prosperi, D., Ronchi, S., & Verderio, P. (2010). HER2 targeting as a two-sided strategy for breast cancer diagnosis and treatment: Outlook and recent implications in nanomedical approaches. *Pharmacol Res,* Vol.62, No.2, pp.150-165.

Coussens, L., Yang-Feng, T. L., Liao, Y. C., Chen, E., Gray, A., McGrath, J., Seeburg, P. H., Libermann, T. A., Schlessinger, J., Francke, U., & et al. (1985). Tyrosine kinase receptor with extensive homology to EGF receptor shares chromosomal location with neu oncogene. *Science,* Vol.230, No.4730, pp.1132-1139.

Crowder, R. J., Lombardi, D. P., & Ellis, M. J. (2004). Successful targeting of ErbB2 receptors—is PTEN the key? *Cancer Cell,* Vol.6, No.2, pp.103-104.

Cully, M., You, H., Levine, A. J., & Mak, T. W. (2006). Beyond PTEN mutations: the PI3K pathway as an integrator of multiple inputs during tumorigenesis. *Nat Rev Cancer,* Vol.6, No.3, pp.184-192.

Debnath, J. (2003a). Akt activation disrupts mammary acinar architecture and enhances proliferation in an mTOR-dependent manner. *J Cell Biol,* Vol.163, No.2, pp.315-326.

———. (2003b). Morphogenesis and oncogenesis of MCF-10A mammary epithelial acini grown in three-dimensional basement membrane cultures. *Methods,* Vol.30, No.3, pp.256-268.

Debnath, J., Mills, K. R., Collins, N. L., Reginato, M. J., Muthuswamy, S. K., & Brugge, J. S. (2002). The role of apoptosis in creating and maintaining luminal space within normal and oncogene-expressing mammary acini. *Cell,* Vol.111, No.1, pp.29-40.

Debnath, J., & Brugge, J. S. (2005). Modelling glandular epithelial cancers in three-dimensional cultures. *Nat Rev Cancer,* Vol.5, No.9, pp.675-688.

Di Fiore, P. P., Pierce, J. H., Kraus, M. H., Segatto, O., King, C. R., & Aaronson, S. A. (1987). erbB-2 is a potent oncogene when overexpressed in NIH/3T3 cells. *Science,* Vol.237, No.4811, pp.178-182.

Downward, J., Yarden, Y., Mayes, E., Scrace, G., Totty, N., Stockwell, P., Ullrich, A., Schlessinger, J., & Waterfield, M. D. (1984). Close similarity of epidermal growth factor receptor and v-erb-B oncogene protein sequences. *Nature,* Vol.307, No.5951, pp.521-527.

Espina, V., & Liotta, L. A. (2010). What is the malignant nature of human ductal carcinoma in situ? *Nat Rev Cancer,* Vol.11, No.1, pp.68-75.

Force, T., Krause, D. S., & Van Etten, R. A. (2007). Molecular mechanisms of cardiotoxicity of tyrosine kinase inhibition. *Nat Rev Cancer,* Vol.7, No.5, pp.332-344.

Garrett, T. P., McKern, N. M., Lou, M., Elleman, T. C., Adams, T. E., Lovrecz, G. O., Kofler, M., Jorissen, R. N., Nice, E. C., Burgess, A. W., & Ward, C. W. (2003). The crystal structure of a truncated ErbB2 ectodomain reveals an active conformation, poised to interact with other ErbB receptors. *Mol Cell,* Vol.11, No.2, pp.495-505.

Gomez, A., Volff, J. N., Hornung, U., Schartl, M., & Wellbrock, C. (2004). Identification of a second egfr gene in Xiphophorus uncovers an expansion of the epidermal growth factor receptor family in fish. *Mol Biol Evol,* Vol.21, No.2, pp.266-275.

Graham, F. L., & van der Eb, A. J. (1973). A new technique for the assay of infectivity of human adenovirus 5 DNA. *Virology,* Vol.52, No.2, pp.456-467.

Gunawardane, R. N. (2005). Novel Role for PDEF in Epithelial Cell Migration and Invasion. *Cancer Res,* Vol.65, No.24, pp.11572-11580.

Guo, H. B., Johnson, H., Randolph, M., Nagy, T., Blalock, R., & Pierce, M. (2010). Specific posttranslational modification regulates early events in mammary carcinoma formation. *Proc Natl Acad Sci U S A,* Vol.107, No.49, pp.21116-21121.

Guo, W., Pylayeva, Y., Pepe, A., Yoshioka, T., Muller, W. J., Inghirami, G., & Giancotti, F. G. (2006). β4 Integrin Amplifies ErbB2 Signaling to Promote Mammary Tumorigenesis. *Cell,* Vol.126, No.3, pp.489-502.

Guy, C. T., Webster, M. A., Schaller, M., Parsons, T. J., Cardiff, R. D., & Muller, W. J. (1992). Expression of the neu protooncogene in the mammary epithelium of transgenic mice induces metastatic disease. *Proc Natl Acad Sci USA,* Vol.89, No.22, pp.10578-10582.

Guy, P. M., Platko, J. V., Cantley, L. C., Cerione, R. A., & Carraway, K. L., 3rd. (1994). Insect cell-expressed p180erbB3 possesses an impaired tyrosine kinase activity. *Proc Natl Acad Sci USA,* Vol.91, No.17, pp.8132-8136.

Hansel, T. T., Kropshofer, H., Singer, T., Mitchell, J. A., & George, A. J. (2010). The safety and side effects of monoclonal antibodies. *Nat Rev Drug Discov,* Vol.9, No.4, pp.325-338.

Heyer, J., Kwong, L. N., Lowe, S. W., & Chin, L. (2010). Non-germline genetically engineered mouse models for translational cancer research. *Nat Rev Cancer,* Vol.10, No.7, pp.470-480.

Hirsch, F. R., Varella-Garcia, M., Franklin, W. A., Veve, R., Chen, L., Helfrich, B., Zeng, C., Baron, A., & Bunn, P. A., Jr. (2002). Evaluation of HER-2/neu gene amplification and protein expression in non-small cell lung carcinomas. *Br J Cancer,* Vol.86, No.9, pp.1449-1456.

Hudis, C. A. (2007). Trastuzumab--mechanism of action and use in clinical practice. *N Engl J Med,* Vol.357, No.1, pp.39-51.

Hudziak, R. M., Schlessinger, J., & Ullrich, A. (1987). Increased expression of the putative growth factor receptor p185HER2 causes transformation and tumorigenesis of NIH 3T3 cells. *Proc Natl Acad Sci USA,* Vol.84, No.20, pp.7159-7163.

Hung, M. C., Schechter, A. L., Chevray, P. Y., Stern, D. F., & Weinberg, R. A. (1986). Molecular cloning of the neu gene: absence of gross structural alteration in oncogenic alleles. *Proc Natl Acad Sci USA,* Vol.83, No.2, pp.261-264.

Hynes, N. E., & Lane, H. A. (2005). ERBB receptors and cancer: the complexity of targeted inhibitors. *Nat Rev Cancer,* Vol.5, No.5, pp.341-354.

Ishizawar, R., & Parsons, S. J. (2004). c-Src and cooperating partners in human cancer. *Cancer Cell,* Vol.6, No.3, pp.209-214.

Jain, R. K. (1990). Physiological barriers to delivery of monoclonal antibodies and other macromolecules in tumors. *Cancer Res,* Vol.50, No.3 Suppl, pp.814s-819s.

Jeselsohn, R., Brown, N. E., Arendt, L., Klebba, I., Hu, M. G., Kuperwasser, C., & Hinds, P. W. (2010). Cyclin D1 kinase activity is required for the self-renewal of mammary stem and progenitor cells that are targets of MMTV-ErbB2 tumorigenesis. *Cancer Cell,* Vol.17, No.1, pp.65-76.

Khazaeli, M. B., Conry, R. M., & LoBuglio, A. F. (1994). Human immune response to monoclonal antibodies. *J Immunother Emphasis Tumor Immunol,* Vol.15, No.1, pp.42-52.

Khazaie, K., Dull, T. J., Graf, T., Schlessinger, J., Ullrich, A., Beug, H., & Vennstrom, B. (1988). Truncation of the human EGF receptor leads to differential transforming potentials in primary avian fibroblasts and erythroblasts. *EMBO J,* Vol.7, No.10, pp.3061-3071.

Kiewe, P., Hasmuller, S., Kahlert, S., Heinrigs, M., Rack, B., Marme, A., Korfel, A., Jager, M., Lindhofer, H., Sommer, H., Thiel, E., & Untch, M. (2006). Phase I trial of the trifunctional anti-HER2 x anti-CD3 antibody ertumaxomab in metastatic breast cancer. *Clin Cancer Res,* Vol.12, No.10, pp.3085-3091.

Kirpotin, D. B., Drummond, D. C., Shao, Y., Shalaby, M. R., Hong, K., Nielsen, U. B., Marks, J. D., Benz, C. C., & Park, J. W. (2006). Antibody targeting of long-circulating lipidic nanoparticles does not increase tumor localization but does increase internalization in animal models. *Cancer Res,* Vol.66, No.13, pp.6732-6740.

Kleinman, H. K., McGarvey, M. L., Liotta, L. A., Robey, P. G., Tryggvason, K., & Martin, G. R. (1982). Isolation and characterization of type IV procollagen, laminin, and heparan sulfate proteoglycan from the EHS sarcoma. *Biochemistry,* Vol.21, No.24, pp.6188-6193.

Kokai, Y., Myers, J. N., Wada, T., Brown, V. I., LeVea, C. M., Davis, J. G., Dobashi, K., & Greene, M. I. (1989). Synergistic interaction of p185c-neu and the EGF receptor leads to transformation of rodent fibroblasts. *Cell,* Vol.58, No.2, pp.287-292.

Konecny, G. E., Pegram, M. D., Venkatesan, N., Finn, R., Yang, G., Rahmeh, M., Untch, M., Rusnak, D. W., Spehar, G., Mullin, R. J., Keith, B. R., Gilmer, T. M., Berger, M., Podratz, K. C., & Slamon, D. J. (2006). Activity of the dual kinase inhibitor lapatinib (GW572016) against HER-2-overexpressing and trastuzumab-treated breast cancer cells. *Cancer Res,* Vol.66, No.3, pp.1630-1639.

Korkaya, H., Paulson, A., Iovino, F., & Wicha, M. S. (2008). HER2 regulates the mammary stem/progenitor cell population driving tumorigenesis and invasion. *Oncogene,* Vol.27, No.47, pp.6120-6130.

Kraus, M. H., Issing, W., Miki, T., Popescu, N. C., & Aaronson, S. A. (1989). Isolation and characterization of ERBB3, a third member of the ERBB/epidermal growth factor receptor family: evidence for overexpression in a subset of human mammary tumors. *Proc Natl Acad Sci USA,* Vol.86, No.23, pp.9193-9197.

Kruser, T. J., & Wheeler, D. L. (2010). Mechanisms of resistance to HER family targeting antibodies. *Exp Cell Res,* Vol.316, No.7, pp.1083-1100.

Lazar, G. A., Dang, W., Karki, S., Vafa, O., Peng, J. S., Hyun, L., Chan, C., Chung, H. S., Eivazi, A., Yoder, S. C., Vielmetter, J., Carmichael, D. F., Hayes, R. J., & Dahiyat, B. I. (2006). Engineered antibody Fc variants with enhanced effector function. *Proc Natl Acad Sci U S A,* Vol.103, No.11, pp.4005-4010.

Lee, E. S., Gao, Z., & Bae, Y. H. (2008). Recent progress in tumor pH targeting nanotechnology. *J Control Release,* Vol.132, No.3, pp.164-170.

Lewis Phillips, G. D., Li, G., Dugger, D. L., Crocker, L. M., Parsons, K. L., Mai, E., Blattler, W. A., Lambert, J. M., Chari, R. V., Lutz, R. J., Wong, W. L., Jacobson, F. S., Koeppen, H., Schwall, R. H., Kenkare-Mitra, S. R., Spencer, S. D., & Sliwkowski, M. X. (2008). Targeting HER2-positive breast cancer with trastuzumab-DM1, an antibody-cytotoxic drug conjugate. *Cancer Res,* Vol.68, No.22, pp.9280-9290.

Livneh, E., Glazer, L., Segal, D., Schlessinger, J., & Shilo, B. Z. (1985). The Drosophila EGF receptor gene homolog: conservation of both hormone binding and kinase domains. *Cell,* Vol.40, No.3, pp.599-607.

Lonberg, N. (2005). Human antibodies from transgenic animals. *Nat Biotechnol,* Vol.23, No.9, pp.1117-1125.

Lu, J., Guo, H., Treekitkarnmongkol, W., Li, P., Zhang, J., Shi, B., Ling, C., Zhou, X., Chen, T., Chiao, P. J., Feng, X., Seewaldt, V. L., Muller, W. J., Sahin, A., Hung, M. C., & Yu, D. (2009). 14-3-3ζ Cooperates with ErbB2 to Promote Ductal Carcinoma In Situ Progression to Invasive Breast Cancer by Inducing Epithelial-Mesenchymal Transition. *Cancer Cell,* Vol.16, No.3, pp.195-207.

Lucs, A. V., Muller, W. J., & Muthuswamy, S. K. (2010). Shc is required for ErbB2-induced inhibition of apoptosis but is dispensable for cell proliferation and disruption of cell polarity. *Oncogene,* Vol.29, No.2, pp.174-187.

Luo, J., Solimini, N. L., & Elledge, S. J. (2009). Principles of cancer therapy: oncogene and non-oncogene addiction. *Cell,* Vol.136, No.5, pp.823-837.

Maeda, H., Bharate, G. Y., & Daruwalla, J. (2009). Polymeric drugs for efficient tumor-targeted drug delivery based on EPR-effect. *Eur J Pharm Biopharm,* Vol.71, No.3, pp.409-419.

Martin-Belmonte, F., Yu, W., Rodriguez-Fraticelli, A. E., Ewald, A. J., Werb, Z., Alonso, M. A., & Mostov, K. (2008). Cell-polarity dynamics controls the mechanism of lumen formation in epithelial morphogenesis. *Curr Biol,* Vol.18, No.7, pp.507-513.

Mattie, M. D., Benz, C. C., Bowers, J., Sensinger, K., Wong, L., Scott, G. K., Fedele, V., Ginzinger, D., Getts, R., & Haqq, C. (2006). Optimized high-throughput microRNA expression profiling provides novel biomarker assessment of clinical prostate and breast cancer biopsies. *Mol Cancer,* Vol.5, p.24.

Miettinen, P. J., Berger, J. E., Meneses, J., Phung, Y., Pedersen, R. A., Werb, Z., & Derynck, R. (1995). Epithelial immaturity and multiorgan failure in mice lacking epidermal growth factor receptor. *Nature,* Vol.376, No.6538, pp.337-341.

Moasser, M. M. (2007). The oncogene HER2: its signaling and transforming functions and its role in human cancer pathogenesis. *Oncogene,* Vol.26, No.45, pp.6469-6487.

Moghal, N., & Sternberg, P. W. (2003). The epidermal growth factor system in Caenorhabditis elegans. *Exp Cell Res,* Vol.284, No.1, pp.150-159.

Moody, S. E., Sarkisian, C. J., Hahn, K. T., Gunther, E. J., Pickup, S., Dugan, K. D., Innocent, N., Cardiff, R. D., Schnall, M. D., & Chodosh, L. A. (2002). Conditional activation of Neu in the mammary epithelium of transgenic mice results in reversible pulmonary metastasis. *Cancer Cell,* Vol.2, No.6, pp.451-461.

Muller, W. J., Sinn, E., Pattengale, P. K., Wallace, R., & Leder, P. (1988). Single-step induction of mammary adenocarcinoma in transgenic mice bearing the activated c-neu oncogene. *Cell,* Vol.54, No.1, pp.105-115.

Muthuswamy, S. K., Gilman, M., & Brugge, J. S. (1999). Controlled dimerization of ErbB receptors provides evidence for differential signaling by homo- and heterodimers. *Mol Cell Biol,* Vol.19, No.10, pp.6845-6857.

Muthuswamy, S. K., Li, D., Lelievre, S., Bissell, M. J., & Brugge, J. S. (2001). ErbB2, but not ErbB1, reinitiates proliferation and induces luminal repopulation in epithelial acini. *Nat Cell Biol,* Vol.3, No.9, pp.785-792.

Muthuswamy, S. K. (2006). ErbB2 Makes β4 Integrin an Accomplice in Tumorigenesis. *Cell,* Vol.126, No.3, pp.443-445.

Nagata, Y., Lan, K.-H., Zhou, X., Tan, M., Esteva, F. J., Sahin, A. A., Klos, K. S., Li, P., Monia, B. P., Nguyen, N. T., Hortobagyi G. N., Hung, M. C., & Yu, D. (2004). PTEN activation contributes to tumor inhibition by trastuzumab, and loss of PTEN predicts trastuzumab resistance in patients. *Cancer Cell,* Vol.6, No.2, pp.117-127.

Nagy, P., Friedlander, E., Tanner, M., Kapanen, A. I., Carraway, K. L., Isola, J., & Jovin, T. M. (2005). Decreased accessibility and lack of activation of ErbB2 in JIMT-1, a herceptin-resistant, MUC4-expressing breast cancer cell line. *Cancer Res,* Vol.65, No.2, pp.473-482.

Nahta, R., & Esteva, F. J. (2006). Herceptin: mechanisms of action and resistance. *Cancer Lett,* Vol.232, No.2, pp.123-138.

Nahta, R., Hung, M. C., & Esteva, F. J. (2004). The HER-2-targeting antibodies trastuzumab and pertuzumab synergistically inhibit the survival of breast cancer cells. *Cancer Res,* Vol.64, No.7, pp.2343-2346.

Nahta, R., Yuan, L. X., Zhang, B., Kobayashi, R., & Esteva, F. J. (2005). Insulin-like growth factor-I receptor/human epidermal growth factor receptor 2 heterodimerization contributes to trastuzumab resistance of breast cancer cells. *Cancer Res,* Vol.65, No.23, pp.11118-11128.

Olayioye, M. A., Neve, R. M., Lane, H. A., & Hynes, N. E. (2000). The ErbB signaling network: receptor heterodimerization in development and cancer. *EMBO J,* Vol.19, No.13, pp.3159-3167.

Overholtzer, M. (2006). Transforming properties of YAP, a candidate oncogene on the chromosome 11q22 amplicon. *Proc Natl Acad Sci USA,* Vol.103, No.33, pp.12405-12410.

Park, J. W., Hong, K., Kirpotin, D. B., Colbern, G., Shalaby, R., Baselga, J., Shao, Y., Nielsen, U. B., Marks, J. D., Moore, D., Papahadjopoulos, D., & Benz, C. C. (2002). Anti-HER2 immunoliposomes: enhanced efficacy attributable to targeted delivery. *Clin Cancer Res,* Vol.8, No.4, pp.1172-1181.

Peer, D., Karp, J. M., Hong, S., Farokhzad, O. C., Margalit, R., & Langer, R. (2007). Nanocarriers as an emerging platform for cancer therapy. *Nat Nanotechnol,* Vol.2, No.12, pp.751-760.

Perera, S. A., Li, D., Shimamura, T., Raso, M. G., Ji, H., Chen, L., Borgman, C. L., Zaghlul, S., Brandstetter, K. A., Kubo, S., Takahashi, M., Chirieac, L. R., Padera, R. F., Bronson, R. T., Shapiro, G. I., Greulich, H., Meyerson, M., Guertler, U., Chesa, P. G., Solca, F., Wistuba, II, & Wong, K. K. (2009). HER2YVMA drives rapid development of adenosquamous lung tumors in mice that are sensitive to BIBW2992 and rapamycin combination therapy. *Proc Natl Acad Sci USA,* Vol.106, No.2, pp.474-479.

Piechocki, M. P., Ho, Y. S., Pilon, S., & Wei, W. Z. (2003). Human ErbB-2 (Her-2) transgenic mice: a model system for testing Her-2 based vaccines. *J Immunol,* Vol.171, No.11, pp.5787-5794.

Plowman, G. D., Culouscou, J. M., Whitney, G. S., Green, J. M., Carlton, G. W., Foy, L., Neubauer, M. G., & Shoyab, M. (1993). Ligand-specific activation of HER4/p180erbB4, a fourth member of the epidermal growth factor receptor family. *Proc Natl Acad Sci USA,* Vol.90, No.5, pp.1746-1750.

Presta, L. G. (2006). Engineering of therapeutic antibodies to minimize immunogenicity and optimize function. *Adv Drug Deliv Rev,* Vol.58, No.5-6, pp.640-656.

Reddy, H. K., Mettus, R. V., Rane, S. G., Graña., X., Litvin, J., Reddy, E. P. (2005). Cyclin-Dependent Kinase 4 Expression Is Essential for Neu-Induced Breast Tumorigenesis. *Cancer Res,* Vol.65, No.22, pp.10174-10178.

Reid, A., Vidal, L., Shaw, H., & de Bono, J. (2007). Dual inhibition of ErbB1 (EGFR/HER1) and ErbB2 (HER2/neu). *Eur J Cancer,* Vol.43, No.3, pp.481-489.

Romond, E. H., Perez, E. A., Bryant, J., Suman, V. J., Geyer, C. E., Jr., Davidson, N. E., Tan-Chiu, E., Martino, S., Paik, S., Kaufman, P. A., Swain, S. M., Pisansky, T. M., Fehrenbacher, L., Kutteh, L. A., Vogel, V. G., Visscher, D. W., Yothers, G., Jenkins, R. B., Brown, A. M., Dakhil, S. R., Mamounas, E. P., Lingle, W. L., Klein, P. M., Ingle, J. N., & Wolmark, N. (2005). Trastuzumab plus adjuvant chemotherapy for operable HER2-positive breast cancer. *N Engl J Med,* Vol.353, No.16, pp.1673-1684.

Santarius, T., Shipley, J., Brewer, D., Stratton, M. R., & Cooper, C. S. (2010). A census of amplified and overexpressed human cancer genes. *Nat Rev Cancer,* Vol.10, No.1, pp.59-64.

Schafer, Z. T., Grassian, A. R., Song, L., Jiang, Z., Gerhart-Hines, Z., Irie, H. Y., Gao, S., Puigserver, P., & Brugge, J. S. (2009). Antioxidant and oncogene rescue of metabolic defects caused by loss of matrix attachment. *Nature,* Vol.461, No.7260, pp.109-113.

Schechter, A. L., Hung, M. C., Vaidyanathan, L., Weinberg, R. A., Yang-Feng, T. L., Francke, U., Ullrich, A., & Coussens, L. (1985). The neu gene: an erbB-homologous gene distinct from and unlinked to the gene encoding the EGF receptor. *Science,* Vol.229, No.4717, pp.976-978.

Schechter, A. L., Stern, D. F., Vaidyanathan, L., Decker, S. J., Drebin, J. A., Greene, M. I., & Weinberg, R. A. (1984). The neu oncogene: an erb-B-related gene encoding a 185,000-Mr tumour antigen. *Nature,* Vol.312, No.5994, pp.513-516.

Scott, G. K., Goga, A., Bhaumik, D., Berger, C. E., Sullivan, C. S., & Benz, C. C. (2007). Coordinate suppression of ERBB2 and ERBB3 by enforced expression of micro-RNA miR-125a or miR-125b. *J Biol Chem,* Vol.282, No.2, pp.1479-1486.

Semba, K., Kamata, N., Toyoshima, K., & Yamamoto, T. (1985). A v-erbB-related protooncogene, c-erbB-2, is distinct from the c-erbB-1/epidermal growth factor-receptor gene and is amplified in a human salivary gland adenocarcinoma. *Proc Natl Acad Sci USA,* Vol.82, No.19, pp.6497-6501.

Seton-Rogers, S. E. (2004). Cooperation of the ErbB2 receptor and transforming growth factor in induction of migration and invasion in mammary epithelial cells. *Proc Natl Acad Sci USA,* Vol.101, No.5, pp.1257-1262.

Shaw, K. R. M., Wrobel, C. N., & Brugge, J. S. (2004). Use of Three-Dimensional Basement Membrane Cultures to Model Oncogene-Induced Changes in Mammary Epithelial Morphogenesis. *J Mammary Gland Biol Neoplasia,* Vol.9, No.4, pp.297-310.

Shih, C., Padhy, L. C., Murray, M., & Weinberg, R. A. (1981). Transforming genes of carcinomas and neuroblastomas introduced into mouse fibroblasts. *Nature,* Vol.290, No.5803, pp.261-264.

Shih, C., Shilo, B. Z., Goldfarb, M. P., Dannenberg, A., & Weinberg, R. A. (1979). Passage of phenotypes of chemically transformed cells via transfection of DNA and chromatin. *Proc Natl Acad Sci USA,* Vol.76, No.11, pp.5714-5718.

Shilo, B. Z. (2003). Signaling by the Drosophila epidermal growth factor receptor pathway during development. *Exp Cell Res,* Vol.284, No.1, pp.140-149.

Sibilia, M., & Wagner, E. F. (1995). Strain-dependent epithelial defects in mice lacking the EGF receptor. *Science,* Vol.269, No.5221, pp.234-238.

Singh, A. P., Chaturvedi, P., & Batra, S. K. (2007). Emerging Roles of MUC4 in Cancer: A Novel Target for Diagnosis and Therapy. *Cancer Res,* Vol.67, No.2, pp.433-436.

Sircoulomb, F., Bekhouche, I., Finetti, P., Adelaide, J., Ben Hamida, A., Bonansea, J., Raynaud, S., Innocenti, C., Charafe-Jauffret, E., Tarpin, C., Ben Ayed, F., Viens, P., Jacquemier, J., Bertucci, F., Birnbaum, D., & Chaffanet, M. (2010). Genome profiling of ERBB2-amplified breast cancers. *BMC cancer,* Vol.10, p.539.

Slamon, D. J., Godolphin, W., Jones, L. A., Holt, J. A., Wong, S. G., Keith, D. E., Levin, W. J., Stuart, S. G., Udove, J., Ullrich, A., & et al. (1989). Studies of the HER-2/neu proto-oncogene in human breast and ovarian cancer. *Science,* Vol.244, No.4905, pp.707-712.

Slamon, D. J., Leyland-Jones, B., Shak, S., Fuchs, H., Paton, V., Bajamonde, A., Fleming, T., Eiermann, W., Wolter, J., Pegram, M., Baselga, J., & Norton, L. (2001). Use of chemotherapy plus a monoclonal antibody against HER2 for metastatic breast cancer that overexpresses HER2. *N Engl J Med,* Vol.344, No.11, pp.783-792.

Soule, H. D., Maloney, T. M., Wolman, S. R., Peterson, W. D., Jr., Brenz, R., McGrath, C. M., Russo, J., Pauley, R. J., Jones, R. F., & Brooks, S. C. (1990). Isolation and characterization of a spontaneously immortalized human breast epithelial cell line, MCF-10. *Cancer Res,* Vol.50, No.18, pp.6075-6086.

Threadgill, D. W., Dlugosz, A. A., Hansen, L. A., Tennenbaum, T., Lichti, U., Yee, D., LaMantia, C., Mourton, T., Herrup, K., Harris, R. C., & et al. (1995). Targeted disruption of mouse EGF receptor: effect of genetic background on mutant phenotype. *Science,* Vol.269, No.5221, pp.230-234.

Timms, J. F., White, S. L., O'Hare, M. J., & Waterfield, M. D. (2002). Effects of ErbB-2 overexpression on mitogenic signalling and cell cycle progression in human breast luminal epithelial cells. *Oncogene,* Vol.21, No.43, pp.6573-6586.

Todaro, G. J., & Green, H. (1963). Quantitative studies of the growth of mouse embryo cells in culture and their development into established lines. *J Cell Biol,* Vol.17, pp.299-313.

Tomizawa, K., Suda, K., Onozato, R., Kosaka, T., Endoh, H., Sekido, Y., Shigematsu, H., Kuwano, H., Yatabe, Y., & Mitsudomi, T. (2011). Prognostic and predictive implications of HER2/ERBB2/neu gene mutations in lung cancers. *Lung Cancer.*

Vargo-Gogola, T., & Rosen, J. M. (2007). Modelling breast cancer: one size does not fit all. *Nat Rev Cancer,* Vol.7, No.9, pp.659-672.

Vennstrom, B., & Bishop, J. M. (1982). Isolation and characterization of chicken DNA homologous to the two putative oncogenes of avian erythroblastosis virus. *Cell,* Vol.28, No.1, pp.135-143.

Visvader, J. E. (2011). Cells of origin in cancer. *Nature,* Vol.469, No.7330, pp.314-322.

Vivanco, I., & Sawyers, C. L. (2002). The phosphatidylinositol 3-Kinase–AKT pathway in human cancer. *Nat Rev Cancer,* Vol.2, No.7, pp.489-501.

Wagner, K. U., Wall, R. J., St-Onge, L., Gruss, P., Wynshaw-Boris, A., Garrett, L., Li, M., Furth, P. A., & Hennighausen, L. (1997). Cre-mediated gene deletion in the mammary gland. *Nucleic Acids Res,* Vol.25, No.21, pp.4323-4330.

Wang, S. E., Narasanna, A., Perez-Torres, M., Xiang, B., Wu, F. Y., Yang, S., Carpenter, G., Gazdar, A. F., Muthuswamy, S. K., & Arteaga, C. L. (2006). HER2 kinase domain mutation results in constitutive phosphorylation and activation of HER2 and EGFR and resistance to EGFR tyrosine kinase inhibitors. *Cancer Cell,* Vol.10, No.1, pp.25-38.

Wang, S.-C., Lien, H.-C., Xia, W., Chen, I. F., Lo, H.-W., Wang, Z., Ali-Seyed, M., Lee, D.-F., Bartholomeusz, G., Ou-Yang, F., Giri, D. K., & Hung, M. C. (2004). Binding at and transactivation of the COX-2 promoter by nuclear tyrosine kinase receptor ErbB-2. *Cancer Cell,* Vol.6, No.3, pp.251-261.

Wolf-Yadlin, A., Kumar, N., Zhang, Y., Hautaniemi, S., Zaman, M., Kim, H.-D., Grantcharova, V., Lauffenburger, D. A., & White, F. M. (2006). Effects of HER2 overexpression on cell signaling networks governing proliferation and migration. *Mol Syst Biol,* Vol.2.

Wrobel, C. N. (2004). Autocrine CSF-1R activation promotes Src-dependent disruption of mammary epithelial architecture. *J Cell Biol,* Vol.165, No.2, pp.263-273.

Wu, A. M., & Senter, P. D. (2005). Arming antibodies: prospects and challenges for immunoconjugates. *Nat Biotechnol,* Vol.23, No.9, pp.1137-1146.

Yamada, K. M., & Cukierman, E. (2007). Modeling Tissue Morphogenesis and Cancer in 3D. *Cell,* Vol.130, No.4, pp.601-610.

Yamamoto, T., Ikawa, S., Akiyama, T., Semba, K., Nomura, N., Miyajima, N., Saito, T., & Toyoshima, K. (1986). Similarity of protein encoded by the human c-erb-B-2 gene to epidermal growth factor receptor. *Nature,* Vol.319, No.6050, pp.230-234.

Yamamoto, T., Nishida, T., Miyajima, N., Kawai, S., Ooi, T., & Toyoshima, K. (1983). The erbB gene of avian erythroblastosis virus is a member of the src gene family. *Cell,* Vol.35, No.1, pp.71-78.

Yang, C., Ionescu-Tiba, V., Burns, K., Gadd, M., Zukerberg, L., Louis, D. N., Sgroi, D., & Schmidt, E. V. (2004). The role of the cyclin D1-dependent kinases in ErbB2-mediated breast cancer. *Am J Pathol,* Vol.164, No.3, pp.1031-1038.

Yarden, Y., & Sliwkowski, M. X. (2001). Untangling the ErbB signalling network. *Nat Rev Mol Cell Biol,* Vol.2, No.2, pp.127-137.

Yu, Q., Geng, Y., & Sicinski, P. (2001). Specific protection against breast cancers by cyclin D1 ablation. *Nature,* Vol.411, No.6841, pp.1017-1021.

Zhang, S., Huang, W. C., Li, P., Guo, H., Poh, S. B., Brady, S. W., Xiong, Y., Tseng, L. M., Li, S. H., Ding, Z., Sahin, A. A., Esteva, F. J., Hortobagyi, G. N., Yu, D. (2011). Combating trastuzumab resistance by targeting SRC, a common node downstream of multiple resistance pathways. *Nat Med,* Vol.17, No.4, pp.461-469.

Zheng, J., Mercado-Uribe, I., Rosen, D. G., Chang, B., Liu, P., Yang, G., Malpica, A., Noara, H., Auersperg, N., Mills, G. B., Bast, R. C., & Liu, J. (2010). Induction of papillary carcinoma in human ovarian surface epithelial cells using combined genetic elements and peritoneal microenvironment. *Cell Cycle,* Vol.9, No.1, pp.140-146.

Zhou, Y., Rideout, W. M., 3rd, Zi, T., Bressel, A., Reddypalli, S., Rancourt, R., Woo, J. K., Horner, J. W., Chin, L., Chiu, M. I., Bosenberg, M., Jacks, T., Clark, S. C., Depinho, R. A., Robinson, M. O., & Heyer, J. (2010). Chimeric mouse tumor models reveal differences in pathway activation between ERBB family- and KRAS-dependent lung adenocarcinomas. *Nat Biotechnol,* Vol.28, No.1, pp.71-78.

Zuo, T., Liu, R., Zhang, H., Chang, X., Liu, Y., Wang, L., & Zheng, P. (2007). FOXP3 is a novel transcriptional repressor for the breast cancer oncogene SKP2. *J Clin Invest,* Vol.117, No.12, pp.3765-3773.

Permissions

All chapters in this book were first published by Springer; hereby published with permission under the Creative Commons Attribution License or equivalent. Every chapter published in this book has been scrutinized by our experts. Their significance has been extensively debated. The topics covered herein carry significant findings which will fuel the growth of the discipline. They may even be implemented as practical applications or may be referred to as a beginning point for another development.

The contributors of this book come from diverse backgrounds, making this book a truly international effort. This book will bring forth new frontiers with its revolutionizing research information and detailed analysis of the nascent developments around the world.

We would like to thank all the contributing authors for lending their expertise to make the book truly unique. They have played a crucial role in the development of this book. Without their invaluable contributions this book wouldn't have been possible. They have made vital efforts to compile up to date information on the varied aspects of this subject to make this book a valuable addition to the collection of many professionals and students.

This book was conceptualized with the vision of imparting up-to-date information and advanced data in this field. To ensure the same, a matchless editorial board was set up. Every individual on the board went through rigorous rounds of assessment to prove their worth. After which they invested a large part of their time researching and compiling the most relevant data for our readers.

The editorial board has been involved in producing this book since its inception. They have spent rigorous hours researching and exploring the diverse topics which have resulted in the successful publishing of this book. They have passed on their knowledge of decades through this book. To expedite this challenging task, the publisher supported the team at every step. A small team of assistant editors was also appointed to further simplify the editing procedure and attain best results for the readers.

Apart from the editorial board, the designing team has also invested a significant amount of their time in understanding the subject and creating the most relevant covers. They scrutinized every image to scout for the most suitable representation of the subject and create an appropriate cover for the book.

The publishing team has been an ardent support to the editorial, designing and production team. Their endless efforts to recruit the best for this project, has resulted in the accomplishment of this book. They are a veteran in the field of academics and their pool of knowledge is as vast as their experience in printing. Their expertise and guidance has proved useful at every step. Their uncompromising quality standards have made this book an exceptional effort. Their encouragement from time to time has been an inspiration for everyone.

The publisher and the editorial board hope that this book will prove to be a valuable piece of knowledge for researchers, students, practitioners and scholars across the globe.

List of Contributors

Hiroko Yamashita, Tatsuya Toyama, Nobuyasu Yoshimoto, Yumi Endo, Mai Iwasa and Yoshitaka Fujii
Oncology, Immunology and Surgery, Nagoya City University Graduate School of Medical Sciences, Japan

Manasi N. Shukla, Donna J. Buckley and Arthur R. Buckley
Division of Pharmaceutical Sciences, James L. Winkle College of Pharmacy, University of Cincinnati, Cincinnati, OH, United States of America

ZhaoYi Wang, XianTian Zhang and LianGuo Kang
Department of Medical Microbiology & Immunology, Creighton University Medical School, Omaha, NE, USA

Soma Mandal, Protiti Khan, Lin Li and James R. Davie
Manitoba Institute of Cell Biology, University of Manitoba, Winnipeg, Manitoba, Canada

In Ah Kim
Department of Radiation Oncology, Seoul National University, Republic of Korea

Ala-Eddin Al Moustafa
Syrian Research Cancer Centre of the Syrian Society against Cancer, Aleppo, Syria
Oncology Department, Faculty of Medicine, McGill University, Montréal, Canada
Department of Mechanical Engineering, Concordia University, Montréal, Canada

Amber Yasmeen
Oncology Department, Faculty of Medicine, McGill University, Montréal, Canada

Lina Ghabreau and Ali H. Mohamed
Department of Pathology, Faculty of Medicine/ University of Aleppo, Aleppo, Syria

Amal Achkhar
Syrian Research Cancer Centre of the Syrian Society against Cancer, Aleppo, Syria
Faculty of Pharmacy, University of Aleppo, Aleppo, Syria

Milos Dokmanovic and Wen Jin Wu
Division of Monoclonal Antibodies, Office of Biotechnology Products, Office of Pharmaceutical Science, Center for Drug Evaluation and Research, U.S. Food and Drug Administration, Bethesda, Maryland, United States of America

Nicole K. Nickerson, Jennifer L. Gilmore and Kah Tan Allen
Medical Sciences Program, Indiana University School of Medicine, Bloomington, IN, United States of America

David J. Riese II
Harrison School of Pharmacy, Auburn University, Auburn, AL, United States of America

Kenneth P. Nephew
Medical Sciences Program, Indiana University School of Medicine, Bloomington, IN, United States of America
Indiana University Cancer Center Indiana University School of Medicine, Indianapolis, IN, United States of America

Samar Azab
Pharmacology and Toxicology Department, Faculty of Pharmacy, Ain Shams University, Cairo, Egypt

John Foley
Medical Sciences Program, Indiana University School of Medicine, Bloomington, IN, United States of America
Indiana University Cancer Center Indiana University School of Medicine, Indianapolis, IN, United States of America
Department of Dermatology, Indiana University School of Medicine, Indianapolis, IN, United States of America

Ayman Al-Hendy
Center for Women Health Research, Department of Obstetrics and Gynecology, Meharry Medical College, Nashville, Tennessee, USA

Tadashi Yamamoto Makoto Saito, Kentaro Kumazawa, Ayano Doi, Atsuka Matsui, Shiori Takebe, Takuya Amari, Masaaki Oyama and Kentaro Semba
The Institute of Medical Science, The University of Tokyo, Japan
Department of Life Science and Medical Bioscience, Waseda University, Japan

Index

www.ingramcontent.com/pod-product-compliance
Lightning Source LLC
LaVergne TN
LVHW062230200926
848484LV00006B/1510